**Diagnosis and Treatment
of Furcation-Involved Teeth**

Diagnosis and Treatment of Furcation-Involved Teeth

Edited by Luigi Nibali

Senior Clinical Lecturer
Centre for Immunobiology and Regenerative Medicine
Centre for Oral Clinical Research, Institute of Dentistry
Barts and the London School of Medicine and Dentistry
Queen Mary University of London (QMUL), London, UK

Honorary Associate Professor, University of Hong Kong

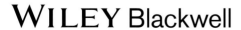

Registered Offices
John Wiley & Sons, Inc., 111 River Street, Hoboken, NJ 07030, USA
John Wiley & Sons Ltd, The Atrium, Southern Gate, Chichester, West Sussex, PO19 8SQ, UK

Editorial Office
9600 Garsington Road, Oxford, OX4 2DQ, UK

For details of our global editorial offices, customer services, and more information about Wiley products visit us at www.wiley.com.

Wiley also publishes its books in a variety of electronic formats and by print-on-demand. Some content that appears in standard print versions of this book may not be available in other formats.

Library of Congress Cataloging-in-Publication Data

Names: Nibali, Luigi, 1978– editor.
Title: Diagnosis and treatment of furcation-involved teeth / edited by Luigi Nibali.
Description: Hoboken, NJ : Wiley, [2018] | Includes bibliographical references and index. |
Identifiers: LCCN 2018010570 (print) | LCCN 2018011380 (ebook) | ISBN 9781119270669 (pdf) |
    ISBN 9781119270676 (epub) | ISBN 9781119270652 (hardback)
Subjects: | MESH: Furcation Defects–diagnosis | Furcation Defects–therapy | Models, Animal
Classification: LCC RK450.P4 (ebook) | LCC RK450.P4 (print) | NLM WU 242 | DDC 617.6/32–dc23
LC record available at https://lccn.loc.gov/2018010570

Cover image: (Main, top left and middle images) © Luigi Nibali; (Top right image) © Roberto Rotundo
Cover design: Wiley

Set in 10/12pt Warnock by SPi Global, Pondicherry, India
Printed and bound in Singapore by Markono Print Media Pte Ltd

10   9   8   7   6   5   4   3   2   1

Contents

List of Contributors

Dr Stephen Barter
Private practice, Eastbourne, UK

Dr Elena Calciolari
Centre for Immunobiology and Regenerative
Medicine
Centre for Oral Clinical Research
Institute of Dentistry
Barts and the London School of Medicine
and Dentistry
Queen Mary University of London (QMUL)
London, UK

Prof. Nikolaos Donos
Centre for Immunobiology and Regenerative
Medicine
Centre for Oral Clinical Research
Institute of Dentistry
Barts and the London School of Medicine
and Dentistry
Queen Mary University of London (QMUL)
London, UK

Prof. Peter Eickholz
Poliklinik für Parodontologie
Zentrum der Zahn- Mund- und
Kieferheilkunde (Carolinum)
Johann Wolfgang Goethe-Universität
Frankfurt
Frankfurt am Main
Germany

Dr Federica Fonzar
Private practice
Udine
Italy

Dr Alberto Fonzar
Private practice
Udine
Italy

Dr Riccardo Fabian Fonzar
Private practice
Udine
Italy

Dr Jia-Hui Fu
Discipline of Periodontics
Faculty of Dentistry
National University of Singapore
Singapore

Dr Christian Graetz
Clinic for Conservative Dentistry and
Periodontology
Christian-Albrechts-University
Kiel
Germany

Dr Karin Jepsen
Department of Periodontology
Operative and Preventive Dentistry
University of Bonn
Germany

Prof. Søren Jepsen
Department of Periodontology
Operative and Preventive Dentistry
University of Bonn
Germany

Dr Nikos Mardas
Centre for Immunobiology and Regenerative
Medicine
Centre for Oral Clinical Research
Institute of Dentistry
Barts and the London School of Medicine
and Dentistry
Queen Mary University of London (QMUL)
London
UK

Dr Luigi Nibali
Centre for Immunobiology and Regenerative
Medicine
Centre for Oral Clinical Research
Institute of Dentistry
Barts and the London School of Medicine
and Dentistry
Queen Mary University of London (QMUL)
London
UK

Dr Iro Palaska
Centre for Immunobiology and Regenerative
Medicine
Centre for Oral Clinical Research
Institute of Dentistry
Barts and the London School of Medicine
and Dentistry
Queen Mary University of London (QMUL)
London
UK

Dr Bernadette Pretzl
Section of Periodontology
Department of Operative Dentistry
University Clinic Heidelberg
Heidelberg
Germany

Dr Roberto Rotundo
Periodontology Unit
UCL Eastman Dental Institute
London
UK

Dr Stefan G. Rüdiger
Department of Periodontology
Public Dental Service/Malmö University
Malmö
Sweden

Dr Falk Schwendicke
Department of Operative and Preventive
Dentistry
Charité-Universitätsmedizin Berlin
Berlin
Germany

Prof. Anton Sculean
Department of Periodontology
School of Dental Medicine
University of Bern
Bern
Switzerland

Dr Yoshinori Shirakata
Department of Periodontology
Kagoshima
University Graduate School of Medical and
Dental Sciences
Kagoshima
Japan

Prof. Clemens Walter
Klinik für Parodontologie
Endodontologie und Kariologie
Universitätszahnkliniken,
Universitäres Zentrum für
Zahnmedizin Basel
Basel
Switzerland

Prof. Hom-Lay Wang
Department of Periodontics and Oral
Medicine
School of Dentistry
University of Michigan
Ann Arbor
MI
USA

Foreword

The preservation of tissues and structures that support the dentition is a major goal of conservative dentistry for the benefit of our patients. As dental practitioners, we are trained to maintain and restore function, aesthetics, and phonetics for the promotion of oral health. In the development of this book, *Diagnosis and Treatment of Furcation-Involved Teeth*, Luigi Nibali and his co-authors have assembled an excellent text that comprehensively examines the management of the most challenging-to-treat teeth in the jaws – the molar and premolar teeth with furcation involvement. It is clear that clinicians are continually tested on which are the best approaches to handle these clinical scenarios that include furcated teeth. The education, skill, and training required to manage furcations are significant given the anatomy, location, and functional biomechanical occlusal forces associated with posterior teeth that make for complex clinical decision-making.

In this text, Dr Nibali has convened international experts providing chapters ranging from the diagnosis of disease to clinical outcomes from the health policy expert's, cariologist's, periodontist's, and endodontist's perspectives on periodontal-endodontic-restorative dilemmas in patient care. It is important to recognize that there is a large evidence base that was initiated from the 'pre–dental implant era' on the long-term success in the maintenance of compromised teeth affected by extensive restorative care, periodontal involvement, and/or pulpal pathology. This text not only focuses on diagnosis and treatment, but includes valuable information from a health economics and treatment algorithms perspectives on long-term tooth preservation.

In the first part of the book, a thorough background on the unique anatomy of multi-rooted teeth and corresponding diagnostic, prognostic, and therapeutic intricacies is presented. The next section provides a strong rationale regarding the concept of tooth preservation from the restorative, periodontal, and endodontic perspectives, which highlights the strong evidence base of treatment success of tooth furcations. This background is important to examine critically, since many oral implantologists in the field are not adequately versed on the ramifications of premature tooth removal versus those teeth that can be predictably retained for the long-term success of the patient. The application in clinical practice by those without adequate training occasionally errs on the expedience of tooth extraction, without pausing to weigh methodically the advantages and disadvantages of embarking on comprehensive therapy for furcated teeth. Those without access to this text on the many options available to increase the lifespan of molar and premolar teeth may not be prepared to treatment plan the complex dental patient appropriately for the comprehensive assessment of restorative, periodontal, endodontic, functional, and aesthetic needs. Given practice trends of more common extractions of furcated periodontally and endodontically compromised teeth, it suggests that 'the time is right' to emphasize the great potential available in the proper assessment and treatment of furcated teeth. This section highlights the long-term success with proper therapy in maintaining furcated teeth.

The next part of the text highlights the many different therapeutic modalities that are clinically available to treat multi-rooted teeth, including non-surgical maintenance, resective procedures (including tunnelling, root resection, and bicuspidization), and reconstructive regenerative therapy using biologics or biomaterials. Other chapters in the book build on our existing evidence base to examine the cases that can genuinely be retained versus those teeth too compromised as 'hopeless' that may benefit from extraction, implant site development (bone grafting and alveolar ridge preservation), followed by dental implant reconstruction. Indeed, dental implant therapy has revolutionized oral care and clinical treatment decision-making paradigms for advanced reconstructive procedures. It is also crucial for the advanced clinician to understand when and when not to attempt to retain advanced disease cases. Large epidemiological studies have demonstrated that dental implant therapy is not a 'panacea' and that, given the significant incidence and prevalence

of peri-implant biological complications in the molar regions, we should re-examine the opportunities for maintaining and treating furcated teeth more diligently and more fully. The concluding chapters scrutinize the health economics opportunities at the patient and clinician levels in terms of tooth preservation of furcated molars, and in which types of cases which treatment planning approach is indicated for such advanced clinical scenarios.

Stimulated by the comprehensive approach in this book, this can be a renaissance period in reconstructive dentistry when we firmly consider the many options available to us as clinicians to better preserve the dentition in treating furcation-involved teeth. This text lays out a contemporary and exciting opportunity for us as clinicians to provide our patients with state-of-the-art therapy for the betterment of oral health!

William V. Giannobile, DDS, MS, DMedSc
Najjar Endowed Professor of Dentistry &
Biomedical Engineering
Departments of Periodontics and Oral
Medicine & Biomedical Engineering,
University of Michigan School of Dentistry and
College of Engineering, Ann Arbor, MI, USA

Preface

Declare the past, diagnose the present, foretell the future.

Hippocrates

Doubt is not a pleasant condition, but certainty is an absurd one.

Voltaire

Young and new to a periodontal clinic, I remember looking at cases of extensive periodontal and bone loss in multi-rooted teeth and wondering how the problem could be solved, and if and how the tooth could be retained. The fascination with the spaces created by inter-radicular bone resorption, called 'furcations', and the struggle over how to manage them in the clinic, continues to occupy large parts of my days and has prompted me to write this book. Here, with the help of several expert colleagues, I have tried to:

- Critically appraise the evidence.
- Present expert opinions.
- Show treated cases.
- Present useful clinical guidelines, step-by step procedures, and treatment algorithms.

The emphasis of the book is to try and maintain molars affected by furcation involvement and regenerate the lost support, when possible, accepting that this is not always possible in the long term. It goes without saying that primary prevention of periodontitis remains the best way to prevent tooth loss. I hope that periodontists, dental/postgraduate students, hygienists, and general dentists might find this book useful for the treatment of molars already affected by periodontitis and furcation involvement.

Immense thanks go to all the expert collaborators and friends, Will Giannobile, Bernadette Pretzl, Peter Eickholz, Clemens Walter, Jia-Hui Fu, Hom-Lay Wang, Federica, Riccardo, and Alberto Fonzar, Roberto Rotundo, Stefan Rüdiger, Nikos Donos, Toni Sculean, Elena Calciolari, Iro Palaska, Yoshinori Shirakata, Søren and Karin Jepsen, Nikos Mardas, Steve Barter, Christian Graetz, and Falk Schwendicke, who all contributed chapters to this book, and to Paul Kletz for kindly proofreading some of the chapters and for his support throughout my career. Special thanks go to the patients who over the years have been a big source of inspiration with their interest and commitment, and who every day make me want to be a better periodontist. I also need to thank my teachers at the University of Catania and at the UCL Eastman Dental Institute, who have all contributed, some with small and some with larger ingredients, to the cauldron of periodontal knowledge from which I drew for the planning and editing of this book. The students and staff at Barts and the London School of Medicine and Dentistry, Queen Mary University of London (QMUL), are gratefully acknowledged. But most of all, I would like to thank my family, Daniela, Domenico, Lorenzo, Delia, and my parents and in-laws, for their continued support of my work.

Luigi Nibali

About the Companion Website

Don't forget to visit the companion website for this book:

www.wiley.com/go/nibali/diagnosis

There you will find valuable material designed to enhance your learning, including:

- video clips
- additional treated cases

Scan this QR code to visit the companion website

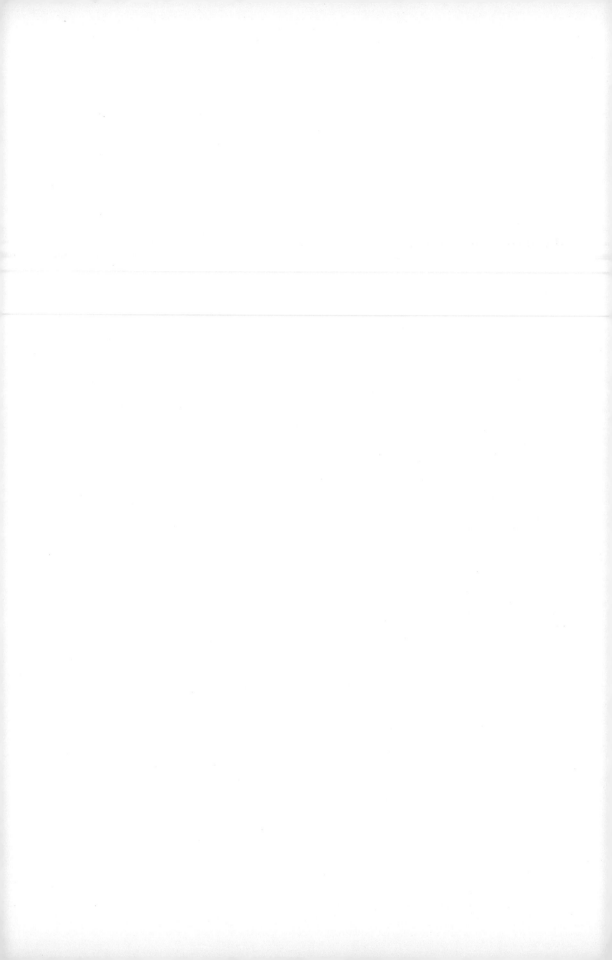

Chapter 1

Anatomy of Multi-rooted Teeth and Aetiopathogenesis of the Furcation Defect

Bernadette Pretzl

Section of Periodontology, Department of Operative Dentistry, University Clinic Heidelberg, Heidelberg, Germany

1.1 Introduction: Why Focus on Molars?

Dentists generally agree on three statements about molars:

- They play an important role in the dentition.
- They are difficult to reach for self-performed as well as professional cleaning due to their posterior position in the mouth.
- They pose some challenges due to their unique anatomy.

The important role of molar teeth in the dentition mainly consists in their contribution to mastication, because they carry a considerable part of the occlusal load. Hiiemäe (1967) focused on the masticatory function in mammals and molars grinding the food, and in 1975 Bates et al. reviewed the literature on the masticatory cycle in natural and artificial dentitions of men, attributing a fundamental role to our posterior teeth regarding the intake and preparation of nutrition. Thus, a focus on molars and the endeavour to retain our posterior teeth in a healthy functional state seems justified.

This chapter will reveal how the posterior position of molars makes them less accessible for cleaning, whether it may be self-performed or carried out by a dental professional. This fact, combined with the unique anatomy of molars, poses a challenge for all dentists focusing on molar retention.

1.2 The 'Special' Anatomy of Molar Teeth

The essential knowledge of molar root anatomy for every periodontist is stressed in a review by Al-Shammari et al. (2001). Due to the higher mortality and compromised diagnoses of furcation-involved molars, and likewise to the reduced efficacy of periodontal therapy in multi-rooted teeth, the authors suggest a thorough engagement with possibly decisive tooth factors such as furcation entrance area, (bi)furcation ridges, root surface area, root separation, and root trunk length, because they may critically affect the diagnosis and therapy of multi-rooted teeth (Leknes 1997; Al-Shammari et al. 2001).

For centuries, scientists have concerned themselves with the human teeth, their anatomy, evolution, function, histology, and histogenesis. Almost 3000 years ago, the Etruscans populating the northern and central part of what is now Italy from 900 to 100 BC recognized the importance of teeth and fabricated quite delicate dental prostheses, which Loevy and Kowitz (1997) compared to prostheses from the mid-twentieth century.

Diagnosis and Treatment of Furcation-Involved Teeth, First Edition. Edited by Luigi Nibali.
© 2018 John Wiley & Sons Ltd. Published 2018 by John Wiley & Sons Ltd.
Companion website: www.wiley.com/go/nibali/diagnosis

The formation and genesis of teeth have been studied in more detail during the last three and a half centuries, starting with the works of the so-called father of microscopic anatomy and histology, Marcello Malpighi (1628–1694) from Italy (Rifkin and Ackerman 2011), who referred to an 'involucrum externum' describing the outer part of the tooth, which is today known as enamel. More than a century later the formation of cementum (1798–1801) and dentine (1835–1839) was described (e.g. Blake 1801; Bell 1835). Written in 1935, *Meyer's Normal Histology and Histogenesis of the Human Teeth and Associated Parts* (Churchill 1935) builds the foundation of our understanding regarding the anatomy of teeth. Orban and Mueller (1929), who studied the development of furcations in multi-rooted teeth, set a focus on molars using graphic reconstructions as early as 1929. Their three-dimensional illustrations allow a detailed impression of the root area comparable to those documented by Svärdström and Wennström (1988). In later years, scientists focused more and more on micro-anatomical and histological research.

Based on the knowledge thus created, the sequence of molar development can be divided into three phases analogous to the development of all teeth (Thesleff and Hurmerinta 1981): initiation, morphogenesis, and cell differentiation. The evolution of more than one root sets molars apart from the rest of the dentition: in multi-rooted teeth the enamel organ expands with projections of Hertwig's root sheath (an epithelial diaphragm). These expansions were described as lobular growing inwards between the lobes. Depending on the number of lobes, two to three (in rarer cases four) roots develop as soon as the projections have fused (Bhussry 1980). In an investigation by Bower (1983) of furcation development, evolving mandibular molars from 13 foetuses between 17 and 38 weeks of gestation were fixed, sectioned, and stained, giving a unique and detailed impression of furcation development. The author measured the base of the dental papilla as well as the buccal and lingual epithelial elements and described the development as follows: The first epithelial elements, which later evolve into the bifurcation, appear at the 24-week stage of gestational age. At that time, the crown formation of the molar is not complete and Hertwig's root sheath has not developed yet (Bhussry 1980; Bower 1983). Thus, the author suggests that the epithelial elements form extensions of the epithelium of the developing crown rather than the root (Bower 1983). Additionally, he detected stellate reticulum (which is essential for the formation of ameloblasts) in the furcation area. The author speculated about a possible mechanism of enamel formation due to the presence of stellate reticulum in the region of the furcation, which develops into ameloblasts, for example resulting in cervical projections of enamel.

1.3 Anatomical Factors in Molar Teeth

In 1988, Svärdström and Wennström plotted three-dimensional contour maps in order to describe the topography of the furcation area and compared drawings of maxillary and mandibular molars. These show a complex area with small ridges, peaks, and pits, and the authors summarize that the complexity of the furcation topography evidently increases the difficulties with respect to proper debridement once the periodontal pocket reaches the furcation entrance and runs into the furcation area. Thus, in addition to the aforementioned potentially decisive factors – furcation entrance area, bifurcation ridges, root surface area, and root trunk length – it has to be kept in mind that the complexity of the furcation area itself poses a challenge to the dental practitioner (Svärdström and Wennström 1988). Figure 1.1 shows a diagram of a mandibular molar, highlighting the main anatomical features.

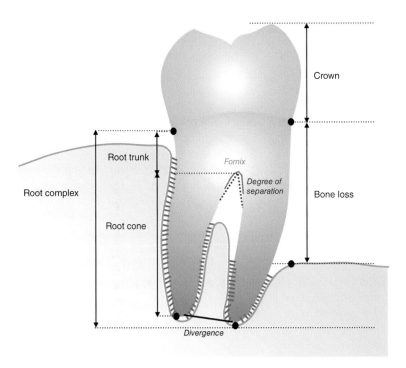

Figure 1.1 Drawing of mandibular molar with furcation involvement, showing the main anatomical features, including root trunk (part of the root from the cemento-enamel junction [CEJ] to the furcation entrance) and root cones, and pointing at root divergence and degree of separation between roots. The 'bone loss' is schematically indicated as the distance between the CEJ and the most apical part of the bone. *Source*: Courtesy of Dr Aliye Akcali.

1.3.1 Furcation Entrance Area

The furcation entrance area was measured by Bower (1979a) in 114 maxillary and 103 mandibular first molars. The diameter of the entrance area was smaller than a curette blade in more than 50% of the examined furcations, with the smallest average diameter in buccal (b) sites of maxillary as well as mandibular first molars. No correlation between the size of the tooth and its furcation entrance area could be detected (Bower 1979a). Hou et al. (1994) studied 89 extracted maxillary and 93 extracted mandibular first and second molars microscopically. In their Chinese population sample, they concurred with the results presented by Bower (1979a) in the maxilla and found a larger diameter in mesio- (mp) and disto-palatal (dp) furcation entrances for first and second molars (mp: 1.04 mm and 0.90 mm; dp: 0.99 mm and 0.67 mm; b: 0.74 mm and 0.63 mm, respectively), which was confirmed by Svärdström and Wennström (1988) and dos Santos et al. (2009).

In mandibular molars the results differed, with wider entrance areas in buccal furcations of first and second molars (b: 0.88 mm and 0.73 mm; l: 0.81 mm and 0.71 mm, respectively). Nonetheless, the furcation entrance area was < 1 mm in the majority of molars and < 0.75 mm in 58%, 49%, and 52% of molars, respectively (Bower 1979a; Chiu et al. 1991; Hou et al. 1994). Thus, the standard width of curettes (0.75–1.0 mm) is mostly too large to access, let alone properly clean, a furcation entrance. Hou et al. (1994) concluded that in order to achieve complete debridement of root surfaces within furcations, an appropriate selection and combination of ultrasonic tips (diameter 0.56 mm) and periodontal curettes should be considered. A recent study by dos Santos et al.

(2009) analysed 50 maxillary and 50 mandibular molars and confirmed the aforementioned findings, concluding that some molar furcation entrances could not be adequately instrumented with curettes and suggesting the use of alternative hand instruments. In a review, Matthews and Tabesh (2004) stressed the importance of the diameter of the furcation entrance in order to judge the effect of professional cleaning, and thus the probable success of periodontal therapy. The challenges of furcation cleaning are discussed by Fu and Wang in Chapter 3.

1.3.2 (Bi)furcation Ridges

In early morphological studies of extracted first molar teeth, cementum was found in the furcation area in a ridge, building the furcation region in mandibular molars, and was called an intermediate bifurcation ridge (IBR), with a high presence of cementum adjacent to the furcation entrance (Everett et al. 1958; Bower 1979a, b; see Figure 1.2). In a study on developing first mandibular molars sectioned at different gestational ages, the lingual element was found to be wider in a mesio-distal dimension comparable

to studies in extracted molars (Bower 1983, 1979b). Secondly, the exclusion of ectomesenchyme between the lobes described by Bhussry (1980) may explain the large quantities of cementum in the furcation area of the mature tooth corresponding to bifurcation ridges (Bower 1983). In general, two types of bifurcation ridge are known: one in the bucco-lingual direction, the other in the mesio-distal direction (intermediate = IBR). Everett et al. (1958) detected buccal and lingual ridges, mainly constituting of dentine, in 63% of mandibular first molars and IBRs, mainly composed of cementum, in 73%. The findings of Burch and Hulen (1974), Dunlap and Gher (1985), and Hou and Tsai (1997a) concur, with a prevalence of 76.3%, 70%, and 67.9%, respectively, in mandibular first molars.

Gher and Vernino (1980) suggest a connection between the presence of an IBR and the progression of the furcation defect due to the morphology and location of IBRs. Hou and Tsai (1997a) confirmed this correlation. Additionally, they stated that an even higher significant correlation exists between the simultaneous presence of IBRs combined with cemento-enamel projections and furcation involvement (FI).

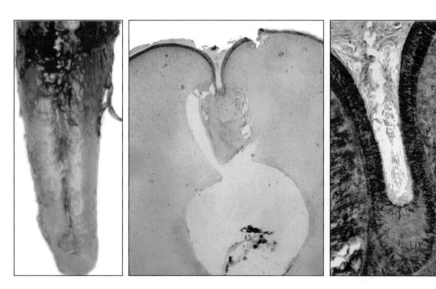

Figure 1.2 Furcation ridge. *Source*: Courtesy of Dr Nicola Perrini.

1.3.3 Root Surface Area

A team of researchers (Hermann et al. 1983; Dunlap and Gher 1985; Gher and Dunlap 1985) focused on the topic of root surface area (RSA) in maxillary and mandibular first molars. In a meta-analysis derived of data from 22 original articles, Hujoel (1994) computed a total RSA (corresponding to the periodontal surface area) for the complete dentition of 65–86 cm^2, excluding third molars. In maxillary first molars a mean of 4.5 cm^2 (second: 4.0 cm^2) and in mandibular first molars a mean of 4.2 cm^2 (second: 3.4 cm^2) were calculated. In molars, it is often difficult to judge the extent of FI clinically (Bower 1979b) and thus to determine the RSA exactly.

1.3.3.1 RSA in the Maxilla

Hermann et al. (1983) as well as Gher and Dunlap (1985) dissected 20 extracted first maxillary molars and cross-sectioned them in 1 mm increments. Molars with fused roots were excluded. They observed that the disto-buccal root had a significantly smaller RSA than either the mesio-buccal or palatal root, confirming the results of Bower (1979b). The root trunk surface area was significantly larger than any surface of the three individual roots, and averaged 32% of the total RSA of the maxillary first molar (Hermann et al. 1983). Gher and Dunlap (1985) measured a mean root length of 13.6 mm (ranging from 10.5 to 16 mm) and a total RSA of 4.77 cm^2 (ranging from 3.36 to 5.84 cm^2). Additionally, a 'ballooning' of the RSA percentage in the furcation area of maxillary molars was described, which could not be detected in other teeth. Accordingly, the importance of periodontal support in the furcation area of maxillary molars was stressed, concluding that a relatively small attachment gain or loss may have a significant impact on the stability of the maxillary first molar (Gher and Dunlap 1985).

1.3.3.2 RSA in the Mandible

For a study on mandibular first molars, 10 teeth were hemisected and measured by Anderson et al. (1983). They concluded that the mesial root showed a statistically significant greater RSA than the distal root, which should be taken into consideration when planning treatment, especially regarding resective approaches. Dunlap and Gher (1985) dissected 20 extracted mandibulary first molars and cross-sectioned them in 1 mm increments. They too observed that the distal root had a significantly smaller RSA than the mesial one, but stressed that the shapes of the roots (conical for the distal one; hour-glass shaped for the mesial one) should be taken into consideration as well. In contrast to their findings in the maxilla, the root trunk surface area was not larger than the surface of the individual roots, and averaged 30.5% of the total RSA of the mandibulary first molar. They found a mean root length of 14.4 ± 1.1 mm and a total RSA of 4.37 ± 0.64 cm^2. In other studies (Jepsen 1963; Anderson et al. 1983), the total RSA varied from 4.31 to 4.7 cm^2.

1.3.4 Root Trunk Length

The portion of multi-rooted teeth located apical to the cemento-enamel junction (CEJ) is called the 'root complex' and is divided into root trunk and root cones. The root trunk is generally defined as the area of the tooth from the CEJ to the furcation fornix. In a study by Gher and Dunlap (1985), the distance between the CEJ and the furcation entrance in maxillary molars differed considerably between the mesial (3.6 ± 0.8 mm) and the distal entrance (4.8 ± 0.8 mm), whereas the buccal entrance was detected 4.2 ± 1.0 mm apical to the CEJ. These findings led to the conclusion that the clinician should suspect a through-and-through furcation (degree III according to Hamp et al. 1975) in maxillary molars once a loss of 6 mm in vertical attachment occurred. In more than 50% of the dissected maxillary molars, the furcation roof was found coronal of the root separations and formed a concave dome between the three roots.

It should be emphasized that the dome-like anatomy further complicates therapy and maintenance of maxillary first molars (Gher and Dunlap 1985). Hou and Tsai (1997b) measured the root trunk in 166 extracted first and second maxillary and 200 extracted first and second mandibular molars of a Taiwanese tooth sample. In the maxilla, short root trunks were more commonly found buccally, whereas long root trunks were more commonly found mesially (Hou and Tsai 1997b). The authors found generally longer root trunks in second molars than in first molars in both jaws, and additionally stated that long root trunks are associated with short root cone length (Hou and Tsai 1997b).

In 134 extracted first and second mandibular molars, Mandelaris et al. (1998) detected longer root trunks in lingual molar surfaces when compared to buccal surfaces (mean: 4.17 mm and 3.14 mm, respectively), confirming the results of Hou and Tsai (1997b). The mean distance between the CEJ and the furcation entrance was 4.0 ± 0.7 mm in mandibular molars (4.6 ± 0.6 mm in maxillary first molars; Dunlap and Gher 1985; Gher and Dunlap 1985), whereas no root trunk of > 6 mm could be found (Dunlap and Gher 1985; Mandelaris et al. 1998). Like in maxillary molars, it can be concluded that a through-and-through furcation (Hamp et al. 1975) should be expected in the mandible once a loss of 6 mm in vertical attachment was reached on both sides (buccal and lingual). On the other hand, it has to be kept in mind that a furcation defect has a horizontal component as well. Santana et al. (2004) measured 100 extracted first and second mandibular molars and their findings suggest that a horizontal attachment loss of 4.3–6.9 mm is essential in order to allow communication between the buccal and lingual furcation entrance. Complete or partial fusion of roots is also not unusual in multi-rooted teeth. Some 40% of maxillary premolars are two-rooted and the entrance to the furcation is located an average 8 mm from the CEJ, well into the middle third of the root complex (Bower 1979a).

A clinically evident FI correlates with the vertical length and type of the root trunk (Carnevale 1995; Hou and Tsai 1997b,

Al-Shammari et al. 2001). Thus, Al-Shammari et al. (2001) summarized that the root trunk length significantly relates to the prognosis and treatment of molars. A short root trunk worsens the prognosis with regard to a more likely FI, but once periodontal destruction has occurred, it improves the chances of a successful treatment (Horwitz et al. 2004).

1.4 Anatomical Aetiological Factors

1.4.1 Cervical Enamel Projections

Enamel surfaces do not allow for the attachment of connective tissue and represent an anatomical abnormality in the root area. Thus, cervical enamel projections (CEP) may contribute to the development of a furcation defect (Al-Shammari et al. 2001). The first to report a possible connection between CEPs and periodontal destruction in molars was Atkinson in 1949. According to Masters and Hoskins (1964), CEPs can be classified in three grades (Table 1.1).

Different prevalences of CEPs have been documented so far. Masters and Hoskins (1964) found CEPs in 29% of mandibular and 17% of maxillary molars. In Egyptian skulls, Bissada and Abdelmalek (1973) detected a CEP prevalence of 8.6%. In the 1138 molars studied, a higher incidence of CEPs in the

Table 1.1 Classification of cervical enamel projections.

Grade I	The enamel projection extends from the cemento-enamel junction of the tooth towards the furcation entrance (<1/3 of the root trunk).
Grade II	The enamel projection approaches the furcation entrance but does not enter it. No horizontal component is present (>1/3 of the root trunk). See Figure 1.3a.
Grade III	The enamel projection extends horizontally into the furcation. Compare Figures 1.3b and 1.3c.

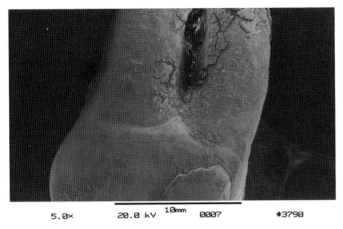

5.0×   20.0 kV   10mm   0007   #3790

Figure 1.3a Cervical enamel projection grade II (>1/3 of root trunk; Masters and Hoskins 1964) on upper right first molar (REM microscope). *Source*: Eickholz and Hausmann 1998.

mandible could be confirmed. A study in 200 East Indian skulls with 2000 molars reported a 32.6% incidence rate of CEPs (Swan and Hurt 1976). They were most often reported in mandibular second molars (51.0%), followed by maxillary second molars (45.6%), mandibular first and maxillary first molars (13.6%). Grade I enamel projections (Masters and Hoskins 1964) were detected most frequently. These could not be significantly related to furcation involvement, as could grade II and III CEPs (Swan and Hurt 1976). An observation in 78 Taiwanese individuals reported detection of CEPs in 49.3% of second and 62.3% of first maxillary and 51.2% of second and 73.9% of first mandibular molars (Hou and Tsai 1987). A study by the same authors in furcation-involved mandibular molars reported even higher CEP percentages: 71% of second and 92.9% of first mandibular molars showed enamel projections (Hou and Tsai 1997b). Mandelaris et al. (1998) documented CEPs in 66.4% of mandibular molars (61.9% of buccal and 50.8% of lingual surfaces) ranging from 0.98 to 1.33 mm in diameter. Current research on CEPs was published in 2013 and 2016. Bhusari et al. (2013) investigated their incidence on the buccal surface of 944 upper and lower first, second and third permanent molars from 89 Indian dry human skulls, and additionally measured FI. Again, it could be

confirmed that CEPs are found more frequently in the mandible and are significantly associated with the occurrence of FI. The incidence ranged from 14.7% in mandibular second molars to 5.5% in wisdom teeth. The most recent study was performed using cone-beam computed tomography data in a Korean population analysing 982 mandibular molars (Lim et al. 2016) and reported an overall prevalence rate of CEP of 76%. Grade I CEPs were the most common, followed by CEPs of grades II and III (Lim et al. 2016).

The huge variations can partly be explained by different study objects: in human skulls healthier periodontal conditions can be assumed, while extracted molars most probably show worse conditions, and Hou and Tsai (1987, 1997a) as well as Mandelaris et al. (1998) studied furcation-involved molars in periodontal patients. Additionally, a higher prevalence of CEPs in Oriental subjects than in Caucasians is suspected (Hou and Tsai 1987; Lim et al. 2016).

Nonetheless, it can be concluded that CEPs are a common problem which must be addressed by clinicians when treating molar teeth. They are more prevalent than enamel pearls and prevent connective tissue attachment, thus contributing to the aetiology of furcation defects, possibly resulting in localized chronic periodontitis and FI in molars (Leknes

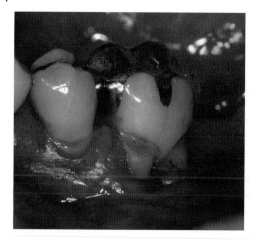

Figure 1.3b Cervical enamel projection on lower left first molar; grade III (reaching furcation entrance area; Masters and Hoskins 1964). *Source*: Eickholz 2005.

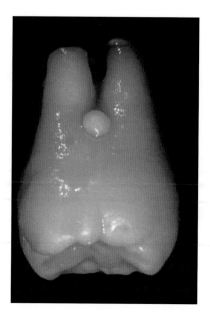

Figure 1.4a Macroscopic image of an enamel pearl on an extracted molar. *Source*: Courtesy of Prof. Dr. H.-K. Albers.

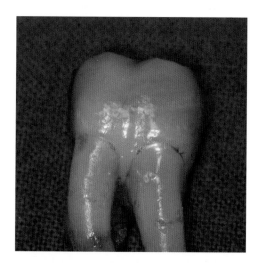

Figure 1.3c Cervical enamel projection on extracted lower right first molar; grade III (reaching furcation entrance area; Masters and Hoskins 1964). *Source*: Eickholz and Hausmann 1998.

1997; Al-Shammari et al. 2001; Bhusari et al. 2013). Additionally, significantly higher plaque and gingivitis index values have been reported in the presence of CEPs (Carnevale et al. 1995).

1.4.2 Enamel Pearls

Enamel pearls (see Figure 1.4) were first described in an article in the *American Journal of Dental Science* in 1841 (Moskow

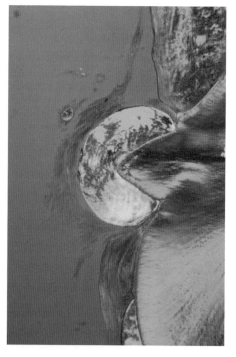

Figure 1.4b Microscopic image of an enamel pearl. *Source*: Courtesy of Prof. Dr. H.-K. Albers.

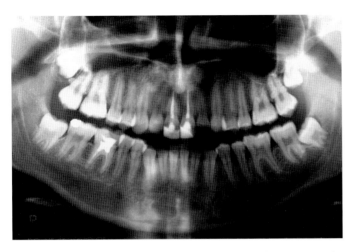

Figure 1.4c Orthopantomogram showing enamel pearls on upper right and left second molars. *Source*: Eickholz and Hausmann 1998.

and Canut 1990). They are ectopic globules consisting mostly of enamel, often containing a core of dentine, and they adhere to the tooth root surface, with a distinct predilection for the furcation areas of molar teeth, particularly maxillary third and second molars. In a review from 1990, an incidence of 2.6% (ranging from 1.1 to 9.7%) was reported, with differences among racial groups and a greater incidence in histological studies (Moskow and Canut 1990). Like CEPs, enamel projections prevent connective tissue attachment and thus contribute to the aetiology of periodontal destruction. They usually occur singularly, but up to four enamel pearls have been observed on the same tooth (Moskow and Canut 1990).

More recent research demonstrates an incidence within the range documented by Moskow and Canut (1990). Darwazeh and Hamasha (2000) evaluated the presence of enamel pearls in a Jordanian patient sample, studying 1032 periapical radiographs. An incidence of 1.6% of enamel pearls in molars and 4.76% per subject with no gender differences was reported. Chrcanovic et al. (2010) evaluated the prevalence of enamel pearls in 45 539 permanent teeth (20 218 molars) from a human tooth bank in Brazil. They confirmed the predominant presence in the maxilla and reported an incidence of 1.71%

in molars. Akgül et al. (2012) evaluated the presence of enamel pearls using cone-beam computed tomography in 15 185 teeth (4334 molars). An incidence of enamel pearls of 0.83% in molars and 4.69% per subject with no gender differences was reported. Again, the incidence was significantly higher in the maxilla. Colak et al. (2014) studied the prevalence of enamel pearls in Turkish dental patients and detected them in 0.85% of teeth and 5.1% of subjects, with a contradictory higher incidence in the mandible and in male patients.

Although lower in incidence than enamel projections, it can be summarized that enamel pearls play an important role in the aetiology of furcation defects, and it is considered essential to diagnose enamel pearls early on to allow for an adequate prognosis of molar retention and probably alter the therapeutic approach.

1.5 Periodontal Aetiological Factors in Molar Teeth

Aetiological factors interact with the previously described anatomical factors and may lead to periodontal destruction and attachment loss in molars, and thus result in a furcation defect. According to Al-Shammari et al. (2001), plaque-associated inflammation, trauma from occlusion, pulpal pathology, vertical root fractures, and iatrogenic factors need to be taken into consideration.

1.5.1 Plaque-associated Inflammation

The reader of this book will surely be well accustomed to plaque formation and the inflammatory component of gingivitis and periodontitis. What is special about molars in this context? In general, it can be stated that furcations are more prone to plaque adhesion and less likely to stay plaque free. The anatomy of the furcation favours retention of bacterial deposits and renders hygiene procedures difficult (Matthews and Tabesh 2004). In 1987, Nordland et al. monitored 2472 sites in 19 periodontal patients for 24 months after periodontal therapy, and reported that furcation sites responded less favourably to therapy and were more likely to exhibit higher plaque and gingivitis scores. Apart from that, it is assumed that furcation areas are an extension of periodontal pockets, because unique histological features are lacking (Glickman 1950; Al-Shammari et al. 2001). Thus, plaque formation follows the same process in molars and their furcations as in the remaining dentition (Leknes 1997).

1.5.2 Occlusal Trauma

Trauma from occlusion is suspected to be another aetiological factor contributing to periodontal destruction in molars. Two groups of researchers, Glickman and co-workers as well as Lindhe and co-workers, focused on this topic in animal studies applying excessive occlusal forces on molars. In their classic studies on beagle dogs, Lindhe and Svanberg (1974) and Nyman et al. (1978) reported significant alterations in tooth mobility combined with angular bony defects and loss of periodontal support in artificially created, gingivally inflamed multi-rooted teeth carrying splints, compared to teeth with inflammation but carrying no addi-

tional occlusal load. Even before that, Glickman et al. (1961) compared the effect of occlusal force on splinted and non-splinted teeth in rhesus monkeys, and suggested that the fibre orientation in the furcation area makes multi-rooted teeth more susceptible to increased functional forces. More recently, Nakatsu et al. (2014) confirmed the aforementioned findings in an observation in rats. On the other hand, Waerhaug (1980) concluded from his observations of 46 human molars (extracted because of advanced periodontal destruction) that increased mobility and occlusal trauma are *not* involved in the aetiology of the FI and are instead a late symptom of periodontal disease. Thus, the impact of occlusal forces in the aetiology of periodontitis in general and FI in particular remains controversial (Al-Shammari et al. 2001; Reinhardt and Killeen 2015). In a review, Harrel (2003) suggest that occlusal interferences should be regarded as a potential risk factor comparable to smoking, rather than a causative or aetiological factor.

1.5.3 Vertical Root Fractures

It is generally agreed that vertical root fractures, which can occur in a longitudinal direction on any surface of the root, are difficult to diagnose because they share symptoms with other dental conditions (Matthews and Tabesh 2004). Additionally, in most cases mild pain or a dull discomfort is the only clinical symptom of a vertical root fracture (Meister at al. 1980). They result in rapid localized loss of attachment and bone (Walton et al. 1984) and can lead to FI depending on their position. Mostly, a poor prognosis is assigned to teeth exhibiting vertical root fractures (Al-Shammari et al. 2001; Matthews and Tabesh 2004).

1.5.4 Endodontic Origin and Pulpal Pathology

Accessory canals are quite common in molar teeth. A study of 46 extracted molars of both jaws found accessory canals in 59% of examined teeth (Lowman et al. 1973). Burch and Hulen (1974) reported 'openings' in 76% of the furcations of maxillary and mandibular molars. These canals allow for products of pulpal necrosis to enter the furcation area and cause an inflammatory lesion (Carnevale et al. 1995). Thus, a pulpal pathosis can result in FI. Carnevale et al. (1995) reported that proximal and inter-radicular bone destruction of endodontic origin is reversible after root canal treatment. Periodontal therapy only becomes necessary in the case of a persistent lesion after the endodontic treatment. A more detailed description of the associations between FI and endodontic pathology is provided in Chapter 4.

1.5.5 Iatrogenic Factors

Generally, overhanging dental restorations or discrepancies of the subgingival margin in any kind of restoration or even orthodontic bands allow for adhesion of plaque and show detrimental effects on adjacent gingival tissues; additionally, the fit of prosthetic restorations is mostly less than perfect (Leknes 1997) and builds a niche, where plaque formation is facilitated and cleansing difficult. According to a study by Lang et al. (1983) in dental students with healthy gingivae who received proximal inlays with 1 mm overhangs, the microbial composition of the subgingival biofilm shifted from healthy to a composition characteristically found in periodontitis. Thus, the authors concluded that the changes observed in the subgingival microflora document a potential mechanism for the initiation of periodontal disease associated with iatrogenic factors. Wang et al. (1993) focused on molars and assessed the correlation between FI and the presence of a crown or proximal restoration in 134 periodontal patients during maintenance therapy. Their results showed a significant association between FI as well as periodontal attachment loss and the presence of a crown or restoration.

Additionally, Matthews and Tabesh (2004) commented that overhangs not only build a plaque retention niche, but also impinge on the biological width (between the depth of a healthy sulcus and the alveolar crest) and thus cause damage. They report ranges of overhangs in restored teeth from 18 to 87% (Matthews and Tabesh 2004). In general, the placement of restorative margins subgingivally results in more plaque, more gingival inflammation and deeper periodontal pockets.

It can be concluded that special care needs to be taken when placing restorations, and overhangs need to be diagnosed and removed as early as possible. Should a restoration margin need to be placed subgingivally, the biological width has to be kept in mind and crown lengthening considered. Thus, a dento-gingival attachment may be achieved (Herrero et al. 1995).

Summary of Evidence

- Numerous anatomical factors like furcation entrance area, bifurcation ridges, root surface area, and root trunk length need to be considered in the diagnosis and periodontal treatment of molars. The periodontist should be aware of these factors because they may have a significant impact on the prognosis and therapeutic outcome of multi-rooted teeth.
- Iatrogenic factors should be tackled early on (at the beginning of periodontal therapy), thus allowing for improvement of gingival and periodontal conditions.

References

Akgül, N., Caglayan, F., Durna, N. et al. (2012). Evaluation of enamel pearls by cone-beam computed tomography (CBCT). *Medicina Oral Patologica Oral y Cirurgia Bucal* 17, e218–e222.

Al-Shammari, K.F., Kazor, C.E., and Wang, H.-L. (2001). Molar root anatomy and management of furcation defects. *Journal of Clinical Periodontology* 28, 730–740.

Anderson, R.W., McGarrah, H.E., Lamb, R.D., and Eick, J.D. (1983). Root surface measurements of mandibular molars using stereophotogrammetry. *Journal of the American Dental Association* 107, 613–615.

Atkinson, S.R. (1949). Changing dynamics of the growing face. *American Journal of Orthodontics* 35, 815–836.

Bates, J.F., Stafford, G.D., and Harrison, A. (1975). Masticatory function – a review of the literature: 1. The form of the masticatory cycle. *Journal of Oral Rehabilitation* 2 (3), 281–301.

Bell, T. (1835). *The Anatomy, Physiology, and Diseases of the Teeth*. London: S. Highley.

Bhusari, P., Sugandhi, A., Belludi, S.A., and Shoyab Khan, S. (2013). Prevalence of enamel projections and its co-relation with furcation involvement in maxillary and mandibular molars: A study on dry skull. *Journal of the Indian Society of Periodontology* 17, 601–604.

Bhussry, B.R. (1980). Development and growth of teeth. In: *Orban's Oral Histology and Embryology* (ed. G.S. Kumar), 23–44. St Louis, MO: C.V. Mosby.

Bissada, N.F., and Abdelmalek, R.G. (1973). Incidence of cervical enamel projections and its relationship to furcation involvement in Egyptian skulls. *Journal of Periodontology* 44, 583–585.

Blake, R. (1801). *An Essay on the Structure and Formation of the Teeth in Man and Various Animals*. Dublin: Porter.

Bower, R.C. (1979a). Furcation morphology relative to periodontal treatment: Furcation entrance architecture. *Journal of Periodontology* 50, 23–27.

Bower, R.C. (1979b). Furcation morphology relative to periodontal treatment: Furcation root surface anatomy. *Journal of Periodontology* 50, 366–374.

Bower, R.C. (1983). Furcation development of human mandibular first molar teeth: A histologic graphic reconstructional study. *Journal of Periodontal Research* 18, 412–419.

Burch, J.G., and Hulen, S. (1974). A study of the presence of accessory foramina and the topography of molar furcations. *Oral Surgery, Oral Medicine, Oral Pathology* 38, 451–455.

Carnevale, G., Pontoriero, R., and Hürzeler, M.B. (1995). Management of furcation involvement. *Periodontology* 2000 9, 69–89.

Chiu, B.M., Zee, K.Y., Corbet, E.F., and Holmgren, C.J. (1991). Periodontal implications of furcation entrance dimensions in Chinese first permanent molars. *Journal of Periodontology* 62, 308–311.

Chrcanovic, B.R., Abreu, M.H.N.G., and Custódio A.L.N. (2010). Prevalence of enamel pearls in teeth from a human teeth bank. *Journal of Oral Science* 52, 257–260.

Churchill, H.R. (1935). *Meyer's Normal Histology and Histogenesis of the Human Teeth and Associated Parts* (trans. and ed. H.R. Churchill). Philadelphia, PA: J.B. Lippincott.

Çolak, H., Hamidi, M.M., Uzgur, R. et al. (2014). Radiographic evaluation of the prevalence of enamel pearls in a sample adult dental population. *European Review for Medical and Pharmacological Sciences* 18, 440–444.

Darwazeh, A., and Hamasha, A.A. (2002). Radiographic evidence of enamel pearls in Jordanian dental patients. *Oral Surgery, Oral Medicine, Oral Pathology, Oral Radiology Endodontology* 89, 255–258.

dos Santos, K.M., Pinto, S.C., Pochapski, M.T. et al. (2009). Molar furcation entrance and its relation to the width of curette blades used in periodontal mechanical therapy. *International Journal of Dental Hygiene* 7, 263–269.

Dunlap, R.M., and Gher, M.E. (1985). Root surface measurements of the mandibular first molar. *Journal of Periodontology* 56 (4), 234–248.

Eickholz, P. (2005). Clinical and radiographic diagnosis and epidemiology of furcation involvement. In: *Parodontologie: Praxis der Zahnheilkunde Band 4* (ed. D. Heidemann), Chapter 2. Munich: Urban & Fischer/Elsevier.

Eickholz, P., and Hausmann, E. (1998). Diagnostik der Furkationsbeteiligung: Eine Übersicht. *Quintessenz* 49 (1), 59–67.

Everett, F.G., Jump, E.B., Holder, T.D., and Williams, G.C. (1958). The intermediate bifurcational ridge: A study of the morphology of the bifurcation of the lower first molar. *Journal of Dental Research* 37, 162–169.

Gher, M.W. Jr, and Dunlap, R.M. (1985). Linear variation of the root surface area of the maxillary first molar. *Journal of Periodontology* 56, 39–43.

Gher, M.E., and Vernino, A.R. (1980). Root morphology: Clinical significance in pathogenesis and treatment of periodontal disease. *Journal of the American Dental Association* 101, 627–633.

Glickman, I. (1950). Bifurcation involvement in periodontal disease. *Journal of the American Dental Association* 40, 528–538.

Glickman, I., Stein, R.S., and Smulow, J.B. (1961). The effect of increased functional forces upon the periodontium of splinted and non-splinted teeth. *Journal of Periodontology* 32, 290–300.

Hamp, S.-E., Nyman, S., and Lindhe, J. (1975). Periodontal treatment of multirooted teeth: Results after 5 years. *Journal of Clinical Periodontology* 2, 126–135.

Harrel, S.K. (2003). Occlusal forces as a risk factor for periodontal disease. *Periodontology* 2000 32, 111–117.

Hermann, D.W., Gher, M.E., Jr, Dunlap, R.M., and Pelleu, G.B., Jr (1983). The potential attachment area of the maxillary first molar. *Journal of Periodontology* 54, 431–434.

Herrero, F., Scott, J.B., Maropis, P.S., and Yukna R.A. (1995). Clinical comparison of desired versus actual amount of surgical crown lengthening. *Journal of Periodontology* 66, 568–571.

Hiiemäe, K.M. (1967). Masticatory function in the mammals. *Journal of Dental Research* 46, 883–893.

Horwitz, J., Machtei, E.E., Reitmeir, P. et al. (2004). Radiographic parameters as prognostic indicators for healing of class II furcation defects. *Journal of Clinical Periodontology* 31, 105–111.

Hou, G.L., and Tsai, C.C. (1987). Relationship between periodontal furcation involvement and molar cervical enamel projections. *Journal of Periodontology* 58, 715–721.

Hou, G.L., and Tsai, C.C. (1997a). Cervical enamel projections and intermediate bifurcational ridge correlated with molar furcation involvements. *Journal of Periodontology* 68, 687–693.

Hou, G.L., and Tsai, C.C. (1997b). Types and dimensions of root trunk correlating with diagnosis of molar furcation involvements. *Journal of Clinical Periodontology* 24, 129–135.

Hou, G.L., Chen, S.F., Wu, Y.M., and Tsai, C.C. (1994). The topography of the furcation entrance in Chinese molars: Furcation entrance dimensions. *Journal of Clinical Periodontology* 21, 451–456.

Hujoel, P.P. (1994). A meta-analysis of normal ranges for root surface areas of the permanent dentition. *Journal of Clinical Periodontology* 21, 225–229.

Jepsen, A. (1963). Root surface measurement and a method for x-ray determination of root surface area. *Acta Odontologica Scandinavica* 21, 35–46.

Lang, N.P., Kiel, R.A., and Anderhalden, K. (1983). Clinical and microbiological effects of subgingival restorations with overhanging or clinically perfect margins. *Journal of Clinical Periodontology* 10, 563–578.

Leknes, K.N. (1997). The influence of anatomic and iatrogenic root surface characteristics on bacterial colonization and periodontal destruction: A review. *Journal of Periodontology* 68, 507–516.

Lim, H.-C., Jeon, S.-K., Cha, J.-K. et al. (2016). Prevalence of cervical enamel projection and its impact on furcation involvement in mandibular molars: A cone-beam computed tomography study in Koreans. *The Anatomical Record* 299, 379–384.

Lindhe, J., and Svanberg, G. (1974). Influence of trauma from occlusion on progression of experimental periodontitis in the beagle dog. *Journal of Clinical Periodontology* 1, 3–14.

Loevy, H.T., and Kowitz, A.A. (1997). The dawn of dentistry: Dentistry among the Etruscans. *International Dental Journal* 47, 279–284.

Lowman, J.V., Burke, R.S., and Pelleu, G.B. (1973). Patent accessory canals: Incidence in molar furcation region. *Oral Surgery Oral Medicine Oral Pathology* 38, 451–455.

Mandelaris, G.A., Wang, H.L., and MacNeil, R.L. (1998). A morphometric analysis of the furcation region of mandibular molars. *Compendium of Continuing Education in Dentistry* 19, 113–120.

Masters, D.H., and Hoskins, S.W. (1964). Projection of cervical enamel into molar furcations. *Journal of Periodontology* 35, 49–53.

Matthews, D., and Tabesh, M. (2004). Detection of localized tooth-related factors that predispose to periodontal infections. *Periodontology* 2000 34, 136–150.

Meister, F., Lommel, T.J., and Gerstein, H. (1980). Diagnosis and possible causes of vertical root fractures. *Oral Surgery, Oral Medicine, Oral Pathology* 49, 243–253.

Moskow, B.S., and Canut, P.M. (1990). Studies on root enamel. *Journal of Clinical Periodontology* 17, 275–281.

Nakatsu, S., Yoshinaga, Y., Kuramoto, A. et al. (2014). Occlusal trauma accelerates attachment loss at the onset of experimental periodontitis in rats. *Journal of Periodontal Research* 49, 314–322.

Nordland, P., Garrett, S., Kiger, R.D. et al. (1987). The effect of plaque control and root debridement in molar teeth. *Journal of Clinical Periodontology* 14, 231–236.

Nyman, S., Lindhe, J., and Ericsson, I. (1978). The effect of progressive tooth mobility on destructive periodontitis in the dog. *Journal of Clinical Periodontology* 5, 213–225.

Orban, B., and Mueller, E. (1929). The development of the bifurcation of multirooted teeth. *Journal of the American Dental Association* 16, 297–319.

Reinhardt, R.A., and Killeen, A.C. (2015). Do mobility and occlusal trauma impact periodontal longevity? *Dental Clinics of North America* 59, 873–883.

Rifkin, B.A., and Ackerman, M.J. (2011). *Human Anatomy: A Visual History from the Renaissance to the Digital Age.* New York, NY: Abrams Books.

Santana, R.B., Uzel, I.M., Gusman, H. et al. (2004). Morphometric analysis of the furcation anatomy of mandibular molars. *Journal of Periodontology* 75, 824–829.

Svärdström, G., and Wennström, J.L. (1988). Furcation topography of the maxillary and mandibular first molars. *Journal of Clinical Periodontology* 15, 271–275.

Swan, R.H., and Hurt, W.C. (1976). Cervical enamel projections as an etiologic factor in furcation involvement. *Journal of the American Dental Association* 93, 342–345.

Thesleff, I., and Hurmerinta, K. (1981). Tissue interactions in tooth development. *Differentiation* 18, 75–88.

Waerhaug, J. (1980). The furcation problem: Etiology, pathogenesis, diagnosis, therapy and prognosis. *Journal of Clinical Periodontology* 7, 73–95.

Walton, R.E., Michelich, R.J., and Smith, G.N. (1984). The histopathogenesis of vertical root fractures. *Journal of Endodontics* 10, 48–56.

Wang, H.L., Burgett, F.G., and Shyr, Y. (1993). The relationship between restoration and furcation involvement on molar teeth. *Journal of Periodontology* 64, 302–305.

Chapter 2

Clinical and Radiographic Diagnosis and Epidemiology of Furcation Involvement

Peter Eickholz[1] and Clemens Walter[2]

[1] Poliklinik für Parodontologie, Zentrum der Zahn- Mund- und Kieferheilkunde (Carolinum), Johann Wolfgang Goethe-Universität Frankfurt, Frankfurt am Main, Germany
[2] Klinik für Parodontologie, Endodontologie und Kariologie, Universitätszahnkliniken, Universitäres Zentrum für Zahnmedizin Basel, Basel, Switzerland

2.1 Introduction

In single-rooted teeth, periodontal destruction proceeds from the cemento-enamel junction (CEJ) apically, predominantly in a vertical direction. The vertical attachment loss is assessed as vertical probing attachment loss (PAL-V) from the CEJ, or if the CEJ is destroyed by a restoration from the restoration margin (RM) to the bottom of the periodontal pocket. Vertical bone loss is assessed radiographically or by vertical probing bone level (PBL-V) from the CEJ or RM to the alveolar crest. If periodontitis affects multi-rooted teeth, the tissues are not only destroyed vertically but also horizontally between the roots, creating furcation involvement. This dimension of periodontal destruction (horizontal attachment and bone loss) may be assessed as horizontal probing attachment loss (PAL-H) or horizontal probing bone level (PBL-H).

Horizontal probing attachment loss and bone loss in the furcation area create a niche (furcation involvement), which impedes accessibility for individual oral hygiene in the molar region (Lang et al. 1973) and professional root debridement (Fleischer et al. 1989). This adds to the factors contributing to more severe disease progression in furcation-involved molars, recurrent periodontal infection, and as a result an inferior long-term prognosis of these teeth (McGuire and Nunn 1996; Dannewitz et al. 2006, 2016; Pretzl et al. 2008; Salvi et al. 2014; Graetz et al. 2015). Furcation-involved molars respond less favourably to periodontal therapy than molars without furcation involvement or single-rooted teeth, and are at greater risk for further attachment loss (Nordland et al. 1987; Loos et al. 1989; Wang et al. 1994) than other teeth. Addressing this issue, Kalkwarf et al. (1988) reported the success of different surgical and non-surgical treatment modalities in 158 molars. Irrespective of the therapy performed, the horizontal defect in the furcation area increased during the two-year follow-up. Thus, reliable diagnosis of incidence and extent of furcation involvement is decisive for prognosis and treatment planning.

2.2 Clinical Furcation Diagnosis

Furcation involvement can only be found in multi-rooted teeth (Table 2.1). More than one root is regularly found in maxillary and mandibular molars as well as in first maxillary

Diagnosis and Treatment of Furcation-Involved Teeth, First Edition. Edited by Luigi Nibali.
© 2018 John Wiley & Sons Ltd. Published 2018 by John Wiley & Sons Ltd.
Companion website: www.wiley.com/go/nibali/diagnosis

Table 2.1 Regularly multi-rooted teeth with location of roots and location of furcation entrances.

Tooth type	Location of roots	Location of furcation entrance
Maxillary molars	Mesio-buccal	Buccal
	Disto-buccal	Mesio-palatal
	Palatal	Disto-palatal
Maxillary premolars	Buccal	Mesial
	Palatal	Distal
Mandibular molars	Mesial	Buccal
	Distal	Lingual

premolars (see Chapter 1). However, two-rooted variants may be found in second maxillary premolars and mandibular anteriors. Rarely, three-rooted variants may be found in mandibular molars and maxillary premolars (Mohammadi et al. 2013). Those sites at which furcation entrances are regularly expected have to be examined for furcation involvement on a regular basis in the course of periodontal examination. Search for and scoring of furcation involvement are fundamental elements of periodontal examination.

Particularly in untreated periodontal patients, furcation entrances do not lie open. In most cases they are covered by gingiva. Thus, furcation involvement cannot be seen simply with the naked eye, but has to be probed below the gingival margin. The

bizarre anatomy of furcations (Schroeder and Scherle 1987), their curved course, and the fact that the furcation entrances of maxillary premolars and molars open into interproximal spaces require the use of particular curved furcation probes in furcation diagnosis (e.g. Nabers probe; Figure 2.1). The probe is placed onto the tooth surface coronally of the gingival margin at the site where a furcation entrance is expected (e.g. lingual of a mandibular molar). Then the probe is pushed apically, gently displacing the gingiva in zigzag movements until the bottom of the sulcus or pocket is reached. If the probe falls into a pit horizontally, in most cases furcation involvement has been detected.

Straight rigid periodontal probes (e.g. PCPUNC15) are inappropriate for furcation

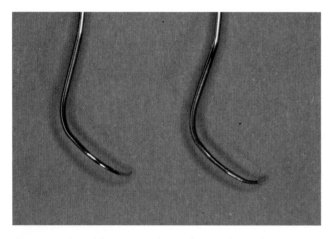

Figure 2.1 Curved furcation probes: Nabers probes (left: without markings; right: marked in 3 mm steps up to 12 mm).

diagnosis because they fail to follow the curved course of most furcations. Their use bears a high risk of underestimating the extent of the furcation involvement (Eickholz and Kim 1998).

2.2.1 Classification of Furcation Involvement

Besides the simple fact of the existence of a furcation involvement and its location, the severity of furcation involvement is of major significance. Severity of furcation involvement is assessed by probing the respective furcation in a horizontal direction using a rigid curved probe (e.g. Nabers probe) and measuring the distance from the probe tip to a virtual tangent to the root convexities adjacent to the furcation (Figure 2.2). Measuring this distance allows assessment of different degrees of furcation involvement or the amount of horizontal attachment loss in millimetres (horizontal probing/clinical attachment level: PAL-H/CAL-H; Figures 2.2–2.4). Whereas assessment of the continuous variable horizontal attachment loss provides information on small changes of inter-radicular tissues (since they are relevant after regenerative therapy), the categorical classification of inter-radicular tissue destruction as degree

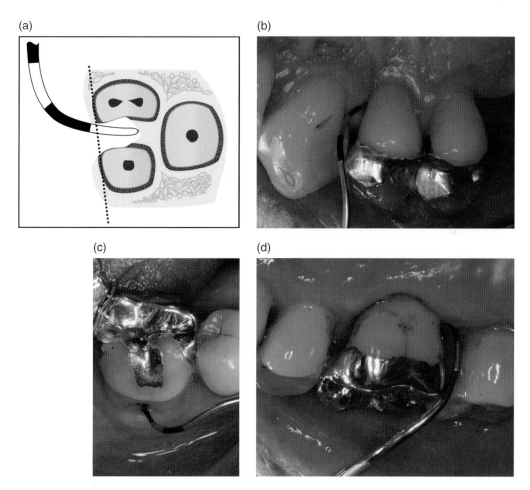

(a)　　(b)

(c)　　(d)

Figure 2.2 Furcation involvement degree I (Eickholz and Staehle 1994; Table 2.4): horizontal loss of periodontal tissue support up to 3 mm: (a) schematic (maxillary molar, buccal furcation entrance): horizontal probing/clinical attachment level 2.5 mm; (b) mesial tooth 24 with neighbouring tooth; (c) buccal tooth 46: the probe does not penetrate more than 3 mm between the two buccal roots; (d) disto-palatal tooth 16 with neighbouring tooth.

(a)

(b)

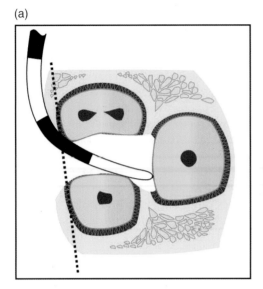
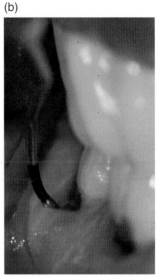

Figure 2.3 Furcation involvement degree II (Hamp et al. 1975; Tables 2.3 and 2.4): horizontal loss of support exceeding 3 mm, but not encompassing the total width of the furcation area: (a) schematic (maxillary molar, buccal furcation entrance): horizontal probing/clinical attachment level 5 mm; (b) tooth 47: the 9 mm marking is at the gingival margin. However, the 6 mm marking is at the height of the virtual tangent placed to the roots adjacent to the furcation. *Source*: Eickholz (2010).

of furcation involvement provides sufficiently relevant information for prognosis and decision regarding therapy of the respective multi-rooted tooth.

The different classifications of furcation involvement basically exhibit differences only in the details (Tables 2.2–2-3). The classification by Glickman (1953) provides somewhat vague criteria to distinguish classes of furcation involvement, and also considers radiographic information which is known to be of low reliability (Table 2.2; Ammons and Harrington 2006). The criteria for the Hamp et al. (1975) classification are based on measurements (threshold: PAL-H = 3 mm). The colour-coded version of the Nabers probe, marked in 3 mm steps (PQ2N; Figure 2.1), is particularly suitable for scoring degrees of furcation involvement, according to Hamp et al. (1975; Eickholz and Kim 1998). However, there exist also furcation probes with 2 mm markings (Zappa probe ZA 2).

The distinction between degrees I and II of the Glickman classification is not as clear or definite as the distinction between degrees I and II according to Hamp et al. (1975); that is, horizontal loss of periodontal tissue support less than 3 mm (degree I) or exceeding 3 mm (degree II). Degrees III and IV of the Glickman classification describe two severity grades of the situation where the desmodontal fibres are detached from the furcation fornix/dome throughout the diameter of the tooth; that is, horizontal 'through-and-through' destruction of the periodontal tissue in the furcation (degree III according to Hamp et al. 1975).

The criteria for assigning a degree III (Hamp et al. 1975) to a furcation have also been modified. For Graetz et al. (2014), it was required to see the tip of the furcation probe (Nabers) at the opposite furcation opening to assign a degree III. For all other cases of deep but not completely penetrating horizontal probing, a degree II was assigned (Graetz et al. 2014). Walter et al. (2009) created a degree II–III for the situation of horizontal probing of more than 6 mm, but not completely penetrating to the opposite furcation entrance (Table 2.3). This at least partially

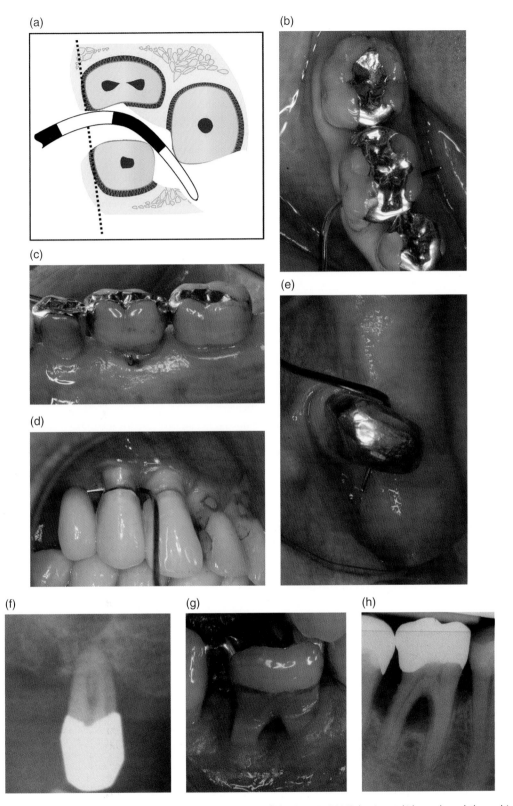

Figure 2.4 Furcation involvement degree III (Ammons and Harrington 2006): horizontal 'through-and-through' destruction of the periodontal tissue in the furcation: (a) schematic (maxillary molar, buccal to interproximal furcation entrance); (b) tooth 46 (occlusal view); (c) lingual view; (d) tooth 14; (e) tooth 16 without neighbouring tooth from mesio-palatal to disto-palatal; (f) respective radiograph; (g) tooth 46: the interdental bone is destroyed, and the soft tissues have receded apically so that the furcation opening is clinically visible. A tunnel therefore exists between the roots of such an affected tooth (Glickman degree IV); (h) respective radiograph. *Source*: d and e, Eickholz (2010).

Table 2.2 Classification of furcation involvement according to Glickman (1953).

Degree 0	No furcation involvement.
Degree I	Early/incipient stage of furcation involvement.
	The pocket is suprabony and primarily affects the soft tissue.
	Early bone loss may have occurred with an increase in probing depth.
	Radiographic changes are not usually found.
Degree II	Can affect one or more of the furcations of the same tooth.
	The furcation lesion is essentially a cul-de-sac with a definite horizontal component.
	If multiple defects are present, they do not communicate with each other because a portion of alveolar bone remains attached to the tooth.
	The extent of the horizontal probing of the furcation determines whether the defect is early or advanced.
	Vertical bone loss may be present and represents a therapeutic complication.
	Radiographs may or may not depict the furcation involvement, particularly with maxillary molars because of the radiographic overlap of the roots. In some views, however, the presence of furcation 'arrows' indicates possible furcation involvement.
Degree III	The bone is not attached to the dome of the furcation.
	In early degree III involvement, the opening may be filled with soft tissue and may not be visible. The clinician may not even be able to pass a periodontal probe completely through the furcation because of interference with the bifurcational ridges or facial/lingual bony margins. However, if the clinician adds the buccal and lingual probing dimensions and obtains a cumulative probing measurement that is equal to or greater than the buccal/lingual dimension of the tooth at the furcation orifice, the clinician must conclude that a degree III furcation exists (Figure 2.5).
	Properly exposed and angled radiographs of early degree III furcations display the defect as a radiolucent area in the crotch of the tooth.
Degree IV	The interdental bone is destroyed, and the soft tissues have receded apically so that the furcation opening is clinically visible.
	A tunnel therefore exists between the roots of such an affected tooth.
	The periodontal probe passes readily from one aspect of the tooth to another.

Source: Ammons and Harrington (2006).

Table 2.3 Classification of furcation involvement according to Hamp et al. (1975).

Degree 0	No furcation involvement.
Degree I	Horizontal loss of periodontal tissue support less than 3 mm (Figure 2.2).
	Modifications by:
	• Eickholz and Staehle (1994): horizontal loss of periodontal tissue support up to 3 mm.
	• Carnevale et al. (1995): horizontal loss of periodontal support not exceeding one-third of the width of the tooth.
Degree II	Horizontal loss of support exceeding 3 mm, but not encompassing the total width of the furcation area (Figure 2.3).
	Modifications by:
	• Carnevale et al. (1995): horizontal loss of periodontal support exceeding one-third of the width of the tooth, but not encompassing the total width of the furcation area.
	• Walter et al. (2009): degree II – horizontal loss of support exceeding 3 mm, but no more than 6 mm.
Degree II–III	• Walter et al. (2009): horizontal loss of support exceeding 6 mm, but no detectable 'through-and-through' destruction.
Degree III	Horizontal 'through-and-through' destruction of the periodontal tissue in the furcation (Figure 2.4).
	Modification by:
	• Graetz et al. (2014): through-and-through furcation (requiring seeing the tip of the Nabers probe at the contralateral furcation opening).

Source: Hamp et al. (1975).

explains the low validity of detecting degree III furcations accurately by clinical probing compared to cone-beam computer tomography (CBCT; Walter et al. 2009) or intrasurgical assessments (Graetz et al. 2014).

Svärdström and Wennström (1996) proposed another classification that does not count millimetres but estimates horizontal probing: degree 0 = the furcation site not probeable; degree 1 = the root trunk coronal to the furcation entrance probeable; degree 2 = the tip of the probe passes horizontally into the furcation but does not reach the centre of the furcation area; degree 3 = the tip of the probe reaches to or beyond the centre of the furcation area (Svärdström & Wennström 1996). The definition of degree 3 is quite similar to Walter et al.'s (2009) degree II–III. However, this classification does not consider the case of a clearly probeable through-and-through furcation.

2.2.2 Distinction Between Degree II and Degree III Furcation Involvement

The distinction between degree II (Hamp et al. 1975; Figure 2.3) and through-and-through furcation (degree III; Figure 2.4) is of decisive significance for either prognosis as well as choice of therapy:

- Molars with degree III furcation defects have a worse long-term prognosis than

degree II lesions (McGuire and Nunn 1996; Dannewitz et al. 2006, 2016; Salvi et al. 2014; Graetz et al. 2015).
- Whereas buccal and lingual degree II lesions at least can be improved by regenerative therapy, there is no clinical evidence for any benefit of regenerative treatment in through-and-through furcations (Sanz et al. 2015; see Chapters 6 and 7).

Particularly from interproximally located furcation entrances in the presence of adjacent teeth, a furcation probe cannot be completely pushed through the whole furcation area involved. Nevertheless, hard and soft tissue may be detached from the furcation fornix; that is, furcation involvement degree III. In the definition of degree III by Graetz et al. (2014), this situation would be rated degree II. Walter et al. (2009) would rate this situation degree II–III. In these cases, it is recommended to follow Ammons and Harrington (2006): in cases where the clinician may not even be able to pass a periodontal probe completely through the furcation because of interference with the bifurcational ridges or facial/lingual bony margins, they may add the buccal and lingual probing dimensions. If a cumulative probing measurement is obtained that is equal to or greater than the buccal/lingual dimension of the tooth at the furcation orifice, the furcation is rated degree III

Table 2.4 Recommended classification of furcation involvement.

Degree 0	No furcation involvement.
Degree I	Horizontal loss of periodontal tissue support up to 3 mm (Eickholz and Staehle 1994).
Degree II	Horizontal loss of support exceeding 3 mm, but not encompassing the total width of the furcation area (Hamp et al. 1975).
Degree III	Horizontal 'through-and-through' destruction of the periodontal tissue in the furcation. In early degree III involvement, the opening may be filled with soft tissue and may not be visible. The clinician may not even be able to pass a periodontal probe completely through the furcation because of interference with the bifurcational ridges or facial/lingual bony margins. However, if the clinician adds the buccal and lingual probing dimensions and obtains a cumulative probing measurement that is equal to or greater than the buccal/lingual dimension of the tooth at the furcation orifice, the clinician must conclude that a degree III furcation exists (Ammons and Harrington 2006).

Sources: Hamp et al. (1975); Eickholz and Staehle (1994); Ammons and Harrington (2006).

(Tables 2.2 and 2.4). Thus, underestimation of furcation involvement as observed by Walter et al. (2009) and Graetz et al. (2014) can be avoided.

2.2.3   The Vertical Dimension of Furcation Involvement

The central problem about furcation involvement is the difficult-to-access horizontal niche between the roots of multi-rooted teeth. Thus, the classifications referred to consider mainly the horizontal component of attachment/bone loss. However, it is plausible that in addition to horizontal attachment/bone loss, vertical attachment/bone loss in the furcation area plays a role. It has been demonstrated that survival of molars after furcation therapy does not only depend on baseline furcation involvement, but also on baseline bone loss (Dannewitz et al. 2006; Park et al. 2009). Thus, a subclassification has been proposed that measures the probeable vertical depth from the roof of the furcation apically. Subclass A indicates a probeable vertical depth of 1–3 mm, B 4–6 mm, and C 7 mm or more of probeable depth from the roof of the furcation apically. Furcations would thus be classified as IA, IB, IC, IIA, IIB, IIC, and IIIA, IIIB, IIIC (Tarnow and Fletcher 1984). The more severe the vertical component the worse is long-term prognosis of molars with degree II furcation involvement (Tonetti et al. 2017). Prognosis also depends on the remaining circular attachment of each root (Walter et al. 2009).

2.2.4   Reproducibility and Validity of the Assessment of Furcation Involvement

Furcation involvement is difficult to access for hygiene. How reliably can furcation lesions be diagnosed; that is, scored? Whereas for buccal, lingual, and mesio-lingual scoring of furcation degrees excellent intrarater reproducibility is reported, disto-lingual furcation lesions provide only moderate reproducibility. Similar results are reported for PAL-H measurements (excluding degree III furcation involvement).

Intrarater reproducibility in disto-lingual furcations is significantly worse than for all other locations. In mesio-buccal furcations, a neighbouring tooth is associated with higher variability (Eickholz and Staehle 1994; Eickholz and Kim 1998). Interproximal furcations, in particular the disto-lingual site and in the presence of a neighbouring tooth, are more difficult to access and to measure than the other locations. This fact has to be kept in mind when the clinical examiner scores maxillary molars in particular.

How accurately does the clinical measurement assess the intrasurgically measured furcation involvement (PBL-H)? Disto-lingual location and a neighbouring tooth are also associated with less accuracy. Furthermore, a curved rigid furcation probe (Nabers probe) demonstrated better accuracy than a straight rigid (PCPUNC 15) and flexible plastic (TPS) probe (Eickholz and Kim 1998). Interestingly, clinical PAL-H measurements on average overestimated intrasurgically measured PBL-H. However, the difference was only significant for measurements with a Nabers probe in degree I furcation lesions (Eickholz 1995; Eickholz and Kim 1998).

2.2.5   Documentation of Furcation Involvement

As documented in Chapter 5, differentiated documentation of furcation involvement according to extent (degree) and location is a prerequisite for proper prognosis and treatment planning (Figure 2.5). In the meantime, many computer programs for dental patient charting provide the necessary differentiated digital documentation (Florida probe chart; Figure 2.6).

2.3   Radiographic Diagnosis of Furcation Involvement

In general, radiographs provide information on the translucency to X-rays of different tissues. The denser a tissue (e.g. compact bone) is, the less translucent it is for X-rays. Thus, both two- and three-dimensional radiographic images primarily provide information

(a)

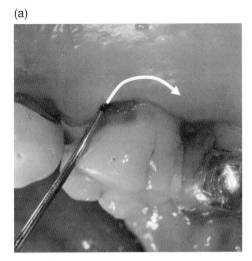

(b)

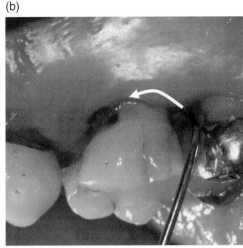

Figure 2.5 Furcation probing at tooth 16: (a) from mesio-palatal – probing (PAL-H)/clinical horizontal attachment loss (CAL-H) = 9 mm; (b) from disto-palatal – probing (PAL-H)/clinical horizontal attachment loss (CAL-H) = 6 mm. In tooth 16 the PAL-H/CAL-H measurements add up to 15 mm. At the furcation entrances tooth 16 has a width less than 15 mm. Thus the furcation is through and through (degree III; Table 2.4). *Source:* Eickholz (2010).

on bone in contrast to soft tissue. However, furcation involvement is not only a matter of bone, but also of connective tissue attachment. Therefore, radiographs tell a substantial part of but not the whole story about furcation involvement. This is particularly true after regenerative treatment, where there may be a new connective tissue attachment without new bone formation within a furcation.

Using two-dimensional radiographic techniques (projection radiography: periapical and panoramic radiographs), reliable diagnosis of furcation involvement is not provided (Topoll et al. 1988). For maxillary premolars, the furcation channel is oriented perpendicularly to the central beam. Thus, furcation involvement in maxillary premolars cannot be visualized using projection radiography. In three-rooted maxillary molars, the furcation channel between mesio- and disto-palatal furcation entrances also runs parallel to the plane of the radiographic film or sensor and perpendicular to the central beam. The buccal furcation entrance is in most cases overlapped by the palatal root. Thus, in maxillary molars inter-radicular bone can be judged

only to a very limited extent. Only in mandibular molars is the furcation channel located perpendicularly to the plane of the film/sensor and parallel to the central beam. Therefore, under conditions of orthoradial projection, inter-radicular bone may be assessed in mandibular molars. However, radiographs only provide information on resorption or density of bone. Reduced bone density may be due to periodontal destruction or reduced bone density caused by loose spongeous structure. Thus, conventional radiographs may only provide hints for a suspicion of furcation involvement; this suspicion has to be confirmed or rejected by furcation probing using a curved probe.

Additional to degree of furcation involvement, radiographs may provide information to judge whether a buccal or lingual degree II furcation may benefit from regenerative therapy. In molars with class II furcation involvement, a long root trunk, a furcation fornix located coronally of the adjacent interproximal alveolar crest, and a wide furcation are associated with less favourable horizontal attachment gain after regenerative therapy (Horwitz et al. 2004).

(a)

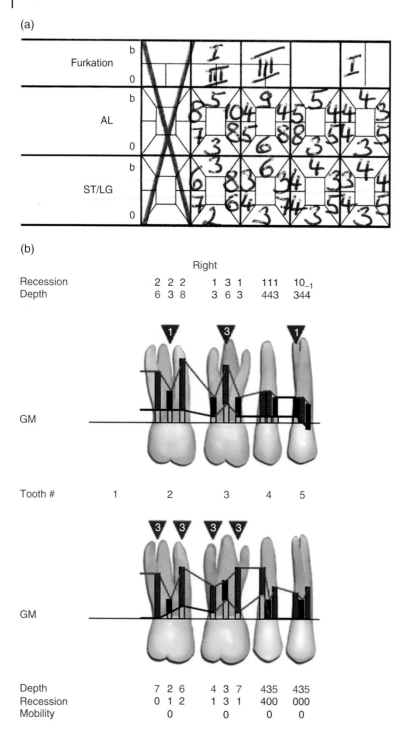

(b)

Right

Recession		2	2	2		1	3	1		111		10$_{-1}$
Depth		6	3	8		3	6	3		443		344

GM

Tooth #   1   2   3   4   5

GM

Depth		7	2	6		4	3	7		435		435
Recession		0	1	2		1	3	1		400		000
Mobility			0				0			0		0

Figure 2.6 Differentiated documentation of furcation scores: (a) periodontal chart from the Department of Periodontology of the Johann Wolfgang Goethe-Universität, Frankfurt am Main: tooth 17 – buccal degree I furcation; through-and-through furcation from mesio-palatal to disto-palatal (Grade III); tooth 16 – through-and-through furcation at all furcation entrances; tooth 14 – distal degree I furcation. (b) Florida Probe: tooth 17 – buccal degree I furcation; through-and-through furcation from mesio-palatal to disto-palatal (Grade III); tooth 16 – through-and-through furcation at all furcation entrances; tooth 14 – distal degree I furcation.

2.3.1 Digital Subtraction Radiography

A highly specialized and technically sensitive radiographic method may be used to follow up changes of inter-radicular bone in molar furcations: digital subtraction radiography (DSR; (Eickholz and Hausmann 1997). Two consecutively obtained radiographs (e.g. prior to and 12 months after therapy) of the same tooth are overlapped in such a way that corresponding structures are positioned exactly over one another. The grey values of the baseline radiograph are inverted (white to black, black to white) and added to those of the follow-up radiograph. In two completely identical radiographs that overlap perfectly, a middle grey value will result. An increase of bone density (bony fill) results in lighter grey values, a decrease of bone density (bone loss) in darker grey values (Eickholz and Hausmann 1997; Figure 2.7). However, DSR requires strict standardization of projection geometry and is highly sensitive to misalignment. Thus, the technique is rarely applied in clinical practice.

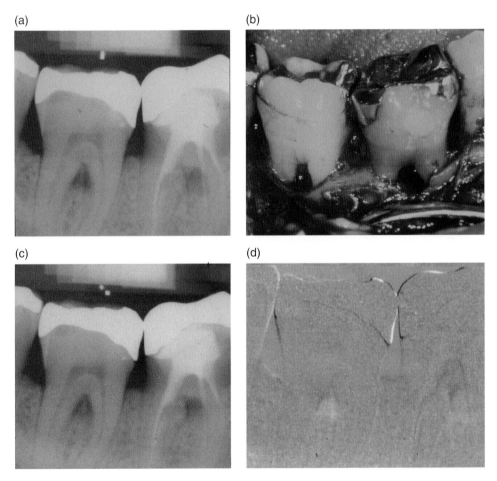

(a)

(b)

(c)

(d)

Figure 2.7 Follow-up of inter-radicular bone at teeth 46 and 47 using digital subtraction radiography (DSR): (a) standardized radiograph of teeth 46 and 47 prior to regenerative therapy; (b) intrasurgical view – buccal degree II furcation involvement at both teeth; (c) standardized radiograph six months after regenerative therapy; (d) subtraction image – increase of bone density within the furcations of 46 and 47. *Source*: Eickholz (2010).

2.3.2 Three-dimensional Radiography

Since conventional two-dimensional radiographic imaging may have some clinically relevant drawbacks, it might be useful to analyse distinct clinical situations, particularly in maxillary molar teeth, with a suitable three-dimensional diagnostic approach with appropriate exposure to radiation (Laky et al. 2013; Walter et al. 2016). Cone Beam Computed Tomography (CBCT) has been validated in vivo for the assessment of furcation-involved maxillary molars (Walter et al. 2016). CBCT data were found to be accurate in assessing the amount of periodontal tissue loss and in classifying the degree of furcation involve-

ment in maxillary molars (Walter et al. 2009, 2010, 2016). In addition, the three-dimensional images revealed several findings, such as the surrounding bony support of each maxillary molar root, fusion or proximity of roots, periapical lesions, root perforations, and/or missing bony walls (Walter et al. 2009). The clinical relevance of these radiographic data was analysed regarding the decision-making process for resective or non-resective therapies (Figures 2.8 and 2.9). These treatment options were classified according to their graduation of invasiveness (GoI), ranging from minimally invasive SPT to maximally invasive extraction and implant restoration: GoI 0 = supportive periodontal treatment

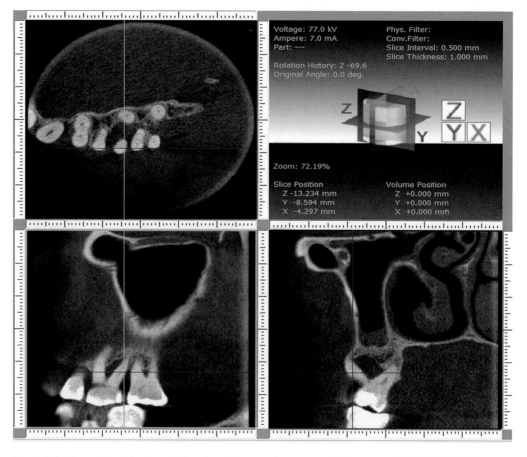

Figure 2.8 Diagnosis and treatment planning using cone-beam computed tomography (CBCT). CBCT images with horizontal, sagittal, and transversal sections of first and second left maxillary molars. According to the bone loss around the disto-buccal root and the remaining periodontal attachment around the mesio-buccal and palatal root, it was decided to extract the distobuccal root. *Source*: Walter et al. (2010).

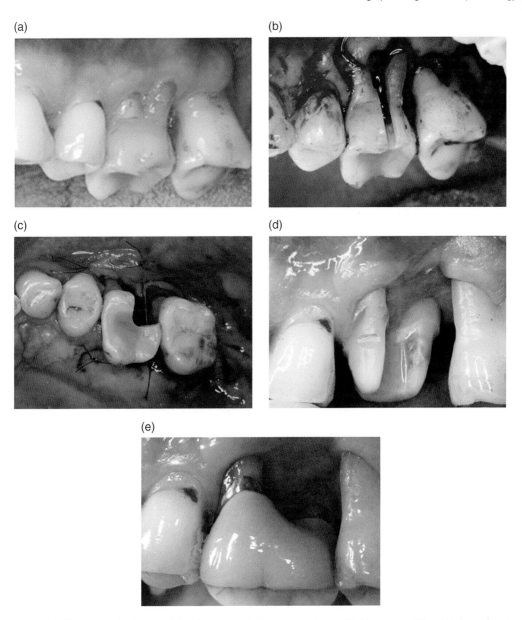

Figure 2.9 Root resection in a maxillary first molar: (a) pre-surgical view; (b) tri-section of the distobuccal root; (c) the flap is fixed with monofil synthetic sutures 5 × 0; (d) four months post-operation, the wound healing was uneventful; (e) a crown with an extended metal margin is placed and the patient is introduced to meticulous oral hygiene.

(SPT); GoI 1 = open flap debridement with or without gingivectomy or apically repositioned flap and/or tunnelling; GoI 2 = root separation; GoI 3 = amputation/trisection of one root (with or without root separation or tunnel preparation; GoI 4 = amputation/trisection of two roots; and GoI 5 = extraction of the entire tooth. Significant discrepancies between conventional and CBCT-based treatment approaches were found in most situations, which possibly necessitates intrasurgical changes in the treatment plan in those cases where no CBCT is available (Walter et al. 2009).

However, the findings from a cost-benefit analysis indicate the need for a critical appraisal of CBCT applications in upper molars (Walter et al. 2012). In most cases with clinically based GoI ≤ 1, CBCT imaging seems to have no or only minor impact on economic benefit and to reduce treatment time only slightly, if at all. With more invasive clinically based treatment decisions (GoI > 1), however, the benefits of using CBCT were greater, probably because the indication for tooth extraction is clarified. On the one hand, a straightforward tooth extraction followed by implant placement and restoration is feasible, thereby avoiding explorative periodontal surgeries when the tooth is not maintainable. On the other hand, unnecessary tooth extractions and implant placement in sites where teeth would be maintainable may be avoided. Moreover, root canal treatments in sites planned for GoI degrees 2, 3, or 4 may be prevented, when CBCT reveals morphological variations such as root proximities or root fusions, which preclude clinically based resective treatment planning.

The main goal of diagnostic radiology is to keep the radiation dose as low as reasonably achievable (ALARA), and this should also be a prerequisite for CBCT application in dentistry, since increased radiation in the dental office may potentially cause malignancies, including thyroid cancer or intracranial meningioma (Hallquist and Näsman 2001; Longstreth et al. 2004; Hujoel et al. 2006). The potential risks associated with additional radiation exposure are only justified in single cases and have to be evaluated in each individual situation.

2.4 Epidemiology of Furcation Involvement

How frequent is furcation involvement? There exists only one population-representative study from the USA on the frequency of furcation involvement. Even in periodontitis patients, studies reporting the frequency of furcation involvement differentiated according to degree are rare and relatively small.

For the third National Health and Nutrition Examination Survey (NHANES III), 9689 individuals representative of the US population received periodontal examinations including furcation scores. Partial furcation involvement was scored in sites where the explorer was definitely catching into but did not pass through the furcation. This represents degrees I and II of the Hamp et al. (1975) classification (Table 2.3). Total furcation involvement was assigned when the explorer could be passed between the roots and through the entire furcation. This represents degree III of the Hamp et al. (1975) classification (Table 2.3). The prevalence of furcation involvement for all age groups was 13.7%, and the extent was 6.8% of posterior teeth per person. The prevalence of through-and-through furcation involvement was 0.9% (extent: 0.5%). The prevalence of furcation-involved teeth (all/through-and-through) increased with age (60–69 years: 27.6/2.1%; 70–79: 31.7/3.2%; 80–89: 37.9/3.4%) and was higher in males (17.8/1.2%) than in females (11.3/0.7%; Albandar et al. 1999).

For a sample of 71 periodontally diseased patients in Germany, Dannewitz et al. (2006) reported tooth-based furcation involvement; that is, they assigned to each molar the most severe furcation involvement that was observed within the particular tooth. Using this mode, the information relevant for prognosis is given for each molar. However, the frequency of less severe furcation degrees is underestimated. They observed degree I furcation lesions in 23%, and degree II and III furcation lesions in 24% and 13% of all molars, respectively. No furcation involvement at all was exhibited in 40% of all molars. Premolars were not scored (Dannewitz et al. 2006).

In a sample of 345 periodontitis patients (Eickholz et al. 2016), the degree of furcation involvement of all sites was reported (site based). This enlarges the proportion of less severe furcation lesions in comparison to reporting tooth-based furcation involvement.

There was no furcation involvement in 45% of all furcation sites, which approximately confirms the frequency reported for molars (Dannewitz et al. 2006). The study observed degree I furcation lesions in 36%, and degree II and III furcation lesions in 13.5% and 5.5% of all molars and first maxillary premolars, respectively. Considering this and the fact that Dannewitz et al. (2006) did not report premolars, the data on frequency of furcation lesions roughly confirm the earlier findings in a much larger sample (Eickholz et al. 2016).

In individuals aged 40 years or older, every second molar was affected by advanced periodontal destruction (score 2–3) in at least one furcation site (Svärdström and Wennström 1996). Furcation involvement was found more frequently in the maxilla than in the mandible (Svärdström and Wennström 1996; Dannewitz et al. 2006). However, this may be due simply to the fact that maxillary molars have more sites at risk than mandibular molars (maxillary molars with three, mandibular with two furcation entrances).

At least in periodontitis patients, furcation involvement is a frequent finding. In periodontally diseased patients, roughly one-third of all molars and almost one-fifth of all furcation sites exhibit degree II and III furcation involvement, which affects prognosis and choice of therapy for the respective multi-rooted teeth.

Summary of Evidence

- Reliable clinical furcation diagnosis requires a rigid curved furcation probe (e.g. colour-coded Nabers probe).
- The distinction between degree II (Hamp et al. 1975) and through-and-through furcation (degree III) is as difficult as it is of decisive significance for either prognosis as well as choice of therapy.
- A modified classification of furcation involvement is recommended.
- Conventional radiographs may only provide hints for a suspicion of furcation involvement. However, this suspicion has to be confirmed or rejected by furcation probing using a curved probe. CBCT may provide additional information for decision-making particularly in maxillary molars if periodontal surgery is required.
- In periodontally diseased patients, roughly one-third of all molars and almost one-fifth of all furcation sites exhibit degree II and III furcation involvement.

References

Albandar, J.M., Brunelle, J.A., and Kingman, A. (1999). Destructive periodontal disease in adults 30 years of age and older in the United States, 1988–1994. *Journal of Periodontology* 70, 13–29.

Ammons, W.F., and Harrington G.W. (2006). Furcation: Involvement and treatment. In: *Carranza's Clinical Periodontology* (ed. M.G. Newman, H.H. Takei, P.R. Klokkevold, and F.A. Carranza), 991–1004. St. Louis, MO: Saunders Elsevier.

Carnevale, G., Pontoriero, R., and Hürzeler, M.B. (1995) Management of furcation involvement. *Periodontology* 2000 9, 69–89.

Dannewitz, B., Krieger, J.K., Hüsing, J., and Eickholz, P. (2006). Loss of molars in periodontally treated patients: A retrospective analysis five years or more after active periodontal treatment. *Journal of Clinical Periodontology* 33, 53–61.

Dannewitz, B., Zeidler, A., Hüsing, J. et al. (2016). Loss of molars in periodontally treated patients: Results ten years and more after active periodontal therapy. *Journal of Clinical Periodontology* 43, 53–62.

Eickholz, P. (1995). Reproducibility and validity of furcation measurements as related to class of furcation invasion. *Journal of Periodontology* 66, 984–989.

Eickholz, P. (2010). Glossar der Grundbegriffe für die Praxis: Parodontologische Diagnostik 6: Furkationsdiagnostik. *Parodontologie* 21, 261–266.

Eickholz, P., and Hausmann, E. (1997). Evidence for healing of class II and III furcations after GTR-therapy: Digital subtraction and clinical measurements. *Journal of Periodontology* 68, 636–644.

Eickholz, P., and Kim, T.-S. (1998). Reproducibility and validity of the assessment of clinical furcation parameters as related to different probes. *Journal of Periodontology* 69, 328–336.

Eickholz, P., and Staehle, H.J. (1994). The reliability of furcation measurements. *Journal of Clinical Periodontology* 21, 611–614.

Eickholz, P., Nickles, K., Koch, R. et al. (2016). Is furcation class involvement affected by adjunctive systemic amoxicillin plus metronidazole? A clinical trial's exploratory subanalysis. *Journal of Clinical Periodontology* 43 (10), 839–848.

Fleischer, H.C., Mellonig, J.T., Brayer, W.K. et al. (1989). Scaling and root planing efficacy in multirooted teeth. *Journal of Periodontology* 60, 402–409.

Glickman, I. (1953). *Clinical Periodontology*. Philadelphia, PA: Saunders.

Graetz, C., Plaumann, A., Wiebe, J.F. et al. (2014). Periodontal probing versus radiographs for the diagnosis of furcation involvement. *Journal of Periodontology* 85, 1371–1379.

Graetz, C., Schützhold, S., Plaumann, A. et al. (2015). Prognostic factors for the loss of molars – an 18-years retrospective cohort study. *Journal of Clinical Periodontology* 42, 943–950.

Hallquist, A., and Näsman, A. (2001). Medical diagnostic X-ray radiation: An evaluation from medical records and dentist cards in a case-control study of thyroid cancer in the northern medical region of Sweden. *European Journal of Cancer Prevention* 10, 147–152.

Hamp, S.-E., Nyman, S., and Lindhe, J. (1975). Periodontal treatment of multirooted teeth: Results after 5 years. *Journal of Clinical Periodontology* 2, 126–135.

Horwitz, J., Machtei, E.E., Reitmeir, P. et al. (2004). Radiographic parameters as prognostic indicators for healing of class II furcation defects. *Journal of Clinical Periodontology* 31, 105–111.

Hujoel, P., Hollender, L., Bollen, A.M. et al. (2006). Radiographs associated with one episode of orthodontic therapy. *Journal of Dental Education* 70, 1061–1065.

Kalkwarf, K.L., Kaldahl, W.B., and Patil, K.D. (1988). Evaluation of furcation region response to periodontal therapy. *Journal of Periodontology* 59, 794–804.

Laky, M., Majdalani, S., Kapferer, I., et al. (2013). Periodontal probing of dental furcations compared with diagnosis by low-dose computed tomography: A case series. *Journal of Periodontology* 84, 1740–1746.

Lang, N.P., Cumming, B., and Löe, H. (1973). Toothbrushing frequency as it relates to plaque development and gingival health. *Journal of Periodontology* 44, 396–405.

Longstreth, W.T., Jr, Phillips, L.E., Drangsholt, M. et al. (2004). Dental X-rays and the risk of intracranial meningioma: A population-based case-control study. *Cancer* 100, 1026–1034.

Loos, B., Nylund, K., Claffey, N., and Egelberg, J. (1989). Clinical effects of root debridement in molar and non-molar teeth: A 2-year follow-up. *Journal of Clinical Periodontology* 16, 498–504.

McGuire, M.K., and Nunn, M.E. (1996). Prognosis versus actual outcome. III: The effectiveness of clinical parameters in developing an accurate prognosis. *Journal of Periodontology* 67, 666–674.

Mohammadi, Z., Shalavi, S., and Jafarzadeh, H. (2013). Extra roots and root canals in premolar and molar teeth: Review of an endodontic challenge. *Journal of Contemporary Dental Practice* 14, 980–986.

Nordland, P., Garrett, S., Kriger, R. et al. (1987). The effect of plaque control and root debridement in molar teeth. *Journal of Clinical Periodontology* 14, 231–236.

Park, S.Y., Shin, S.Y., Yang, S.M., and Kye, S.B. (2009). Factors influencing the outcome of root-resection therapy in molars: A 10-year retrospective study. *Journal of Periodontology* 80, 32–40.

Pretzl, B., Kaltschmitt, J., Kim, T.-S. et al. (2008). Tooth loss after active periodontal therapy. 2: Tooth-related factors. *Journal of Clinical Periodontology* 35, 175–182.

Salvi, G.E., Mischler, D.C., Schmidlin, K. et al. (2014). Risk factors associated with the longevity of multi-rooted teeth: Long-term outcomes after active and supportive periodontal therapy. *Journal of Clinical Periodontology* 41, 701–707.

Sanz, M., Jepsen, K., Eickholz, P., and Jepsen, S. (2015). Clinical concepts for regenerative therapy in furcations. *Periodontology* 2000 68, 308–332.

Schroeder, H.E., and Scherle, W.F. (1987). Warum die Furkation menschlicher Zähne so unvorhersehbar bizarr gestaltet ist. *Schweizerische Monatsschrift für Zahnmedizin* 97, 1495–1508.

Svärdström, G., and Wennström, J.L. (1996). Prevalence of furcation involvements in patients referred for periodontal treatment. *Journal of Clinical Periodontology* 23, 1093–1099.

Tarnow, D., and Fletcher, P. (1984). Classification of the vertical component of furcation involvement. *Journal of Periodontology* 55, 283–284.

Tonetti, M.S., Christiansen A.L., and Cortellini, P. (2017). Vertical subclassification predicts survival of molars with class II furcation involvement during supportive periodontal care. *J Clin Periodontol* 44, 1140–1144.

Topoll, H.H., Streletz, E., Hucke, H.P., and Lange, D.E. (1988). Furkationsdiagnostik: Ein Vergleich der Aussagekraft von OPG, Röntgenstatus und intraoperativem Befund. *Deutsche Zahnärztliche Zeitschrift* 43, 705–708.

Walter, C., Kaner, D., Berndt, D.C. et al. (2009). Three-dimensional imaging as a pre-operative tool in decision making for furcation surgery. *Journal of Clinical Periodontology* 36, 250–257.

Walter, C., Schmidt, J.C., Dula, K. et al. (2016). Cone beam computed tomography (CBCT) for diagnosis and treatment planning in periodontology: A systematic review. *Quintessence International* 47, 25–37.

Walter, C., Weiger, R., Dietrich, T. et al. (2012). Does three-dimensional imaging offer a financial benefit for the treatment of maxillary molars with furcation involvement? A pilot clinical case series. *Clinical Oral Implants Research* 23, 351–358.

Walter, C., Weiger, R., and Zitzmann, N.U. (2010). Accuracy of three-dimensional imaging in assessing maxillary molar furcation involvement. *Journal of Clinical Periodontology* 37, 436–441.

Wang, H.L., Burgett, F.G., Shyr, Y., and Ramfjord, S. (1994). The influence of molar furcation involvement and mobility on future clinical periodontal attachment loss. *Journal of Periodontology* 65, 25–29.

Chapter 3

How Good are We at Cleaning Furcations? Non-surgical and Surgical Studies

Jia-Hui Fu[1] and Hom-Lay Wang[2]

[1] Discipline of Periodontics, Faculty of Dentistry, National University of Singapore, Singapore
[2] Department of Periodontics and Oral Medicine, School of Dentistry, University of Michigan, Ann Arbor, MI, USA

3.1 Introduction

An experimental gingivitis model in humans established that microbial plaque is the aetiological factor of gingivitis (Loe et al. 1965). A 26-year longitudinal study on well-maintained Norwegian males found that sites with persistent plaque-induced gingival inflammation had 70% more clinical attachment loss (odds ratio [OR] = 3.22) compared to sites that were always healthy, thereby supporting the concept that gingivitis is a prerequisite for the inception of periodontitis (Schatzle et al. 2003). Microbial plaque exists in the oral cavity as biofilms, which are consortia of micro-organisms interacting with the surrounding environment in a dynamic manner. Subgingival plaque samples from 588 patients with chronic periodontitis demonstrated that with increasing probing depth, there was a significant increase in the 'orange' and 'red complex' microbes (Socransky and Haffajee 2005). These Gram-negative bacteria release molecules such as lipopolysaccharide and extracellular proteolytic enzymes, which interact with the innate host inflammatory surveillance system to mount an immune response against the invading bacteria (Darveau et al. 1997). The inflammatory response results in breakdown of the connective tissue attachment and supporting bone, leading to established periodontitis lesions (Page and Kornman 1997). The microbial nature of periodontitis is very complex; it is thought that alterations in the composition of the subgingival biofilm (dysbiosis) involving 'accessory' and 'keystone' pathogens and pathobionts drive periodontitis in a susceptible host (Hajishengallis and Lamont 2012).

In order to arrest the initiation and progression of periodontitis, its management is predominantly focused on removing microbial plaque and its retentive factors from root surfaces and gingival sulci. This is primarily achieved by professional supra- and subgingival mechanical debridement, with the aim of disrupting the microbial biofilm growing on the root surface. Subgingival tooth debridement has traditionally been referred to as 'scaling and root planing', although the importance of necessarily planing or smoothening the root surface has been questioned (Checchi and Pelliccioni 1988; Smart et al. 1990). Microbial biofilm disruption leads to a reduction of the host response cascade, which halts periodontal destruction and thus results in improvement of the clinical signs of disease. Immediately after scaling and root planing, the denuded root surface will be partially covered by fibrin and polymorphonuclear leukocytes. The junctional epithelium will start to migrate apically towards the periodontal ligament. Granulation tissue will form in the transseptal fibre region. By the third week, the apical migration of the junctional epithelium will terminate at the apical end of the root instrumentation, with the periodontal ligament fibres oriented parallel to the root surface. Some root resorption or even crestal bone loss may occur along the root surface at areas that are not covered by the long junctional epithelium. As a result, the healing after scaling and root planing is therefore mainly by periodontal repair, with the formation of the long junctional epithelium and gingival recession (Tagge et al. 1975; Biagini et al. 1988).

It is relatively straightforward to debride single-rooted teeth; however, in multi-rooted teeth the furcal areas are anatomically challenging to access because of their configurations. Several anatomical factors related to furcations and roots, covered by Pretzl in Chapter 1, contribute to the aetiology and compromised prognoses of furcation-involved teeth. These factors include furcation entrance width, root trunk length, and the presence of root concavities, cervical enamel projections, bifurcation ridges, and enamel pearls. An evaluation of 50 mandibular molars revealed variations in the furcation area, with 48%, 34%, and 18% having flat, convex, and concave domes, respectively (Matia et al. 1986). Therefore, it has been reported that complete plaque and calculus removal in the furcation is highly unlikely (Matia et al. 1986; Parashis et al. 1993a, b; Kocher et al. 1998a, b). The imperfect debridement can be attributed to the presence of difficult-to-reach root concavities, which are commonly found in the furcal areas, with an incidence of 100% in maxillary premolars, 17–94% in maxillary molars, and 99–100% in mandibular molars (Bower 1979a, b; Booker and Loughlin 1985). In addition, furcation entrances are generally narrower (less than 0.75 mm) than the blade of conventional curettes (0.75–1.10 mm; Bower 1979a, b; Chiu et al. 1991; dos Santos et al. 2009). Therefore, this chapter attempts to provide an overview of the efficacy of non-surgical and surgical debridement of furcal areas, using instruments such as curettes, ultrasonic scalers, lasers, photodynamic therapy, and interdental brushes.

3.2 Longitudinal Studies on Management of Furcation-involved Teeth

Ramfjord and colleagues first introduced the concept of longitudinal studies in 1968, where they compared different treatment modalities in a large subject population over time using the split-mouth design. This approach allowed clinicians to better appreciate the possible treatment outcomes that will arise over time with minimal host variability. Subsequently, several research groups have adopted this approach to evaluate the treatment outcomes of non-surgical and surgical debridement of single- and multi-rooted teeth. These studies are generally described based on geographical locations and treatment modalities performed, including scaling and root planing, subgingival curettage, modified Widman flap, modified Kirkland's flap, pocket elimination, and apically positioned flap with and without osseous resection. Clinical parameters, such as clinical attachment level gain, probing depth reduction, bleeding on probing, and plaque index, were used to determine the outcome of the treatment rendered. Table 3.1 shows a summary of longitudinal studies that reported data on multi-rooted teeth. The results described the treatment outcomes specific to multi-rooted teeth.

Results from the Michigan longitudinal studies reported more tooth loss in teeth with baseline furcation involvement (FI) despite surgical interventions, thus implying that the quality of surgical debridement or post-surgical home or professional care did not deter disease progression in the long term (Ramfjord et al. 1968, 1987; Wang et al. 1994). The authors believed that although flap elevation would improve access to the furcation areas, complete

Table 3.1 Summary of some longitudinal studies that evaluated multi-rooted teeth.

Group	Author/ Year	Sample Size	No. of Teeth	Treatment Modalities	Follow-Up Years	SPT Protocol	Results
Michigan	Ramfjord et al. 1968	32	729	Initial SRP with curettes. Subgingival curettage vs gingivectomy/APF with osseous resection as needed.	2	3 months	Baseline FI did not significantly affect CAL in molars in the short term.
	Ramfjord et al. 1987	72	1881	Initial SRP with curettes. Surgical pocket elimination vs MWF vs subgingival curettage vs SRP	5	3 months	Out of 17 teeth that were lost due to periodontal reasons: • 16 had FI at baseline. • 15 were treated with surgical interventions and 2 were treated with SRP.
	Wang et al. 1994	24	165	Initial SRP with curettes. Surgical pocket elimination vs MWF vs subgingival curettage vs SRP.	8	3 months	FI molars had 2.54 times greater risk of being lost.
Minnesota	Pihlstrom et al. 1984	10	266	SRP alone vs SRP with MWF vs subgingival curettage vs SRP	6.5	3–4 months	Compared to non-molars: • Molars with baseline PPD 4–6 mm: significantly deeper residual PPD (1.05 mm) and greater apical CAL (0.54 mm) after SRP alone. • Molars with baseline PPD of 4–6 mm: significantly deeper residual PPD (1.02 mm) and greater apical CAL (1.27 mm) after SRP with MWF. • Molars with baseline PPD ≥7 mm: no significant difference in PPD or CAL, for both treatment modalities. 9/11 teeth lost after completion of treatment were molars.
Loma Linda	Nordland et al. 1987	19		Initial SRP with curettes and ultrasonic scaler	2	3 months	Compared to non-molar or non-furcation sites, molar FI sites had: • More bleeding on probing. • Higher bleeding scores of 60% to 70% and > attachment loss (1 out of 5 molars) when PPDs were 7 mm or more. • Lowest post-treatment reduction was in PPD (1.0 mm). • 0.5 mm loss of CAL instead of attachment gain.

(Continued)

Table 3.1 (Continued)

Group	Author/Year	Sample Size	No. of Teeth	Treatment Modalities	Follow-Up Years	SPT Protocol	Results
	Loos et al. 1988	11	43	Initial SRP with ultrasonic scaler.	1.1	3 months	Compared to non-molar sites, molar FI sites had: • Greater tendency to rebound after treatment. • Mean probing attachment level gain of 0.1 mm (0.7 mm at non-molar sites). • Significantly higher microbial count.
	Loos et al. 1989	12	1682	Initial SRP with ultrasonic or sonic scaler.	2	3 months	Molar FI sites: • Similar PPD and CAL pre- and post-treatment. • With at least 7.0 mm PPD had lower PPD reduction after treatment. • Did not have significant changes in CAL. • Had greater percentage of sites worsening over time (38.5%).
Nebraska	Kalkwarf et al. 1988	82	1394	Initial scaling with curettes and ultrasonic scaler. Coronal scaling only vs SRP vs SRP with MWF vs SRP with flap and osseous resection.	2	3 months	• FI sites tended to progress with horizontal probing attachment loss irrespective of treatment. • Periodontal breakdown rate was 2.6% for sites that had osseous resection, 5.9% for sites that had MWF, 8.4% for sites that had SRP, and 8.3% for sites that had coronal scaling only.
North Carolina	Hirschfeld and Wasserman 1978	600	15 666	SRP, gingivectomy, gingivoplasty, and APF with osseous surgery.	15	4–6 months	• 19.3% of FI molars were lost compared to 1.7% of incisors in a well-maintained population.
	McFall 1982	100	2627	SRP, curettage, gingivectomy, gingivoplasty, and APF with osseous surgery.	15	3–6 months	• 27.3% of FI molars were lost compared to 0.6% of incisors in a well-maintained population.
	Wood et al. 1989	63	1607	SRP.	13.6	6–9 months	• 23.2% of FI molars were lost compared to 0.8% of incisors in a well-maintained population.

Location	Study			Treatment	Time	Maintenance	Findings

New Jersey	Ross and Thompson 1978	100	387	Scaling, curettage, gingivectomy, gingivoplasty, and APF	5–24	–	• 12% of FI maxillary molars were extracted, of which 22% had been present for at least 6 years and 33% for 11–18 years.
							• Changes in bone support of FI maxillary molars at 5–24 years post-treatment:
							  – 75% had no significant change.
							  – 11% had bone loss.
							  – 2% had slight improvement.
							  – 12% were extracted.

Sweden	Lindhe et al. 1982	15	–	SRP vs MWF.	2	2 weeks for 6 months, followed by once every 3 months	• Reduction in mean plaque index scores was greater in non-molars. • In surgically treated sites, greater PPD reduction in non-molars, but in non-surgically treated sites it was comparable between non-molars and molars.
Germany	Dannewitz et al. 2006	71	505	Initial SRP, followed by OFD, GTR, root resection or separation, or tunnelling procedure.	>5 years	–	• 3.8% of FI molars lost after active therapy. • 31.8% of FI molars lost over time after SRP. • 34.6% of FI molars lost over time after SRP and flap surgery. • Molars with class III FI tended to deteriorate significantly over time.
	Dannewitz et al. 2016	136	–	Initial SRP	13.2	–	• Molars with class III furcations had 4.68 times higher risk of being lost compared to non-FI molars.

APF = apically positioned flap; CAL = clinical attachment level; FI = furcation involvement; GTR = guided tissue regeneration; MWF = modified Widman flap; OFD = open-flap debridement; PPD = probing pocket depth; SRP = scaling and root planning; SPT = supportive periodontal therapy.

debridement was difficult to achieve and maintain post-surgically due to the complex configurations of the furcal area; therefore, furcation-involved teeth had a poorer long-term prognosis. In addition, it was hard to maintain furcated molars, thus they had a 2.54 times greater susceptibility of being lost during the periodontal maintenance phase (Wang et al. 1994). A longitudinal study by the Minnesota group demonstrated that molars compared to non-molars had significantly greater post-treatment pocket depth and clinical attachment level changes at sites with baseline pocket depths of 4–6 mm, regardless of the treatment rendered. However, at deeper sites (pocket depth of 7 mm or more), no significant differences were detected between molars and non-molars in the long term. Although the authors did not report the severity of FI in the molars in their study, 9 out of the 11 teeth that were extracted at the end of treatment were molars (Pihlstrom et al. 1984).

The Loma Linda group evaluated the effectiveness of plaque control and subgingival root debridement of non-molar, molar non-furcation, and molar furcation sites over a two-year period and found that molar furcation sites had persistent inflammation, the poorest response to treatment in terms of pocket depth reduction and clinical attachment gain, and a significant tendency to rebound to baseline status after treatment (Nordland et al. 1987; Loos et al. 1988, 1989). The Nebraska group compared coronal scaling alone, complete scaling and root planing alone and followed by modified Widman flap or osseous-respective surgery in the management of molars with FI. Their results showed that osseous resection had the greatest probing depth reduction with the least tendency for further breakdown (Kalkwarf et al. 1988). The North Carolina group evaluated patients over 13–15 years and found that molars with FI were lost 10–27 times more frequently compared to incisors, despite having non-surgical and surgical periodontal treatment with regular maintenance (Hirschfeld and Wasserman 1978; McFall 1982; Wood et al. 1989).

A group in New Jersey evaluated 384 maxillary molars with varying degrees of FI over 5–24 years. They used a combination of scaling, curettage, gingivectomy and/or gingivoplasty, and apically positioned flap to manage the furcation-involved maxillary molars. Their results showed that the therapies rendered were able to maintain maxillary molars with FI over that period, with only 12% of molars being lost over time. However, the therapies did not have any effect on the bone support, as 75% of the molars had no significant changes in bone levels. On the contrary, 11% had detectable bone loss and 12% were extracted (Ross and Thompson 1978). A German group evaluated only molars in 136 patients over a mean follow-up period of 13 years. They reported that similar percentages of molars were lost when treated with both closed- and open-flap scaling and root planing (Dannewitz et al. 2006, 2016). A group in Sweden too found that reduction in the mean plaque index score was greater in non-molars compared to molars (Lindhe et al. 1982).

A review of the longitudinal studies seemed to show that debridement of the furcation areas during root planing or with a surgical procedure, for instance apically positioned flap with osseous surgery, did not significantly improve the long-term prognosis of these teeth. Although furcation-involved teeth might survive in the long term, their survival rates were substantially lower than single-rooted teeth such as incisors. The authors alluded that the anatomy of the furcation area complicated both professional debridement and patient home care, implying that the quality of debridement might not be ideal and thereby indicating that molar teeth are tougher to maintain successfully over time. A summary on the long-term survival of molars with FI is provided in Chapter 5.

3.3 Professional Debridement

Conventionally, scaling and root planing are carried out using manual instruments, such as curettes, sickles, chisels, hoes, and files, or power-driven scalers, for example sonic or ultrasonic scalers. These instruments can be used in both the non-surgical and surgical phases of periodontal therapy. Curettes, for instance universal and Gracey, are double-ended instruments with customized cutting edges, shank lengths, blade lengths, and angulations. Therefore, each one of the nine standard Gracey curettes is designed to scale and root plane a specific area in the mouth. These curettes have a blade width of at least 0.76 mm and a blade length of 5 mm (Oda et al. 2004).

Powered scalers are either sonic or ultrasonic. In sonic scalers, compressed air causes the working tip to vibrate in an elliptical fashion at frequencies of 2000 to 6000 Hz under a water spray. Ultrasonic scalers, on the other hand, are subclassified into magnetostrictive and piezoelectric scalers. The magnetostrictive scalers, such as Cavitron® (Dentsply, USA), work by creating a magnetic field where an expanding and contracting coil, together with an alternating current, results in vibrations that are transmitted to the working tip. The tip moves in an elliptical motion, thus all sides of the tip are active. In the piezoelectric scalers, such as Piezon Master® (EMS, Switzerland), reactive ceramic crystals undergo dimensional changes when subjected to an alternating electrical current. The expansion and contraction result in vibrations that are transmitted to the working tip, which moves in a linear manner, thus only the lateral sides of the tip act as the active sides. The average ultrasonic scaler tip width is 0.55 mm (Oda et al. 2004).

A comparison between the use of hand instruments and ultrasonic scalers showed that the latter were better suited for the debridement of narrow furcation areas, as their tips were narrower than curettes and thus could debride the hard-to-reach areas (Matia et al. 1986; Sugaya et al. 2002). In addition, they were able to significantly reduce the bacterial counts for all degrees of FI and were more effective in debriding the class II and III furcations compared to curettes (Leon and Vogel 1987). A study that evaluated the efficacy of four ultrasonic sharp tips (Cavitron TFI 10 tip, Cavitron EWPP [Probe] tip, Titan-S Universal tip, and Titan-S Sickle tip) showed that there were no significant differences in calculus removal when different tips were used (Patterson et al. 1989). When sharp tips were compared to ball tips, the Titan sonic scaler with universal tip and Cavitron with ball tip were the most efficient at debriding both maxillary and mandibular molars, especially the furcation roofs (Takacs et al. 1993). Other similar studies evaluated modified sonic tips with different angulations, and found that angulated tips provided a more thorough debridement because the tips could better access the furcations (Kocher et al. 1996, 1998a, b). In addition, some of the sonic tips had an ellipsoidal terminal end of 0.8 mm in diameter, which would provide more intimate contact with the root concavities and the furcation dome, thus improving the quality of the instrumentation. Diamond-coated ultrasonic and sonic scaler tips were found to remove calculus 2–3.3 times faster than manual curettes, but they were prone to remove cementum and dentine during debridement (Kocher and Plagmann 1999; Scott et al. 1999).

A study that investigated the quality of the mechanical and chemical debridement of root surfaces on 90 periodontally involved extracted teeth found that with unlimited access to the root surfaces, all mechanical debridement methods – that is, curettes, and ultrasonic with regular or diamond-coated P-10 tip – were equally effective. Thus, this study suggested that access was the main critical factor that affected the quality of root surface debridement (Eschler and Rapley 1991). In addition, it was reported that interproximal

FIs responded less favourably to mechanical debridement compared to their buccal and lingual counterparts. This phenomenon could be due to the increased difficulty in accessing the interproximal furcations for debridement (Del Peloso Ribeiro et al. 2007).

Besides modifying the scaler tips, root surface debridement can be performed through a non-surgical (closed) or surgical (open) approach. It was reported that significantly more residual calculus was found in groups that had the closed approach (34.1–37.0%) compared to the open approach (1.0–2.7%; Matia et al. 1986). In addition, clinical experience and proficiency did significantly affect the quality of debridement at the furcations. Less experienced residents left significantly more calculus-free surfaces with the open approach (43%) compared to the closed approach (8%). This percentage of only 8% calculus-free furcation surfaces for less experienced operators with a closed approach was particularly striking. On the other hand, there was no significant difference between the open and closed approaches for experienced periodontists (Fleischer et al. 1989). Using the open approach, experienced periodontists had 68% calculus-free furcation surfaces compared to 44% with a closed approach. Although the percentages were not statistically significant, they were clinically important, because almost a quarter of the root surfaces had residual calculus when the closed approach was used. However, despite the increased visibility with the open approach, the use of hand instruments at the furcal areas was ineffective (Fleischer et al. 1989; Wylam et al., 1993).

Figure 3.1 shows an extracted maxillary first molar which had received what was defined as 'deep cleaning' by a general dental practitioner. The tooth was extracted, since it was deemed hopeless due to bone loss to the apex and mobility degree III. The images show very extensive deposits of calculus in the furcation region.

Table 3.2 shows a summary of the studies that evaluated the effectiveness of mechanical and chemical debridement at multi-rooted teeth. It is obvious that there is a paucity of available literature on the effectiveness of mechanical debridement in furcation areas. A systematic review of 13 randomized controlled clinical trials revealed that there

(a)

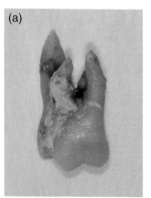

(b)

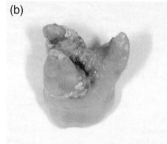

(c)

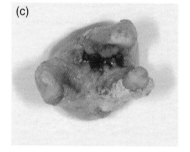

Figure 3.1 The upper right maxillary molar (UR6) of a 53-year-old female patient affected by generalized advanced chronic periodontitis, extracted as deemed hopeless due to bone loss to the apex and mobility degree III. This tooth had received what was defined as 'deep cleaning' by a general dental practitioner. However, the images show very extensive deposits of calculus in the furcation region, testifying to the difficulty of achieving good subgingival debridement in furcation regions.

Table 3.2 Summary of studies that evaluated efficacy of mechanical debridement.

Author/ Year	Sample Size	No. of Teeth	Study Design	Results
Matia et al. 1986	48	50 mandibular molars with class II or III FI	Curette (closed approach) vs curette (open approach) vs ultrasonic (closed approach) vs ultrasonic (open approach) vs no treatment.	• Closed approach: ultrasonic scaler and curette had 37.7% and 34.1% of residual calculus, respectively. • Open approach: ultrasonic scaler and curette had 1.0% and 2.7% of residual calculus, respectively. • More calculus was removed with the open approach. • Ultrasonic scaling removed more calculus in narrow furcations (<2.3 mm) compared to curette.
Leon and Vogel 1987	6	33 maxillary and mandibular molars (class I, II, and III FI)	Gracey curettes vs ultrasonic scaler (Cavitron® with P-10 tip) vs no treatment.	• Ultrasonic scaling was significantly more effective than curettes in reducing the bacterial counts for all degrees of FI. • Ultrasonic scaling was more effective in the class II and III FI.
Oda and Ishikawa 1989	—	120 extracted maxillary and mandibular molars	Gracey curettes #11/12 and #13/14 vs standard tip for ultrasonic scaler (ST-08) vs newly designed spherical tip (0.8 mm diameter).	• Mean % of residual marks that represents calculus: 15.1%, 50.3%, and 61.1% for newly designed tip, conventional ultrasonic scaler tip, and Gracey curettes, respectively, in maxillary molars (16.7%, 44.1%, and 39.5%, respectively, in mandibular molars). • The newly designed tip produced surfaces that were as smooth as those produced by the Gracey curettes. • The newly designed tip was more effective in debriding the furcation area.
Patterson et al. 1989	—	24 extracted mandibular molars mounted on a typodont	Cavitron TFI 10 tip vs Cavitron EWPP (Probe) tip vs Titan-S Universal tip vs Titan-S Sickle tip.	• Mean % of residual calculus: 13 mm^2, 11 mm^2, 9 mm^2, and 8 mm^2 for Cavitron TFI 10 tip, Cavitron EWPP (Probe) tip, Titan-S Universal tip, and Titan-S Sickle tip (no significant differences). • On average 25–30% of calculus remained after debridement. • No significant differences between the efficacy of the four ultrasonic tips.

(Continued)

Table 3.2 (Continued)

Author/Year	Sample Size	No. of Teeth	Study Design	Results
Scott et al. 1999	–	60 extracted mandibular molars	Cavitron TFI-10 tip vs Gracey curettes vs fine- or medium-grit diamond-coated ultrasonic tips.	• Ultrasonic scaling was significantly faster than hand curettes in calculus removal.
Parashis et al. 1993b	23	30 mandibular molars (60 furcations)	SRP with closed approach vs SRP with open approach vs SRP with open approach + rotary diamond instrumentation.	• The use of the rotary diamond tip significantly removed more calculus in the furcation area.
Kocher et al. 1996	–	24 acrylic molars	Universal curettes vs sonic scaler vs modified sonic scaler with bud-shaped tips and different angulations vs modified sonic scaler tips with plastic coating.	• Ultrasonic scaling was more effective than hand instrumentation. • Specific angulations of the scaler tips were more suited for distal furcations or the root of the furcations. • Sonic scaler tips with plastic coatings appeared to remove only plaque and thus were not suitable for furcation debridement.
Kocher et al. 1998a	–	15 extracted maxillary and mandibular molars placed in a dummy model	Curettes vs diamond bur and curettes vs ultrasonic scaler vs sonic scaler vs diamond-coated sonic scaler tips (angulated like Gracey curette #13/14 with 1.5 mm diameter and 45 microns diamond grit size).	• Ultrasonic and sonic scalers cleaned only 70% of the root surfaces compared to the other groups (85%). • Only the diamond-coated sonic scaler managed to effectively clean the maxillary molars (85% of the root surfaces were clean compared to 75% by curettes).
Kocher et al. 1998b	–	15 extracted maxillary and mandibular molars placed in a dummy model	Curettes vs diamond-coated sonic scaler tips (angulated like Gracey curette #13/14 and universal curette, with 1 mm diameter and 15 microns diamond grit size).	• Mandibular molars were better debrided compared to maxillary molars. • Diamond-coated sonic scalers do damage the root surfaces to the same degree as hand curettes (more definitive notches were seen on the palatal roots). • Diamond-coated sonic scaler tips with varying angulations did improve root surface debridement.

Study				Results
Kocher and Plagmann 1999	15	45 maxillary and mandibular molars	OFD with hand curettes (Barnhart curette #5/6 and Gracey curettes #7/8, #11/12, and #13/14) vs diamond-coated sonic scaler.	• Diamond-coated sonic scalers cleaned two times faster than hand curettes. • The initial reduction in probing depths at the furcations was not maintained over time in both groups.
Auplish et al. 2000	–	Acrylic molars in dummy head	Curettes (Gracey #11/12 and #13/14) vs diamond-coated sonic scaler vs sonic scaler.	• Diamond-coated sonic scaler took the least time to complete the debridement. • Diamond-coated sonic scaler significantly removed more calculus compared to the sonic scalers or curettes.
Fleischer et al. 1989	36	61	Curette (closed approach) by experienced periodontist vs curette (open approach) by experienced periodontist vs ultrasonic (closed approach) by less experienced residents vs ultrasonic (open approach) by less experienced residents vs no treatment.	• Experienced periodontists: significantly greater calculus-free area (78%) in open approach vs closed approach (36%). • Less experienced residents: significantly greater calculus-free area (45%) in open approach vs closed approach (18%). • At the furcal areas, less experienced residents: significantly greater calculus-free surface with open approach (43%) vs closed approach (8%). • At the furcal areas, no significant difference between the open (68%) and closed (44%) approaches for experienced periodontists.
Eschler and Rapley 1991	–	90 extracted teeth	Grouping (1) curette (Columbia #13/14) vs (2) curette (Columbia #13/14), antiformin-citric acid vs (3) ultrasonic with P-10 tip vs (4) ultrasonic with diamond-coated P-10 tip vs (5) ultrasonic with diamond-coated P-10 tip + antiformin-citric acid vs (6) ultrasonic with diamond-coated P-10 tip and curette (Columbia #13/14) vs (7) ultrasonic with diamond-coated P-10 tip and curette (Columbia #13/14) + antiformin-citric acid vs (8) antiformin-citric acid vs (9) no treatment.	• All groups that had mechanical debridement had significantly less residual stains compared to groups that had no treatment and antiformin-citric acid treatment (chemical root preparation did not improve stain removal). • Debridement with ultrasonic with P-10 tip: significantly greater residual stains vs debridement with diamond-coated P-10 tip and curette. • With unlimited access, all mechanical debridement methods appeared to be equally effective.

(Continued)

Table 3.2 (Continued)

Author/ Year	Sample Size	No. of Teeth	Study Design	Results
Takacs et al. 1993	–	100 extracted molars with FI	Cavitron® ultrasonic with 0.8 mm ball tip vs Cavitron ultrasonic with EWP12R/12 L pointed tip vs ENAC ultrasonic with furcation 0.8 mm ball tip vs EVA contra-angle reciprocating handpiece with Per-Io-Tor #1 and #2 tips (similar to threaded fissure bur) vs Titan-S sonic scaler with universal tip.	• On average 74.2% of calculus was left behind at the furca roof of mandibular molars after debridement (the pointed tip and universal tip removed the most calculus). • On average 76.4% of calculus was left behind at the furca roof of maxillary molars after debridement (Cavitron ball tip and universal tip removed the most calculus). • Titan sonic scaler with universal tip and Cavitron with ball tip were the most efficient at debriding molars.
Wylam et al. 1993	26	60 molars with class II or III FI	Curettes (closed approach) vs curettes (open approach) vs no treatment.	• Molars after non-surgical SRP: significantly greater residual calculus (54.3%) vs open approach (33.0%). • At the furcal area, molars after non-surgical SRP: slightly greater residual calculus (93.2%) vs open approach (91.1%). • Hand instrumentation was unable to effectively clean the furcal area.
Otero-Cagide and Lang 1997	–	100 artificial teeth	Curettes (Vision curvettes #11/12 and #13/14) vs ultrasonic with EWP-12 L-R scaler tip.	• Debridement with curettes had significantly less residual calculus compared to ultrasonics.

FI = furcation involvement; OFD = open-flap debridement; SRP = scaling and root planing.

was no evidence on the efficacy of powered scalers in debriding multi-rooted teeth. This outcome needs to be interpreted with caution, because out of the 13 studies, 7 evaluated only single-rooted teeth, and the remaining 6 studies focused on patient healing outcomes. In addition, the instruments used in the studies were conventional Gracey and Columbia curettes and Cavitron ultrasonic tips, which have thicker blade widths than the instruments that are available today. The evidence, however, did show that powered scalers debride faster than hand curettes (Tunkel et al. 2002).

In recent years, advancements in material science have allowed curettes and ultrasonic tips to be stronger and thinner than in past decades. Gracey curettes are available in different angulations, for example Gracey curette #17/#18, or blade widths, for instance Micro Mini Five® Gracey curettes. The newer Micro Mini Five curettes have a shorter blade length (2 mm) and thinner blade width (0.6 mm) compared to regular Gracey curettes, with a blade length and width of 5mm and 0.9mm respectively. A study of 100 artificial teeth used Vision curvettes that had 50% shorter blades and increased blade curvature to debride the furcation of mandibular molars. The authors reported that the modified blades were more effective than ultrasonic scalers in the debridement of the furcation area (Otero-Cagide and Long 1997). Besides curettes, ultrasonic tips are now slimmer with improved angulations. For example, the Cavitron ultrasonic tips THINserts® are 47% thinner than the Slimline® inserts (diameter 0.5 mm), with an additional 9° backbend to gain better access to the subgingival areas. The EMS Piezon Master universal ultrasonic tips are 0.6 mm in diameter, and are thus able to access most furcation areas (<0.75 mm). Certain systems, such as Kavo®, have an inbuilt light-emitting diode (LED) to improve visibility in the more posterior areas of the oral cavity. All these modifications aim to improve the access of instruments into the furcation area (Figures 3.2–3.5).

Other authors have also proposed the use of chemotherapeutics, such as chlorhexidine, essential oils, locally delivered tetracycline, and doxycycline, to facilitate microbial biofilm removal at the furcation areas, with contradictory results. A more detailed review of this topic is provided in Chapter 10.

Figures 3.6 and 3.7 show two cases of FI with pre-, intra-, and post-treatment views, showing limitations in non-surgical debridement of furcation defects and tools used for intrasurgical furcation debridement.

3.4 Patient Home Care

It has been shown that poor plaque control results in suboptimal treatment outcome (Rosling et al. 1976). The clinician can perform effective instrumentation, but the patient must be able to maintain the root surface free of microbial biofilm. Numerous tools are available for the patient to clean their furcation-involved multi-rooted teeth. These are manual and powered toothbrushes, interspace brushes, interdental brushes, and the WaterPik®. A recent Cochrane systematic review conducted a meta-analysis on 51 clinical trials concluded that powered toothbrushes, compared to manual ones, were more effective in reducing plaque and gingival inflammation in both the short and long term (Yaacob et al. 2014). Powered toothbrushes have different modes of action, namely side to side, counter-oscillation, rotation oscillation, multi-dimensional, and circular. The rotating oscillating powered toothbrushes were found to significantly reduce plaque and gingivitis in the short and long term, with the greatest benefit at the lingual surfaces (Klukowska et al. 2014a, b). Another Cochrane review evaluated 17 randomized controlled trials comparing the efficacy of powered toothbrushes with different modes of action (Deacon et al. 2010). It was reported that powered toothbrushes with the rotation oscillation motion performed better than those with the side-to-side action. However, limited studies with short follow-up

(a)   (b)

(c)

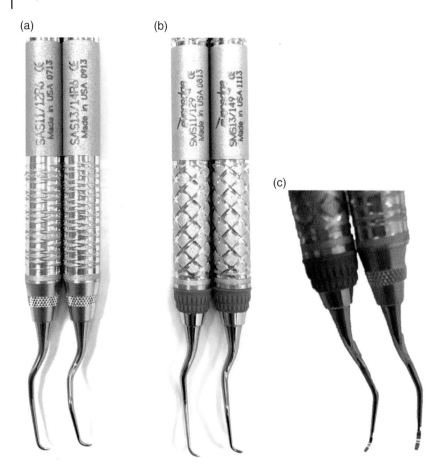

Figure 3.2 (a) Mini Five® Gracey curettes #11/12 and #13/14 with blade width of 0.76 mm; (b) Micro Mini Five® Gracey curettes #11/12 and #13/14 with blade width of 0.6 mm; (c) difference in the blade widths of the Micro Mini Five Gracey curette #11/12 (left) and Mini Five Gracey curette #11/12 (right).

periods (three months or less) and unclear risk of bias were included. Therefore, the results of the review should be interpreted with caution.

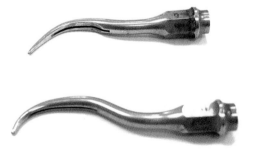

Figure 3.3 Traditional piezoelectric ultrasonic scaler tips with a diameter of 0.7–0.8 mm.

There is only one study that evaluated the efficacy of brushing instruments at the furcal areas (Bader and Williams 1997). The authors compared a pointed-end tufted powered brush and a small-head powered toothbrush, and found that the former was more effective in removing plaque at the furcal area. The pointed tip is able to fit into the furcal area to remove the plaque. As the end-tufted brush looks similar to the interspace brush, it might be inferred that the interspace brush will be effective in maintaining the furcation area free of biofilm.

Interdental brushes come in various sizes and shapes. They can be conical or cylindrical in shape, have angled or straight handles, have regular nylon bristles or rubber bristles, and be of different sizes. They are used to

Figure 3.4 EMS Piezon® Master ultrasonic scaler and tips: (a) PL1 tip with a diameter of 0.5 mm for debridement of hard-to-reach interproximal areas; (b) PL5 tip with a ball end of diameter 0.8 mm for debridement of furcations and concavities; (c) PS universal tip with a diameter of 0.6 mm for debridement of deep pockets.

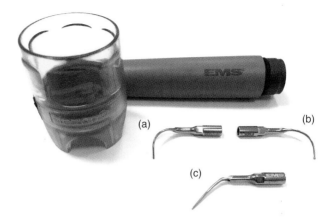

(a) (b)

(c)

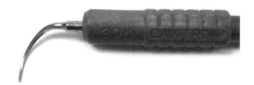

Figure 3.5 Cavitron® Slimline™ insert with a diameter of 0.5 mm.

clean the interproximal surfaces or furcation areas. A comparison between dental floss and the interdental brush showed that the latter was significantly more effective in removing plaque (mean proximal plaque score: 1.22 for interdental brush and 1.71 for dental floss; Kiger et al. 1991), hence it is better suited for cleaning proximal surfaces. As evidenced by the significantly higher bleeding and plaque scores, a short-term study found that conical interdental brushes did not clean the lingual proximal surface as well as their cylindrical counterparts (Larsen et al. 2017). Also, straight brushes can clean better than angled ones (Jordan et al. 2014). It seemed that rubber-bristled interdental brushes were as effective as regular interdental brushes in terms of plaque removal and patients found them more comfortable to use (Abouassi et al. 2014). Therefore, in patients with periodontitis, and possibly interproximal FI, interdental brushes remove more plaque than flossing or brushing alone (Christou et al. 1998).

The WaterPik is an oral irrigator introduced in 1962 that uses pulsating hydrodynamic force to remove food debris from the tooth surface. Its clinical benefits include removal of subgingival bacteria, clinical and histological reduction in gingival inflammation, down-regulation of pro-inflammatory cytolines, reduction of probing depths, improvement of clinical attachment loss, being safe for gingival tissues, and minimal bacteremia (Jolkovsky and Lyle 2015; Cutler et al. 2000). Therefore, in patients with less than ideal oral hygiene, supragingival irrigation will flush out the subgingival bacteria, reducing gingival inflammation to a degree greater than toothbrushing alone (Research, Science and Therapy Committee of the American Academy of Periodontology 2001). In comparison to the Sonicare Airfloss®, which uses a fluid spray of micro-bubbles to disrupt the plaque, the WaterPik may be more effective in terms of removing plaque and consequently reducing the bleeding score (Goyal et al. 2015).

Evidence on home care of furcations is scarce. As such, results from studies that assessed interproximal cleaning was used to infer the effectiveness of these brushes in removing plaque from the tooth surfaces. It appears that powered toothbrushes with the rotation oscillation action, interspace brushes, straight cylindrical interdental brushes with rubber or nylon bristles, and the WaterPik are effective in cleaning interproximal areas and potentially furcations.

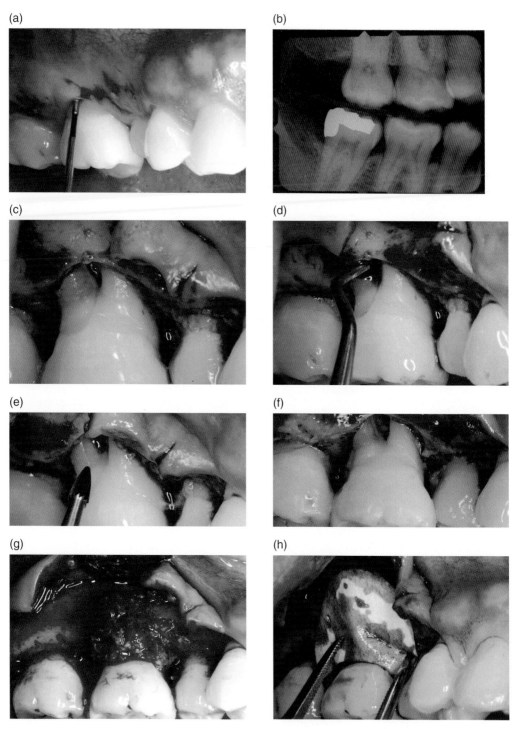

Figure 3.6 (a) The maxillary right first molar presented with a Grade I cervical enamel projection, 6 mm pockets, and a class II furcation. (b) Periapical radiograph showed radiolucency in the furcation area. (c) Cervical enamel projection was evident and seen protruding into the furcation. (d) Furcal area was debrided with After-5 Gracey curettes (Hu-Friedy, USA) and Piezo ultrasonic scalers (EMS, Switzerland). (e) Newmeyer's rotary bur was used to remove the cervical enamel projection and any remaining granulomatous tissue. (f) Clinical photo showed the defect after cleaning. (g) Defect was grafted with human cancellous allograft (LifeNet, USA). (h) The graft was then protected with a well-trimmed collagen membrane (2–3 mm beyond the defect margin all around).

(i)

(j)

(k)

(l)

(m)

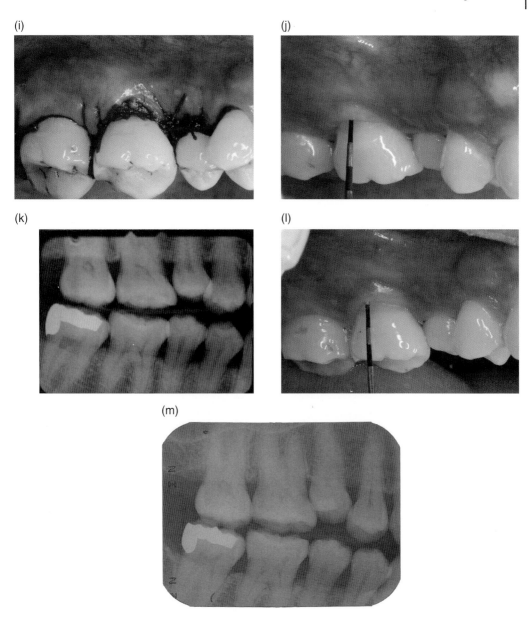

Figure 3.6 (Continued) (i) The flap was then coronally advanced and sutured. (j) At the two-year post-surgery follow-up visit, the probing pocket depth at the furcation area was reduced to 3 mm and (k) radiographic bone fill was observed. (l) The furcation area remained stable clinically and (m) radiographically even at the four-year post-surgery follow-up visit. Further details and indications of furcation regenerative therapy are given in Chapter 7.

(a)   (b)

(c)   (d)

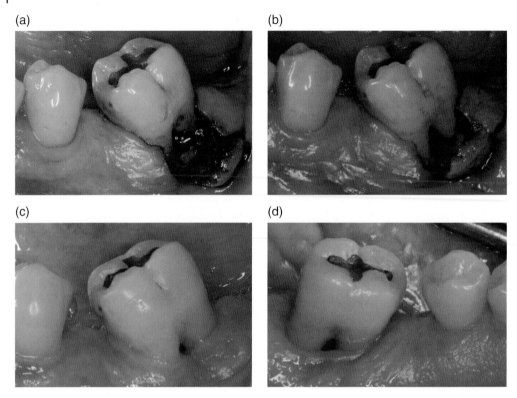

Figure 3.7 The mandibular left second molar presented with a grade III cervical enamel projection, 6–8 mm pockets, and a class III furcation. (a) Residual calculus observed on flap elevation, reflecting the ineffectiveness of non-surgical debridement. (b) Surgical open-flap scaling and root planing with fine ultrasonic inserts (Cavitron®, Dentsply, USA) and Gracey curettes (Hu-Friedy, USA) were performed to achieve a smooth root surface. The flap was repositioned and sutured apically, exposing the class III furcation involvement. (c) At the two-year post-surgery follow-up visit, there was recurrence of the pocket to 5 mm at the midlingual site (d) with bleeding on probing, despite the patient using an interdental brush of the appropriate size and being on a strict three-monthly periodontal maintenance regimen. This therefore concurs with the literature that plaque removal at the furcation area is unpredictable, even when exposed and visible.

Summary of Evidence

- Longitudinal studies show that, compared to single-rooted teeth, furcation-involved teeth respond poorly to non-surgical and surgical treatment. Improvements in the furcation area, if any, are also less sustainable over time.
- Finer and angulated ultrasonic tips can better debride the furcation area than hand instruments, e.g. Gracey curettes.
- There is limited evidence on home care of furcations, however tools such as powered toothbrushes, interspace brushes, interdental brushes, and the WaterPik may be useful in removing plaque from the furcation area.

References

Abouassi, T., Woelber, J.P., Holst, K. et al. (2014). Clinical efficacy and patients' acceptance of a rubber interdental bristle: A randomized controlled trial. *Clinical Oral Investigations* 18, 1873–1880. doi: 10.1007/s00784-013-1164-3.

Auplish, G., Needleman, I.G., Moles, D.R., and Newman, H.N. (2000). Diamond-coated sonic tips are more efficient for open debridement of molar furcations: A comparative manikin study. *Journal of Clinical Periodontology* 27, 302–307.

Bader, H., and Williams, R. (1997). Clinical and laboratory evaluation of powered electric toothbrushes: Comparative efficacy of two powered brushing instruments in furcations and interproximal areas. *Journal of Clinical Dentistry* 8, 91–94.

Biagini, G., Checchi, L., Miccoli, M.C. et al. (1988). Root curettage and gingival repair in periodontitis. *Journal of Periodontology* 59, 124–129. doi: 10.1902/jop.1988.59.2.124.

Booker, B.W., III, and Loughlin, D.M. (1985). A morphologic study of the mesial root surface of the adolescent maxillary first bicuspid. *Journal of Periodontology* 56, 666–670. doi: 10.1902/jop.1985.56.11.666.

Bower, R.C. (1979a). Furcation morphology relative to periodontal treatment: Furcation entrance architecture. *Journal of Periodontology* 50, 23–27. doi: 10.1902/jop.1979.50.1.23.

Bower, R.C. (1979b). Furcation morphology relative to periodontal treatment: Furcation root surface anatomy. *Journal of Periodontology* 50, 366–374. doi: 10.1902/jop.1979.50.7.366.

Checchi, L., and Pelliccioni, G.A. (1988). Hand versus ultrasonic instrumentation in the removal of endotoxins from root surfaces in vitro. *Journal of Periodontology* 59, 398–402. doi: 10.1902/jop.1988.59.6.398.

Chiu, B.M., Zee, K.Y., Corbet, E.F., and Holmgren, C.J. (1991). Periodontal implications of furcation entrance dimensions in Chinese first permanent molars. *Journal of Periodontology* 62, 308–311. doi: 10.1902/jop.1991.62.5.308.

Christou, V., Timmerman, M.F., Van der Velden, U., and Van der Weijden, F.A. (1998). Comparison of different approaches of interdental oral hygiene: Interdental brushes versus dental floss. *Journal of Periodontology* 69, 759–764. doi: 10.1902/jop.1998.69.7.759.

Cutler, C.W., Stanford, T.W., Abraham, C. et al. (2000). Clinical benefits of oral irrigation for periodontitis are related to reduction of pro-inflammatory cytokine levels and plaque. *Journal of Clinical Periodontology* 27, 134–143.

Dannewitz, B., Krieger, J.K., Husing, J., and Eickholz, P. (2006). Loss of molars in periodontally treated patients: A retrospective analysis five years or more after active periodontal treatment. *Journal of Clinical Periodontology* 33, 53–61. doi: 10.1111/j.1600-051X.2005.00858.x.

Dannewitz, B., Zeidler, A., Husing, J. et al. (2016) Loss of molars in periodontally treated patients: Results 10 years and more after active periodontal therapy. *Journal of Clinical Periodontology* 43, 53–62. doi: 10.1111/jcpe.12488.

Darveau, R.P., Tanner, A., and Page, R.C. (1997). The microbial challenge in periodontitis. *Periodontology* 2000 14, 12–32.

Deacon, S.A., Glenny, A.M., Deery, C. et al. (2010). Different powered toothbrushes for plaque control and gingival health. *Cochrane Database of Systematic Reviews* 12 (Art. No. CD004971). doi: 10.1002/14651858.CD004971.pub2.

Del Peloso Ribeiro, E., Bittencourt, S., Nociti, F.H., Jr. et al. (2007). Comparative study of ultrasonic instrumentation for the non-surgical treatment of interproximal and non-interproximal furcation involvements. *Journal of Periodontology* 78, 224–230. doi: 10.1902/jop.2007.060312.

dos Santos, K.M., Pinto, S.C., Pochapski, M.T. et al. (2009). Molar furcation entrance and its relation to the width of curette blades used in periodontal mechanical therapy. *International Journal of Dental Hygiene* 7,

263–269. doi: 10.1111/j.1601-5037. 2009.00371.x.

Eschler, B.M., and Rapley, J.W. (1991). Mechanical and chemical root preparation in vitro: Efficiency of plaque and calculus removal. *Journal of Periodontology* 62, 755–760. doi: 10.1902/jop.1991.62.12.755.

Fleischer, H.C., Mellonig, J.T., Brayer, W.K. et al. (1989). Scaling and root planing efficacy in multirooted teeth. *Journal of Periodontology* 60, 402–409. doi: 10.1902/jop.1989.60.7.402.

Goyal, C.R., Lyle, D.M., Qaqish, J.G., and Schuller, R. (2015). Efficacy of two interdental cleaning devices on clinical signs of inflammation: A four-week randomized controlled trial. *Journal of Clinical Dentistry* 26, 55–60.

Hajishengallis, G., and Lamont, R.J. (2012). Beyond the red complex and into more complexity: The polymicrobial synergy and dysbiosis (PSD) model of periodontal disease etiology. *Molecular and Oral Microbiology* 27, 409–419.

Hirschfeld, L., and Wasserman, B. (1978). A long-term survey of tooth loss in 600 treated periodontal patients. *Journal of Periodontology* 49, 225–237. doi: 10.1902/jop.1978.49.5.225.

Jolkovsky, D.L., and Lyle, D.M. (2015). Safety of a water flosser: A literature review. *Compendium of Continuing Education in Dentistry* 36, 146–149.

Jordan, R.A., Hong, H.M., Lucaciu, A., and Zimmer, S. (2014). Efficacy of straight versus angled interdental brushes on interproximal tooth cleaning: A randomized controlled trial. *International Journal of Dental Hygiene* 12, 152–157. doi: 10.1111/idh.12042.

Kalkwarf, K.L., Kaldahl, W.B., and Patil, K.D. (1988). Evaluation of furcation region response to periodontal therapy. *Journal of Periodontology* 59, 794–804. doi: 10.1902/jop.1988.59.12.794.

Kiger, R.D., Nylund, K., and Feller, R.P. (1991). A comparison of proximal plaque removal using floss and interdental brushes. *Journal of Clinical Periodontology* 18, 681–684.

Klukowska, M., Grender, J.M., Conde, E. et al. (2014a). A randomized 12-week clinical comparison of an oscillating-rotating toothbrush to a new sonic brush in the reduction of gingivitis and plaque. *Journal of Clinical Dentistry* 25, 26–31.

Klukowska, M., Grender, J.M., Conde, E. et al. (2014b). A six-week clinical evaluation of the plaque and gingivitis efficacy of an oscillating-rotating power toothbrush with a novel brush head utilizing angled CrissCross bristles versus a sonic toothbrush. *Journal of Clinical Dentistry* 25, 6–12.

Kocher, T., and Plagmann, H.C. (1999). Root debridement of molars with furcation involvement using diamond-coated sonic scaler inserts during flap surgery: A pilot study. *Journal of Clinical Periodontology* 26, 525–530.

Kocher, T., Gutsche, C., and Plagmann, H.C. (1998a). Instrumentation of furcation with modified sonic scaler inserts: Study on manikins, part I. *Journal of Clinical Periodontology* 25, 388–393.

Kocher, T., Ruhling, A., Herweg, M., and Plagman, H.C. (1996). Proof of efficacy of different modified sonic scaler inserts used for debridement in furcations: A dummy head trial. *Journal of Clinical Periodontology* 23, 662–669.

Kocher, T., Tersic-Orth, B., and Plagmann, H.C. (1998b). Instrumentation of furcation with modified sonic scaler inserts: A study on manikins, part II. *Journal of Clinical Periodontology* 25, 451–456.

Larsen, H.C., Slot, D.E., Van Zoelen, C. et al. (2017). The effectiveness of conically shaped compared with cylindrically shaped interdental brushes: A randomized controlled clinical trial. *International Journal of Dental Hygiene* 13 (3), 211–218. doi: 10.1111/idh.12189.

Leon, L.E., and Vogel, R.I. (1987). A comparison of the effectiveness of hand scaling and ultrasonic debridement in furcations as evaluated by differential dark-field microscopy. *Journal of Periodontology* 58, 86–94. doi: 10.1902/jop.1987.58.2.86.

Lindhe, J., Westfelt, E., Nyman, S. et al. (1982). Healing following surgical/non-surgical treatment of periodontal disease: A clinical study. *Journal of Clinical Periodontology* 9, 115–128.

Loe, H., Theilade, E., and Jensen, S.B. (1965). Experimental gingivitis in man. *Journal of Periodontology* 36, 177–187. doi: 10.1902/jop.1965.36.3.177.

Loos, B., Claffey, N., and Egelberg, J. (1988). Clinical and microbiological effects of root debridement in periodontal furcation pockets. *Journal of Clinical Periodontology* 15, 453–463.

Loos, B., Nylund, K., Claffey, N., and Egelberg, J. (1989). Clinical effects of root debridement in molar and non-molar teeth: A 2-year follow-up. *Journal of Clinical Periodontology* 16, 498–504.

Matia, J.I., Bissada, N.F., Maybury, J.E., and Ricchetti, P. (1986). Efficiency of scaling of the molar furcation area with and without surgical access. *International Journal of Periodontics and Restorative Dentitry* 6, 24–35.

McFall, W.T., Jr (1982). Tooth loss in 100 treated patients with periodontal disease: A long-term study. *Journal of Periodontology* 53, 539–549. doi: 10.1902/jop.1982.53.9.539.

Nordland, P., Garrett, S., Kiger, R. et al. (1987). The effect of plaque control and root debridement in molar teeth. *Journal of Clinical Periodontology* 14, 231–236.

Oda, S., and Ishikawa, I. (1989). In vitro effectiveness of a newly-designed ultrasonic scaler tip for furcation areas. *Journal of Periodontology* 60, 634–639. doi: 10.1902/jop.1989.60.11.634.

Oda, S., Nitta, H., Setoguchi, T. et al. (2004). Current concepts and advances in manual and power-driven instrumentation. *Periodontology* 2000 36, 45–58. doi: 10.1111/j.1600-0757.2004.03674.x.

Otero-Cagide, F.J., and Long, B.A. (1997). Comparative in vitro effectiveness of closed root debridement with fine instruments on specific areas of mandibular first molar furcations. II. Furcation area. *Journal of Periodontology* 68, 1098–1101. doi: 10.1902/jop.1997.68.11.1098.

Page, R.C., and Kornman, K.S. (1997). The pathogenesis of human periodontitis: An introduction. *Periodontology 2000* 14, 9–11.

Parashis, A.O., Anagnou-Vareltzides, A., and Demetriou, N. (1993a). Calculus removal from multirooted teeth with and without surgical access. I: Efficacy on external and furcation surfaces in relation to probing depth. *Journal of Clinical Periodontology* 20, 63–68.

Parashis, A.O., Anagnou-Vareltzides, A., and Demetriou, N. (1993b). Calculus removal from multirooted teeth with and without surgical access. II: Comparison between external and furcation surfaces and effect of furcation entrance width. *Journal of Clinical Periodontology* 20, 294–298.

Patterson, M., Eick, J.D., Eberhart, A.B. et al. (1989). The effectiveness of two sonic and two ultrasonic scaler tips in furcations. *Journal of Periodontology* 60, 325–329. doi: 10.1902/jop.1989.60.6.325.

Pihlstrom, B.L., Oliphant, T.H., and McHugh, R.B. (1984). Molar and nonmolar teeth compared over 6½ years following two methods of periodontal therapy. *Journal of Periodontology* 55, 499–504. doi: 10.1902/jop.1984.55.9.499.

Ramfjord, S.P., Caffesse, R.G., Morrison, E.C. et al. (1987). 4 modalities of periodontal treatment compared over 5 years. *Journal of Clinical Periodontology* 14, 445–452.

Ramfjord, S.P., Nissle, R.R., Shick, R.A., and Cooper, H., Jr (1968). Subgingival curettage versus surgical elimination of periodontal pockets. *Journal of Periodontology* 39, 167–175.

Research, Science and Therapy Committee of the American Academy of Periodontology (2001). Treatment of plaque-induced gingivitis, chronic periodontitis, and other clinical conditions. *Journal of Periodontology* 72, 1790–1800. doi: 10.1902/jop.2001.72.12.1790.

Research, Science and Therapy Committee of the American Academy of Periodontology (2005). Position paper: The role of supra- and subgingival irrigation in the treatment of periodontal diseases. *Journal of Periodontology* 76, 2015–2027. doi: 10.1902/jop.2005.76.11.2015.

Rosling, B., Nyman, S., and Lindhe, J. (1976). The effect of systematic plaque control on bone regeneration in infrabony pockets. *Journal of Clinical Periodontology* 3, 38–53.

Ross, I.F., and Thompson, R.H., Jr (1978). A long term study of root retention in the treatment of maxillary molars with furcation involvement. *Journal of Periodontology* 49, 238–244. doi: 10.1902/jop.1978.49.5.238.

Schatzle, M., Loc, H., Burgin, W. et al. (2003). Clinical course of chronic periodontitis. *I: Role of gingivitis. Journal of Clinical Periodontology* 30, 887–901.

Scott, J.B., Steed-Veilands, A.M., and Yukna, R.A. (1999). Improved efficacy of calculus removal in furcations using ultrasonic diamond-coated inserts. *International Journal of Periodontics and Restorative Dentistry* 19, 355–361.

Smart, G.J., Wilson, M., Davies, E.H., and Kieser, J.B. (1990). The assessment of ultrasonic root surface debridement by determination of residual endotoxin levels. *Journal of Clinical Periodontology* 17, 174–178.

Socransky, S.S., and Haffajee, A.D. (2005). Periodontal microbial ecology. *Periodontology 2000* 38, 135–187. doi: 10.1111/j.1600-0757.2005.00107.x.

Sugaya, T., Kawanami, M., and Kato, H. (2002). Effects of debridement with an ultrasonic furcation tip in degree II furcation involvement of mandibular molars. *Journal of the International Academy of Periodontology* 4, 138–142.

Tagge, D.L., O'Leary, T.J., and El-Kafrawy, A.H. (1975). The clinical and histological response of periodontal pockets to root planing and oral hygiene. *Journal of Periodontology* 46, 527–533. doi: 10.1902/jop.1975.46.9.527.

Takacs, V.J., Lie, T., Perala, D.G., and Adams, D.F. (1993). Efficacy of 5 machining instruments in scaling of molar furcations. *Journal of Periodontology* 64, 228–236. doi: 10.1902/jop.1993.64.3.228.

Tunkel, J., Heinecke, A., and Flemmig, T.F. (2002). A systematic review of efficacy of machine-driven and manual subgingival debridement in the treatment of chronic periodontitis. *Journal of Clinical Periodontology* 29 (Suppl. 3), 72–81; discussion 90–91.

Wang, H.L., Burgett, F.G., Shyr, Y., and Ramfjord, S. (1994). The influence of molar furcation involvement and mobility on future clinical periodontal attachment loss. *Journal of Periodontology* 65, 25–29. doi: 10.1902/jop.1994.65.1.25.

Wood, W.R., Greco, G.W., and McFall, W.T., Jr (1989). Tooth loss in patients with moderate periodontitis after treatment and long-term maintenance care. *Journal of Periodontology* 60, 516–520. doi: 10.1902/jop.1989.60.9.516.

Wylam, J.M., Mealey, B.L., Mills, M.P. et al. (1993). The clinical effectiveness of open versus closed scaling and root planing on multi-rooted teeth. *Journal of Periodontology* 64, 1023–1028. doi: 10.1902/jop.1993.64.11.1023.

Yaacob, M., Worthington, H.V., Deacon, S.A. et al. (2014). Powered versus manual toothbrushing for oral health. *Cochrane Database of Systematic Reviews* 6 (Art. No.: CD002281). doi:10.1002/14651858.CD002281.pub3.

Chapter 4

Furcation: The Endodontist's View

Federica Fonzar and Riccardo Fabian Fonzar

Private practice, Udine, Italy

4.1 Introduction

To avoid contact with the exogenous substances of the oral cavity, pulp and dentine are genetically protected by the overlying enamel and cementum. Despite these defensive physical barriers, the pulp can be threatened by manifold insults, such as caries, restorative procedures, and mechanical, chemical, and thermal trauma. In periodontitis-affected patients, periodontal pathogens can induce pulp infection because of the vascular interconnections between periodontium and endodontium. Through the accessory canals or exposed dentinal tubules, bacteria and toxins might gain the access to the pulp. The effect is generally atrophy and is comparable with 'pulp aging'. Likewise, endodontic infections can influence periodontal health. When the *noxae* of degenerated pulp involve the supporting periodontium, rapid inflammatory responses, characterized by bone loss, tooth mobility, and/or sinus tract formation, might develop. These clinical conditions where both endodontium and periodontium are simultaneously affected in what appears to be a single periodontal lesion are known as endodontic-periodontal lesions.

Despite the topic of the book regarding exclusively furcation pathology, the ethiopathogenesis of endodontic-periodontal disease cannot be described by merely considering the inter-radicular space only. Therefore, the present chapter aims to comprehensively detail the aetiology and development of endodontic-periodontal lesions, with particular emphasis on the diagnosis, management, and long-term prognoses of the affected teeth, especially when the furcation region is involved.

4.2 Pathways Between Endodontium and Periodontium: Anatomical Considerations

Because of the anatomical and vascular interconnections, periodontium and endodontium can influence each other during function and should therefore be considered as one biological unit. The main pathways involved in the development of endodontic-periodontal lesions are the dentinal tubules, the lateral and accessory canals, and the apical foramen or foramina (Seltzer et al. 1963).

4.2.1 Dentinal Tubules

Crown and root dentinal tubules, which extend from the pulp to the amelodentinal and dentinocemental junctions, respectively, are permeable structures. Their permeability varies with regard to the dentine type, tooth

Diagnosis and Treatment of Furcation-Involved Teeth, First Edition. Edited by Luigi Nibali.
© 2018 John Wiley & Sons Ltd. Published 2018 by John Wiley & Sons Ltd.
Companion website: www.wiley.com/go/nibali/diagnosis

area, and functional tubular diameter (Pashley 1990).

The root dentine is less patent than the coronal. The number of tubules generally ranges from approximately 42 000/mm^2 in the cervical area to about 8000/mm^2 in the radicular. By the lower permeability, roots and furcation dentine act as a real protective barrier (Rapp et al. 1992). From the outer to the closer surfaces to the pulp, tubules, which follow an S-shaped path, are denser, wider, more patent, and therefore greater in flow rate (Ghazali 2003). With ageing or as a response to continuous low-grade stimuli, diameters and patency might decrease through the apposition of highly mineralized peritubular dentine.

On healthy teeth, enamel and cementum usually prevent the pulpo-dentinal complex from contact with the oral cavity microorganisms. Owing to developmental defects, caries, trauma, restorative procedures, or periodontal disease, cementum might not cover the underlying dentine any longer, and the exposed dentinal tubules might serve as communication pathways between the endodontium and periodontium (Adriaens et al. 1988; Love and Jenkinson 2002). Bacteria and bacterial products can therefore induce pulpal reactions by migrating towards the pulp (Langeland et al. 1974; Bergenholtz 1981; Adriaens et al. 1988). By colonizing the root dentine tubules of periodontally diseased teeth, pathogens might act as a reservoir for pocket recolonization after debridement (Adriaens et al. 1987). As proof of this, microbiological investigations revealed the presence of Gram-negative and Gram-positive species in the root dentine (Adriaens et al. 1988; Guiliana et al. 1997).

While it has been proved that bacteria are able to invade radicular dentine from the periodontal pocket, it remains unclear whether bacteria invade the healthy cementum before penetrating the dentine, or reach the root dentine through breaches in the cementum layer (Adriaens et al. 1987, 1988; Guiliana et al. 1997; Love and Jenkinson 2002). Cementum is a thin, often discontinuous

layer that commonly shows surface defects, for instance in the sites where Sharpey's fibres attach to its matrix (Adriaens et al. 1987). Its exposure to crevicular fluid, bacterial enzymes, or acidic metabolites might induce physicochemical and structural alterations, such as localized resorptive lacunae or demineralization (Daly et al. 1982; Adriaens et al. 1987). It can be speculated, therefore, that cementum might be structurally damaged by physiological, bacterial, and environmental factors, and that this alteration might facilitate bacterial penetration within the exposed root of periodontally diseased teeth.

The vitality of the tooth is another variable that might play an important role in hindering bacteria migration towards the pulp. By exposing the dentine surface to the oral environment for 150 days, bacterial invasion occurs faster in non-vital rather than vital teeth (Nagaoka et al. 1995). A possible explanation of this finding might be sought in the resistance offered by outward dentinal fluid movement and the presence of odontoblast processes in the tubules of vital teeth (Vongsavan and Matthews 1991, 1992; Pashley et al. 2002). In addition, antibodies and anti-microbial components contained within the dentinal fluid might also help the vital teeth to be more properly defended (Hahn and Overton 1997).

4.2.2 Lateral and Accessory Canals

An accessory canal is any branch starting from the pulp chamber or the main root canal that communicates with the external surface of the root. When the location is the coronal or middle third of the root, and the orientation is horizontal with respect to the main canal, accessory canals are named lateral canals (American Association of Endodontists 2015).

It is estimated that 30–40% of teeth exhibit accessory canals, most of which are found in the apical third of the root (De Deus 1975). Their prevalence might vary within the teeth, and was seen to be greater in mandibular molars and premolars than in maxillary molars and lateral incisors (Kirkham 1975). In addition, it can also change according to the root third analysed. In fact, De Deus (1975) found that 17%, 9%, and less than 2% of teeth showed accessory canals in the apical, middle, and coronal third, respectively. With regard to the number of accessory canals per tooth, 17% and 6% of teeth have one or two accessory canals (Kirkham 1975). Despite these anatomical considerations, the prevalence of periodontal disease associated with accessory canals seems to be relatively low (Rotstein and Simon 2004).

In multi-rooted teeth, furcation dentine might represent a communication pathway between endodontium and periodontium. In fact, the vascular system of the pulp is connected to that of periodontium through the accessory canals. At the furcation, their prevalence generally ranges from 23 to 76% (Lowman et al. 1973; Burch and Hulen 1974; Goldberg et al. 1987), but the extension rarely covers the entire distance between the pulp chamber and the furcation floor (Goldberg et al. 1987) and only 30–60% of molars have patent canals connecting the main root canal system and the periodontal ligament (see Figure 4.1). In particular, mandibular molars have a higher incidence (56%) than maxillary (48%) (Lowman et al. 1973; Gutmann 1978; Vertucci 2005). Because of these interconnections, pulp inflammation might have detrimental consequences on the furcation by inducing inflammatory responses on the inter-radicular periodontal tissues (Seltzer et al. 1963).

4.2.3 Apical Foramen or Foramina

The major connections between periodontal and pulp tissues are the apical foramina. The

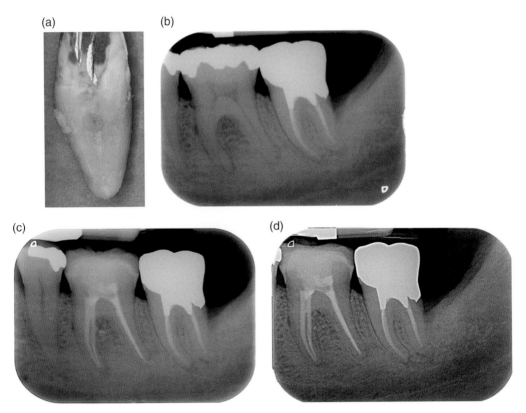

Figure 4.1 Accessory canal located distally to the mesial root on 4.6 (LR6) (a). Interradicular radiolucency on 3.6 (LL6) (b). After root canal therapy, the accessory canal located distally to the mesial root was filled with cement (c). Complete remineralization after four-year follow-up (d).

morphology of the apex might be quite variable. All the teeth have at least one accessory foramen. Generally, there are fewer primary dentinal tubules in the apical root third than in the coronal dentine. Their direction and density might be somewhat irregular, and some areas can be completely free of tubules (Mjör et al. 2001). Maxillary premolars have the most complicated apical morphology with the largest accessory foramina, followed by maxillary and mandibular molars (Marroquin et al. 2004), and this makes the prognosis of endodontic therapy in premolars and molars more uncertain than for other teeth.

4.2.4 Non-physiological Communications

Root perforation, vertical root fracture, and inflammatory root resorption are artificial pathways between periodontal and pulpal tissues.

Iatrogenic root canal perforations are serious complications that originate from manual/rotatory instrumentation or post-space preparation, and can threaten the prognosis of the tooth (Tsesis et al. 2010; Gorni et al. 2016). The treatment outcome depends on several factors that should be evaluated early, such as the size and position of the root perforation, the time elapsed before making the diagnosis and treatment, the degree of periodontal involvement, and the sealing ability and biocompatibility of the sealant. The faster the sealing, the more controlled the infection. Hence, time elapsed before treatment seems to be crucial for success. Among sealants, reinforced zinc oxide-eugenol cements and bioceramic materials, such as mineral trioxide aggregate, are used most for this purpose (Weldon et al. 2002; Parirokh and Torabinejad 2010; Haapasalo et al. 2015; Gorni et al. 2016).

Vertical root fractures (see Figures 4.2 and 4.3) are generally caused by loading trauma and occur more frequently in non-vital teeth (Chan et al. 1999; Sugaya et al. 2015). In vital teeth, vertical fractures can initiate coronally in 'cracked tooth syndrome' (Cameron 1964) or can involve the root only (Chan et al. 1999; Sugaya et al. 2015). While in the past endodontically treated teeth were considered to be weaker due to structural changes in dentine composition, such as water and collagen cross-linking loss, currently it is believed that the greater brittleness is linked to the loss of structural integrity. In fact, the extension of cavity access might influence the degree of cuspal deflection during function, increasing the risk of fracture. Furthermore, a history of extensive restorations, especially in mandibular posterior teeth, might make the tooth even more susceptible to fracture, especially in elderly patients (Lewinstein and Grajower 1981; Huang et al. 1992; Cheron et al. 2011; Faria et al. 2011).

Root resorption is a pathological process associated with dentine, cementum, and/or

(a)

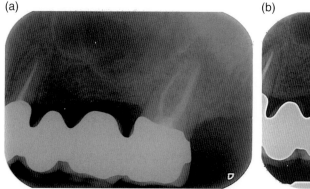

(b)

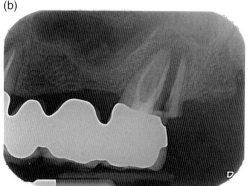

Figure 4.2 Vertical root fracture starting from the apex on 2.7 (UL7). The lesion resembled an endodontic infection (a). Complete failure after two years follow-up (b). Root resection was not possible due to unfavourable anatomy.

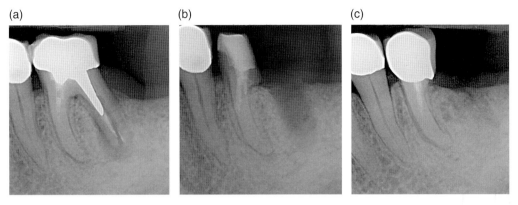

Figure 4.3 Vertical fracture of the distal root on 3.6 (LL6) (a). Rizectomy of the distal root (b) and after healing (c).

bone loss. It can be external or internal, depending on whether the origin is the periodontium or the pulp. The aetiopathogenesis is far from being completely understood. Mechanical and infective factors such as orthodontic treatment, trauma, intracoronal bleaching, periodontitis, and thermal stimuli might be considered as predisposing factors. The presence of profuse bleeding on probing, granulation tissue, and hard cavity bottom might confirm the diagnosis of external inflammatory root resorption. Electric and cold pulp tests might be positive. However, sensitivity tests alone do not differentiate this pathological process from dental caries or internal resorption. Radiographic evaluation reveals that the canal profile is well defined in internal resorption, and rather undefined and faded in external. External resorption progression (see Figure 4.4) can lead to the invasion of the pulp space as a last resort. Likewise, untreated internal resorption can establish a communication between endodontium and periodontium by breaking the external root surface (Tronstad 1988; Trope 1998; Andreasen and Andersson 2007; Patel et al. 2010).

4.3 Bacteria Involved in Endodontic-periodontal Disease

Periodontal diseases are mixed anaerobic infections, modulated by a complex interplay between local and host factors (Page 1999).

Similarly, endodontic infection has an anaerobic nature. Most of the species found in infected root canals are also present in periodontal pockets. However, the endodontic biofilm seems to be less complex than the periodontal biofilm (Trope et al. 1988; Kobayashi et al. 1990; Sundqvist 1994; Kurihara et al. 1995; Zehnder et al. 2002). Root canal infection is a dynamic process, and different bacterial species can apparently prevail at different stages. The most prevalent named species detected in primary endodontic infections, including abscessed cases, belong to diverse genera of Gram-negative (*Fusobacterium*, *Dialister*, *Porphyromonas*, *Prevotella*, *Tannerella*, *Treponema*, *Campylobacter*, and *Veillonella*) and Gram-positive bacteria (*Parvimonas*, *Filifactor*, *Pseudoramibacter*, *Olsenella*, *Actinomyces*, *Peptostreptococcus*, *Streptococcus*, *Propionibacterium*, and *Eubacterium*). Conversely, the microflora changes if endodontic therapy fails. Several culture and molecular biology studies revealed that *Enterococcus faecalis* is the most frequent species in root canal–treated teeth, with a prevalence of up to 90% of cases and a strong association with persistent infections (Rôças et al. 2004; Mohammadi et al. 2013). Canals that are apparently well treated might contain from 1 to 5 bacterial species; however, in those not properly treated, the number might vary from 10 to 30, which is very similar to that of untreated canals (Sundqvist et al. 1998; Pinheiro et al. 2003; Sakamoto et al. 2008).

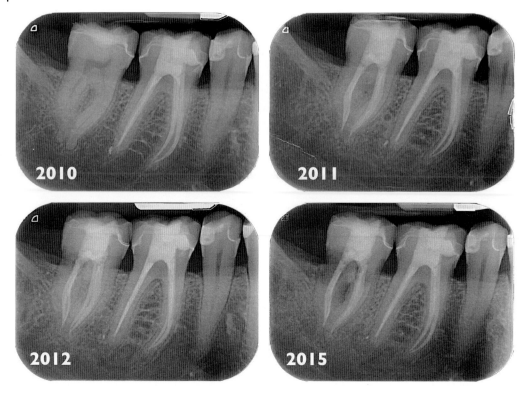

Figure 4.4 Disto-lingual external progressive root resorption on 4.7 (LR7). Initally, the invisible resorption induced pulpitis and root canal therapy was performed.

4.4 Relationship Between Periodontal Disease and Histological Pulp Changes

Many controversies still exist about the relationship between periodontal inflammation and pulp health (see Table 4.1). However, it seems to be widely accepted that periodontitis and periodontal therapy can induce pathological changes in the pulp. Periodontal disease progression can lead to the exposure and bacterial contamination of the accessory canals, more frequent in the apical third of the tooth and at the furcation (Seltzer et al. 1963; Rubach and Mitchell 1965), or it can reach the root apex with subsequent neuro-vascular bundle damage (Langeland et al. 1974; De Deus 1975). Cementum removal, resulting from scaling and root planing, can expose the dentinal tubules and accessory canals (Adriaens et al. 1988), therefore the micro-organisms can migrate towards the pulp, inducing hystological changes (Rubach and Mitchell 1965; see Figure 4.5). However, the deposition of reparative dentine (Bergenholtz and Lindhe 1978; Nilvéus and Selvig 1983; Hattler and Listgarten 1984), the outward movement of the dentinal fluid (Vongsavan and Matthews 1991, 1992; Pashley et al. 2002), the presence of odontoblast processes in the tubules (Nagaoka et al. 1995; Pasley et al. 2002), and the presence of antibodies and anti-microbial components within the dentinal fluid (Hahn and Overton 1997) can act as a defense system, preventing the bacteria from reaching the pulp. In reference to this, we should stress that, as mentioned in Chapter 3, subgingival debridement is now moving away from the concept of 'root planing' and 'removal of all diseased cementum' (Aleo et al. 1974) towards an emphasis on disruption of the subgingival biofilm, with minimal alteration to the cementum (Nibali et al. 2015).

Table 4.1 Effect of periodontal disease on pulp tissue.

Do progressive periodontitis and periodontal treatment affect the pulp?			Pulp damage		Pulp response	
Progressive periodontal disease	Yes	Apex Apical foramen (Langeland et al. 1974; Harrington et al. 2002; Sheykhrezaee et al. 2007; Aguiar et al. 2014; Rathod et al. 2014)	Neuro-vascular bundle damage Main canal involved	Irreversible	Inflammatory Degenerative (Rubach and Mitchell 1965; Zehnder 2001; Sheykhrezaee et al. 2007; Aguiar et al. 2014; Rathod et al. 2014)	Complete necrosis
		Apical root third (Rubach and Mitchell 1965; Adriaens et al. 1988; Sheykhrezaee et al. 2007; Zuza et al. 2012)	Bacteria and toxins migrate towards the pulp through the accessory canals	Irreversible or Reversible	Inflammatory Degenerative (Rubach and Mitchell 1965; Sheykhrezaee et al. 2007; Rathod et al. 2014)	Fibrosis Calcification Inflammation Odontoblast integrity loss Neuro-vascular alteration Partial/complete necrosis
		Furcation (Rubach and Mitchell 1965; Bender and Seltzer 1972; Adriaens et al. 1988; Zuza et al. 2012)			Reparative (Mazur and Massler 1964; Bender and Seltzer 1972; Langeland et al. 1974; Lantelme et al. 1976; Bergenholtz and Lindhe 1978; Ross and Thompson 1978; Czarnecki and Schilder 1979; Torabinejad and Kiger 1985; Cortellini and Tonetti 2001; Harrington et al. 2002; Aguiar et al. 2014)	Calcification Fibrosis Vascular alteration Nerve alteration $\approx$ pulp ageing
Periodontal treatment (scaling and root planing)	Yes (Rubach and Mitchell 1965; Adriaens et al. 1988)		Neuro-vascular bundle damage Main canal involved	Irreversible	Inflammatory Degenerative (Rubach and Mitchell 1965; Sheykhrezaee et al. 2007; Rathod et al. 2014)	Complete necrosis

(Continued)

Table 4.1 (Continued)

Do progressive periodontitis and periodontal treatment affect the pulp?	Pulp damage		Pulp response	
	Cementum removal: bacteria and toxins migrate towards the pulp through the accessory canals and the exposed dentinal tubules	Irreversible or Reversible	Inflammatory Degenerative (Rubach and Mitchell 1965; Sheykhrezaee et al. 2007; Rathod et al. 2014)	Fibrosis Calcification Inflammation Odontoblast integrity loss Vascular alteration Partial/complete necrosis
			Reparative (Mazur and Massler 1964; Bender and Seltzer 1972; Langeland et al. 1974; Lantelme et al. 1976; Bergenholtz and Lindhe 1978; Ross and Thompson 1978; Czarnecki and Schilder 1979; Torabinejad and Kiger 1985; Cortellini and Tonetti 2001; Harrington et al. 2002; Aguiar et al. 2014)	Calcification Fibrosis Vascular alteration Nerve alteration ≈ pulp ageing
No (Bergenholtz and Lindhe 1978; Nilvéus and Selvig 1983; Hattler and Listgarten 1984; Nagaoka et al. 1995; Hahn and Overton 1997; Pashley et al. 2002)	No bacteria and toxins migrate towards the pulp through the accessory canals and the exposed dentinal tubules	Reversible	Reparative dentine (Bergenholtz and Lindhe 1978; Hattler and Listgarten 1984; Vongsavan and Matthews 1991) + Dentinal fluid (Vongsaven and Matthews 1991, 1992; Pashley et al. 2002) + Odontoblast processes (Nagaoka et al. 1995; Pashley et al. 2002) Antibodies/antimicrobial components within the dentinal fluids (Hahn and Overton 1997)	

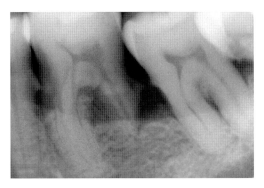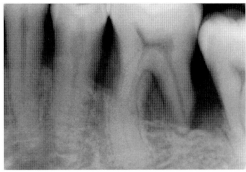

Figure 4.5 Pulp necrosis on 3.6 (LL6) after deep root debridement. *Source*: Courtesy Dr Cristiano Luciano.

Pulp response might vary, from normal (Mazur and Massler 1964; Smukler and Tagger 1976; Czarnecki and Schilder 1979; Torabinejad and Kiger 1985) to reparative (Mazur and Massler 1964; Langeland et al. 1974; Czarnecki and Schilder 1979; Torabinejad and Kiger 1985; Harrington et al. 2002) or degenerative (Rubach and Mitchell 1965; Sheykhrezaee et al. 2007; Zuza et al. 2012; Aguiar et al. 2014; Rathod et al. 2014). Repaired vital pulp is calcificated, fibrotic, and has fewer blood vessels and nerve fibres (Mazur and Massler 1964; Langeland et al. 1974; Czarnecki and Schilder 1979; Torabinejad and Kiger 1985; Harrington et al. 2002). Conversely, degenerated pulp exhibits fibrosis, calcification, inflammation, vascular alteration, loss of odontoblast integrity, and partial necrosis (Rubach and Mitchell 1965; Aguiar et al. 2014; Rathod et al. 2014). Complete necrosis seems to only occur if the apical neuro-vascular bundle is involved (Langeland et al. 1974; Zehnder 2001; Harrington et al. 2002; Sheykhrezaee et al. 2007; Aguiar et al. 2014; Rathod et al. 2014).

The lack of randomized clinical trials with test and control groups prevents a clear association between progressive periodontal disease and pulp alterations being established. Data have to be carefully interpreted, since pulpal alterations might be the result of multiple factors, such as periodontal disease, history of caries, physiological pulp ageing, previous ignored trauma, or pulp tissue fixation. Indeed, pulp fixation is challenging and artifacts resulting from improper specimen preparation might lead to misjudgements (Harrington et al. 2002; Sheykhrezaee et al. 2007).

At the current stage of scientific knowledge, we could summarize that periodontal disease might induce reparative or degenerative pulp changes. Pulp necrosis is rather rare and occurs when the defect is up to the apical third of the tooth and the neuro-vascular bundle is involved. If the blood supply through the apical foramen remains intact, the pulp is usually able to withstand the physiological insults induced by both periodontal disease and therapy.

4.5 Endodontic-periodontal Disease

Because of their anatomical and functional interconnection, pulp and periodontium can be simultaneously affected in what appears to be a single periodontal lesion. This clinical scenario, known as 'endodontic-periodontal lesion' (Bergenholtz and Hasselgreen 2008) was first described by Simring and Goldberg in 1964.

4.5.1 Classification

Despite the many attempts to classify endodontic-periodontal lesions, the Simon, Glick, and Frank (1972) classification remains the most widely accepted point of reference (see also Gargiulo 1984; Guldener 1985; Abbott and Salgado 2009; Kerns and Glickman 2011). According to Simon et al., endodontic-periodontal lesions are classified as:

- Primary endodontic lesion.
- Primary periodontal lesion.
- Primary endodontic lesion with secondary periodontal involvement.
- Primary periodontal lesion with secondary endodontic involvement.
- True combined lesion.

4.5.1.1 Primary Endodontic Lesion

Primary endodontic lesions (Box 4.1 and Table 4.2) mostly involve decayed, restored, or traumatized teeth. As a result of the endodontic inflammatory process, bone resorption occurs at the apex, along the lateral aspect of the root, or at the furcation area when multi-rooted teeth are affected (see Figures 4.6 and 4.7). Because of the suppurative process, the sinus tract can develop through the periodontal ligament space or the cortical bone in accordance with the *locus minoris resistentiae* (place of least resistance) principle. For multi-rooted teeth, the tract can drain off into the furcation area, resembling a class III periodontal defect.

Pain, tooth mobility, tenderness to pressure and percussion, and periodontal abscess-like swelling can be the related clinical inflammatory signs.

Sensitivity tests show necrotic pulp, even though in multi-rooted teeth the response can be positive because of the partial necrosis. As the lesion has an endodontic origin, root canal treatment (European Society of Endodontology 2006) is mandatory for sinus tract resolution without any associated periodontal therapy (Zehnder et al. 2002; Bergenholtz and Hasselgreen 2008; Shenoy and Shenoy 2010; Kerns and Glickman 2011). Sometimes, a period of up to four or five years might be required for the complete radiographic healing of the periapical lesion (Ng et al. 2007; Zitzmann et al. 2009). Incongruous root canal treatment or untreated canals (i.e. MB2 in first maxillary molars or D2 in lower molars) might prevent the lesion from healing, because of the high residual bacterial load within the endodontium.

4.5.1.2 Primary Periodontal Lesion

Periodontitis (Box 4.2 and Table 4.3) is a progressive inflammatory process that starts in the sulcus and moves towards the apex due to the accumulation of plaque and calculus on the root surface. The final effect is the loss of alveolar bone and supporting tissues around the teeth. This process can also be accompanied by periodontal abscess in the acute phases of the disease (Toto and Gargiulo 1970; Hoffman and Gold 1971). Clinical examination reveals soft-tissue inflammation, tooth mobility, bleeding on probing, and the presence of wide pockets (i.e. accessible at different points on the

---

Box 4.1 Primary endodontic lesion.

- Tooth history: caries, cracks, extensive restoration, crown or bridge abutment, incongruous root canal treatment, dental trauma,* root resorption.**
- Root surface: smooth on probing. No presence of subgingival calculus.
- Pocket conformation: narrow if the pocket is present.
- Sensitivity pulp test response: generally negative. However, it might be positive in multi-rooted teeth.
- Radiographic sign: lateral, apical and/or inter-radicular radiolucency.
- Treatment: root canal treatment.

---

* Post-traumatic pulp healing, especially after luxation injuries, is characterized by temporary loss of sensitivity. All sensitivity tests show low reliability right after the trauma (Bastos et al. 2014).
** Root resorption might affect the external surfaces of the tooth (external resorption) or the internal dentine (internal resorption) after being started in the periodontium or within the pulp space, respectively.

Table 4.2 Primary endodontic lesions.

Diagnostic Elements	Findings	Clinical Management
Presence of caries/restorations/cracks	+	Anamnesis
Subgingival calculus	–	Clinical examination
		Periodontal probing
History of trauma	+/–	Radiographic examination
Abscess	+*	Sensitivity tests
		Endodontic treatment
Narrow deep pocket	+/–	Re-evaluation after a few months
Bleeding on probing	–	
Thermal test	–/+**	
Electric test	–/+**	
Radiolucency	+	
Mobility	+/–	
Palpation test	+	
Percussion test	+	

* In the acute phase.
** The test is negative if all the pulp tissue is necrotic, except in case of gases-related thermal expansion. The test could be positive in case of partial necrosis.

Differential Diagnosis	Vertical root fractures
	Primary periodontal lesions
Favourable Endodontic Prognostic Factors	Congruous endodontic treatment
	No symptoms
	No probing within 30 days
	Fistular track closure within 30 days
	Radiolucency improvement within 6 months

Source: Adapted from AIE – Collana di Monografie Piccin Nuova Libraria S.p.A 2014.

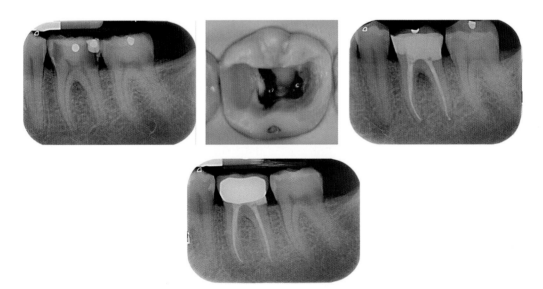

Figure 4.6 Pulpitis on 3.6 (LL6). Inter-radicular and periapical radiolucencies due to bacterial toxins. Five-year follow-up after root canal therapy.

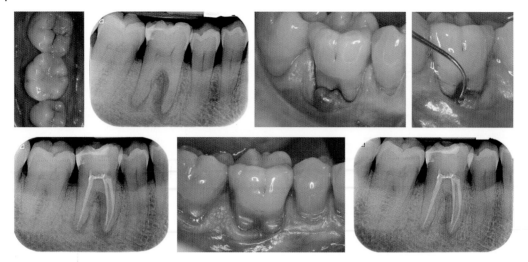

Figure 4.7 Primary endodontic lesion with inter-radicular and apical involvement on 4.6 (LR6). No furcation probing after three months and partial healing after one-year follow-up.

Box 4.2 Primary periodontal lesion.

- Tooth history: periodontal pocket, attachment loss, bleeding on probing.
- Root surface: rough on probing because of subgingival plaque and calculus.
- Pocket conformation: wide, often multiple pockets.
- Sensitivity pulp test response: generally positive.
- Radiographic sign: lateral and/or inter-radicular radiolucency, apical radiolucency in advanced disease.
- Treatment: oral hygiene instructions (OHI) and root debridement.

---

tooth) supported by plaque and calculus along the root. It should be noted that periodontal pockets might also originate from anomalies in the root development (Rotstein and Simon 2004). During the diagnostic phase, pulp sensitivity tests generally reveal positive responses. However, negative responses can also be recorded and do not necessarily account for pulp necrosis. Owing to dystrophic calcifications, the pulp space might be reduced and the tooth might not respond to the sensitivity tests despite its vitality (Abou-Rass 1982).

On the basis of the previous considerations, the prognosis would mainly depend on the extension of the periodontal disease, the outcome of the periodontal therapy, and the patient's ability to comply with potential long-term maintenance (Bergenholtz and Hasselgreen 2008; Kerns and Glickman 2011).

Primary Endodontic Lesion with Secondary Periodontal Involvement

Periodontal pathogens might induce periodontitis by migrating apically into the patent sinus tract when the endodontic infection is not treated or persists after root canal therapy. At the radiographic evaluation, angular intrabony or inter-radicular osseous defects are appreciated. Plaque and calculus are detected on probing, therefore healing requires both endodontic and periodontal therapies for necrotic pulp removal and root debridement. Since root canal treatment resolves only a part of the defect (European Society of Endodontology 2006; Shenoy and Shenoy 2010), dental prognosis relies on the extent and severity of the osseous defect, and on the efficacy of the periodontal therapy.

For suppurative processes fistulizing through the cortical bone, bacteria from the oral cavity might colonize first the fistula and

Table 4.3 Primary periodontal lesions.

Diagnostic Elements	Findings	Clinical Management
Presence of caries/restorations/cracks	+/−	Anamnesis
Subgingival calculus	+	Clinical examination
History of trauma	+/−	Periodontal probing
		Radiographic examination
Abscess	+*	Sensitivity tests
Wide, not isolated, deep pocket/furcation	+	Splinting of mobile teeth (if needed)
Bleeding on probing	+	Oral hygiene instructions and periodontal non-surgical therapy
Thermal test	+	Periodontal re-evaluation after a few months
Electric test	+	Periodontal surgical therapy (if needed)
Lateral/interradicular radiolucency	+	
Mobility	+	
Palpation test	+*	
Percussion test	+*	

* In the acute phase.

Differential Diagnosis	Endodontic-periodontal lesions
Favourable Prognostic Factors	No symptoms
	Pulpal vitality
	No bleeding on probing
	Probing pocket depth reduction
	Mobility reduction
	Radiographic bone remineralization in the apical part of the defect

Source: Adapted from AIE – Collana di Monografie Piccin Nuova Libraria S.p.A 2014.

then the apex, affecting the tooth prognosis. Primary endodontic lesion with secondary periodontal involvement (Box 4.3 and Table 4.4) might also occur in endodontically treated teeth because of root perforation and/or fracture. Once the communication between endodontium and periodontium is established, the secondary periodontal lesion can develop as a result of the micro-organisms' migration from the root canal to the periodontium.

The clinical signs may range from local periodontal pocket deepening to abscess formation associated with pain, exudate, and tooth mobility. In single-rooted teeth, the prognosis is usually poor if the defect is close to the apex. In multi-rooted teeth, the prognosis might be better, since the tooth can be maintained by resecting the affected root, if the anatomy is indicated for this procedure

---

Box 4.3 Primary endodontic lesion with secondary periodontal involvement.

- Tooth history: caries, cracks, extensive restoration, crown or bridge abutment, incongruous root canal treatment, dental trauma.
- Root surface: rough on probing because of subgingival plaque and calculus.
- Pocket conformation: narrow to wide, depending on the exposition time of the sinus tract to periodontal pathogens.
- Sensitivity pulp test response: negative.
- Radiographic sign: lateral, apical, and/or inter-radicular radiolucency.
- Treatment: root canal treatment, oral hygiene instructions (OHI), and root debridement.

Table 4.4 Primary endodontic lesions with secondary periodontal involvement.

Diagnostic Elements	Findings	Clinical Management
Presence of caries/restorations/cracks	+	Anamnesis
Subgingival calculus	+	Clinical examination
		Periodontal probing
History of trauma	+/−	Radiographic examination
Abscess	+*	Sensitivity tests
		Splinting of mobile teeth (if
Narrow to wide deep pocket	+	needed)
Bleeding on probing	+	Oral hygiene instructions and
		non-surgical periodontal therapy§
Thermal test	−	Endodontic treatment
Electric test	−	Re-evaluation after a few months
Radiolucency	+	Surgical periodontal therapy (if
		needed)
Mobility	+	
Palpation test	+	
Percussion test	+	

* In the acute phase

§ **Deep Root Debridement Should Be Avoided Before Determining The Endodontic Component Of The Defect (See Section 4.5.3)**

Differential Diagnosis	Primary periodontal lesion with secondary endodontic involvement
	Vertical root fracture
	Root/furcation perforation in endodontically treated teeth
Favourable Endodontic Prognostic Factors	Congruous endodontic treatment
	No symptoms
	Partial probing depth reduction within 30 days
	Fistular track closure within 30 days
	Mobility reduction
	Partial radiolucency improvement within 6 months

Source: Adapted from AIE – Collana di Monografie Piccin Nuova Libraria S.p.A 2014.

(Cameron 1964; Chan et al. 1999; Zehnder et al. 2002; Sunitha et al. 2008; Kerns and Glickman 2011; Sugaya et al. 2015; see also Chapter 8).

Primary Periodontal Lesion with Secondary Endodontic Involvement

Primary periodontal lesion with secondary endodontic involvement (Box 4.4 and Table 4.5) differs from primary endodontic lesion with secondary periodontal involvement only in the temporal sequence of the disease processes. If periodontitis remains untreated, periodontal pathogens can reach the pulp through the accessory canals or

---

Box 4.4 Primary periodontal lesion with secondary endodontic involvement.

- Tooth history: probing pocket depth deepening, bleeding on probing.
- Root surface: rough on probing because of subgingival plaque and calculus.
- Pocket conformation: wide, often multiple pockets.
- Sensitivity pulp test response: generally negative.
- Radiographic sign: lateral, apical, and/or inter-radicular radiolucency.
- Treatment: root canal treatment, oral hygiene instructions (OHI), and root debridement.

Table 4.5 Primary periodontal lesions with secondary endodontic involvement.

Diagnostic Elements	Findings	Clinical Management
Presence of caries/restorations/cracks	+/−	Anamnesis
Subgingival calculus	+	Clinical examination
History of trauma	+/−	Periodontal probing
Abscess	+*	Radiographic examination
Not isolated, wide deep pocket/furcation	+	Sensitivity tests
Bleeding on probing	+	Splinting of mobile teeth (if needed)
Thermal test	−**	Oral hygiene instructions and non-surgical periodontal therapy[§]
Electric test	−**	Endodontic treatment
Lateral/apical/inter-radicular radiolucency	+	Periodontal re-evaluation after a few months
Mobility	+	Surgical periodontal therapy (if needed)
Palpation test	+	
Percussion test	+	

* In the acute phase.
** The test is negative if all the pulp tissue is necrotic, except in case of gases-related thermal expansion. The test could be positive in the case of partial necrosis.

[§] **Deep Root Debridement Should Be Avoided Before Determining The Endodontic Component of The Defect (See Section 4.5.3)**

Differential Diagnosis	Primary endodontic lesions with secondary periodontal involvement
Favourable Endodontic Prognostic Factors	Congruous endodontic treatment No symptoms Partial probing depth reduction within 30 days Fistular track closure within 30 days Mobility reduction Partial radiolucency improvement within 6 months

Source: Adapted from AIE – Collana di Monografie Piccin Nuova Libraria S.p.A 2014.

apical foramina. Pulp necrosis occurs and an endodontic-periodontal lesion develops (Rubach and Mitchell 1965; Aguiar et al. 2014). Periodontal therapy can also lead to secondary pulp involvement. By exposing lateral canals and dentine during scaling and root planing or surgical flap procedures, blood supply might be interrupted and micro-organisms might penetrate into the tubules, resulting in pulp inflammation and/or necrosis (Adriaens et al. 1988).

To differentiate between endodontic-periodontal lesions with primary periodontal and endodontic origin, anamnesis and clinical examination have to be exhaustively performed (see Figure 4.8). A history of generalized periodontitis might suggest a primary periodontal origin. The number and conformation of pockets can help in the diagnosis. Wider or narrower defects generally suggest a periodontal or endodontic origin of the lesions, respectively (Zehnder et al. 2002; Sunitha et al. 2008; Kerns and Glickman 2011). In addition, periodontal probing may reveal the presence of calculus on the root surface. Pulp sensitivity tests are generally negative when the endodontium is involved, whereas the radiographic evaluation does not prove the primary origin of the lesion.

Once the endodontic therapy is properly performed (European Society of Endodontology

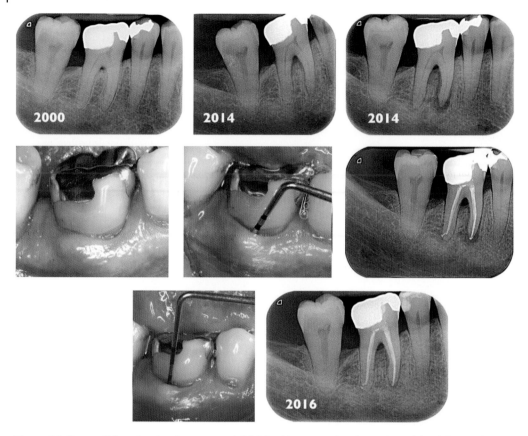

Figure 4.8 Degree III furcation involvement on 4.6 (LR6) with progressive deepening of the defect and secondary pulp necrosis after 14 years. Root canal therapy led to resolution of the endodontic component of the defect. Besides scaling and root planing and oral hygiene instructions, no further periodontal treatment was performed.

2006; Shenoy and Shenoy 2010), clinical success basically depends on the outcome of the periodontal therapy and the patient's ability to comply with potential long-term maintenance. As previously mentioned, multi-rooted teeth might have a better prognosis than single-rooted teeth, since root resection represents an alternative for tooth survival.

True Combined Lesion

A true combined lesion (Box 4.5 and Table 4.6) means that the endodontic and periodontal infections simultaneously exist as independent, separated, or merging lesions. When the periodontal pocket deepens up to the periapical lesion, the endodontic and periodontal components of the defect are unidentifiable. Symptoms are similar to

---

Box 4.5 True combined lesions.

- Tooth history: caries, cracks, extensive restoration, crown or bridge abutment, incongruous root canal treatment, dental trauma, probing pocket depth deepening, bleeding on probing.
- Root surface: rough on probing because of subgingival plaque and calculus.
- Pocket conformation: wide and conical pocket.
- Sensitivity pulp test response: negative.
- Radiographic signs: communicating or non-communicating extensive apical, lateral, and/or inter-radicular radiolucencies.
- Treatment: root canal treatment, oral hygiene instructions (OHI), and root debridement.

Table 4.6 True periodontal-endodontic combined lesions.

Diagnostic Elements	Findings	Clinical Management
Presence of caries/restorations/cracks	+	Anamnesis
		Clinical examination
Subgingival calculus	+	Periodontal probing
History of trauma	+/−	Radiographic examination
Abscess	+*	Sensitivity tests
		Splinting of mobile teeth (if needed)
Not isolated, wide deep pocket/furcation	+	Oral hygiene instructions and
Bleeding on probing	+	non-surgical periodontal therapy§
		Endodontic treatment
Thermal test	−	Periodontal re-evaluation after a
Electric test	−	few months
Lateral/apical/inter-radicular radiolucency	+	Surgical periodontal therapy (if
		needed)
Mobility	+	
Palpation test	+	
Percussion test	+	

* It depends on whether the phase is acute or chronic.

§ **Deep Root Debridement Should Be Avoided Before Determining The Endodontic Component Of The Defect (see Section 4.5.3)**

Differential Diagnosis	Vertical root fracture
Favourable Endodontic Prognostic Factors	Congruous endodontic treatment
	No symptoms
	Partial probing depth reduction within 30 days
	Fistular track closure within 30 days
	Mobility reduction
	Partial radiolucency improvement within 6 months

Source: Adapted from AIE – Collana di Monografie Piccin Nuova Libraria S.p.A 2014.

those previously mentioned for the combined lesions with primary endodontic or periodontal origin. The radiographic evaluation shows extensive osseous radiolucencies, communicating or not, similar to those of vertically fractured teeth. Indeed, pulp space invasion through vertical root fracture might also be considered as a true combined lesion.

Prior to endodontic therapy, mobile teeth should be splinted and carefully debrided. Once the root canal treatment is properly performed (European Society of Endodontology 2006), the endodontic component of the defect is expected to heal within a couple of months (Shenoy and Shenoy 2010; see Figure 4.9). Tooth prognosis would entirely depend on both the periodontal pocket depth and the related periodontal therapy. Uncertain prognosis concerns more single-rooted that

multi-rooted teeth, since root resection might be a treatment option if not all the roots are severely involved and tooth anatomy is indicative for this procedure (Zehnder et al. 2002; Rotstein and Simon 2004; Sunitha et al. 2008).

4.5.2 Diagnosis of Endodontic-periodontal Disease

Diagnosis of endodontic-periodontal lesions can be easily performed when the patient has been monitored over time. Similar clinical and radiographic findings might make the differential diagnosis somewhat challenging. To avoid any misinterpretation, comprehensive information can be obtained through detailed anamnesis and clinical examination, and by the use of specific tests aimed to assess the vitality of the pulp. Primary endodontic

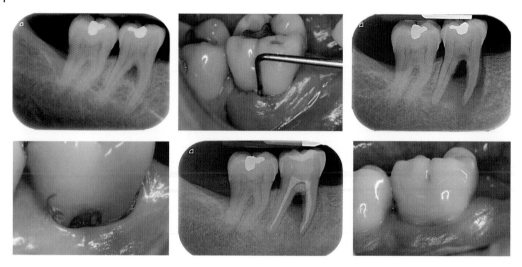

Figure 4.9 Class 3 inter-radicular defect and concomitant decay of the furcation roof on 4.7 (LR7). The caries progression led to pulp necrosis. Tunnelling spontaneously occurred after non-surgical periodontal treatment. One-year follow-up after root canal therapy.

lesions generally originate from infected and non-vital pulp, whereas vital teeth are more characteristic of primary periodontal disease (Rotstein and Simon 2004; Bergenholtz and Hasselgreen 2008; Sunitha et al. 2008; Parolia et al. 2013).

4.5.2.1 Clinical Examination

Pulpal and periodontal diseases might have many clinical signs in common, such as gingival swelling, pus discharge, probing, tooth mobility, and tenderness to percussion. Teeth have to be evaluated for caries, incongruous under- or over-contoured restorations, loss of marginal seal, erosions, abrasions, cracks, and fractures. All these situations are more related to endodontic disease.

4.5.2.2 Palpation

Palpation is performed by applying firm digital pressure in correspondence with the root and the apex, with the index finger pressing the mucosa against the underlying cortical bone. A positive response might indicate an active periradicular inflammatory process. However, this test does not indicate whether the origin is endodontic or periodontal. The test should be compared to control teeth.

4.5.2.3 Percussion

This test indicates the presence of periradicular inflammation without revealing the status of the pulp. An abnormal positive response shows inflammation of the periodontal ligament, but it does not indicate whether the origin is endodontic or periodontal. The test should be compared to control teeth.

4.5.2.4 Bite Test

This test does not disclose the condition of the pulp. However, it might be positive in vital teeth affected by cracked tooth syndrome (Cameron 1964) and in non-vital teeth with periradicular inflammation.

4.5.2.5 Mobility

This clinical sign does not prove whether the origin of the lesion is primarily periodontal or endodontic. It might be speculated that its primary cause is periodontitis. In fact, tooth mobility depends on the amount and inflammation of the residual supporting tissues. The greater the bone loss, the higher the mobility. However, periradicular oedema or trauma, with or without tooth fracture, can also lead to similar mobility (Biancu et al. 1995; Séguier et al. 2000).

The Endodontist's View | 73

4.5.2.6 Fistula Tracking

Endodontic and periodontal diseases can lead to the formation of a fistulous sinus track. Following a minor resistance path, inflammatory exudate drains off into the oral mucosa through the attached buccal gingiva or the vestibule. The track is generally more representative of the endodontic infection rather than the periodontal disease, which often drains through the periodontal pocket without any fistulous sinus track formation. Fistula tracking is performed by inserting a semirigid radiopaque material, commonly a gutta-percha cone, into the sinus track until resistance is met (see Figure 4.10). A radiograph is taken to identify the course of the sinus tract and, therefore, the tooth involved.

4.5.2.7 Cracked Tooth Testing

Cracked teeth (Cameron 1964) or vertical root fractures can be diagnosed through the observation of incomplete or complete cracks by transillumination. The fibre-optic light source is directly placed on the cleaned tooth. Cracks can be appreciated with a magnification source by evaluating the disruption of the light transmission (Liewehr 2001; Liewehr et al. 2010). Unlike a vertical root fracture with a 'tear-shaped' radiographic radiolucency, cracked teeth do not generally show any pathognomonic radiographic signs.

4.5.2.8 Radiographs

Despite the benefits of radiographs, consisting in the detection of caries, over- or under-contoured restorations, pulp caps, periradicular radiolucencies, periodontal ligament widening, calculus, alveolar bone loss, and root fractures, this examination alone does not indicate whether the radiolucency has an endodontic, periodontal, or any additional origin. It is important to consider that some other pathologies, such as cysts and neoplasia, can resemble periodontal or endodontic lesions in radiographic appearance.

Occlusal trauma may also lead to radiographic radiolucencies on the lateral, apical, or inter-radicular aspect of the root. In periodontally involved teeth suffering from occlusal trauma, the amount of demineralization is not quantitatively reflected in the probing pocket depth, which is less deep than could be guessed radiographically. Occlusal adjustment might be necessary and must always precede any endodontic or periodontal therapy. Demineralization resolves within a few months when the occlusal interferences and the mobility are eliminated by grinding and splinting, respectively [75,81,96,97] (Bergenholtz and Hasselgreen 2008; Carnevale et al. 2008; Lindhe et al. 2008; Kerns and Glickman 2011; see Figures 4.11 and 4.12).

4.5.2.9 Pocket Probing

To assess whether the origin of the lesion is endodontic or periodontal, probing can be crucial in the diagnosis (Harrington and Steiner 2002). Defects are evaluated for

(a)

(b)

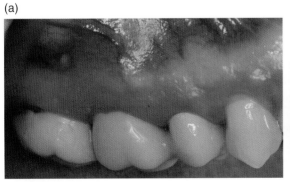 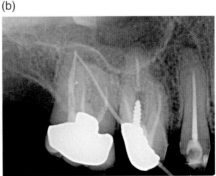

Figure 4.10 Fistulous sinus track between 1.6 (UR6) and 1.7 (UR7) (a). Fistula tracking revealed the origin of the endodontic infection on 1.7 (b).

(a)   (b)

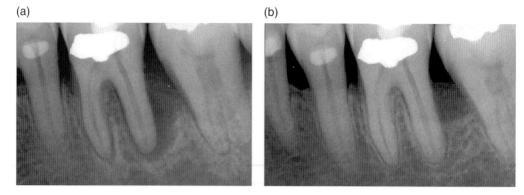

Figure 4.11 Radiographic radiolucency on 3.6 (LL6) affected by secondary occlusal trauma without furcation involvement (a). Six-month follow-up after root debridement and occlusal adjustment (b). *Source*: AIE—Collana di Monografie Piccin Nuova Libraria S.p.A 2014, p. 139.

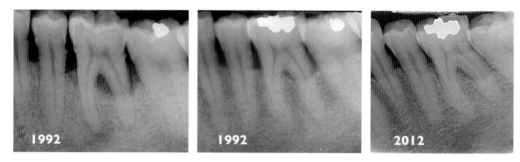

Figure 4.12 Degree II furcation defect (lingual) on 3.6 (LL6) affected by secondary occlusal trauma. Being the possible result of jiggling movements, the apical radiolucency present on the mesial root disappeared after the occlusal adjustment. Twenty-year follow-up after non-surgical periodontal therapy and oral hygiene instructions. *Source*: AIE—Collana di Monografie Piccin Nuova Libraria S.p.A 2014, p. 140.

extent, severity, and shape by means of a calibrated periodontal probe. The presence of plaque and calculus, detected by sounding the root surface with the tip of the probe, explains the periodontal involvement, although this may not be necessarily easy to detect. Primary periodontal lesions are frequently characterized by wide calculus-induced defects in patients with further periodontal pockets, whereas primary endodontic lesions typically show narrow solitary calculus-free defects. Inter-radicular involvement without further signs of periodontal disease might indicate the endodontic origin of the lesion.

Periodontal probing can be considered as a prognostic indicator in the short term. In fact, early fistulous sinus track resolution after root canal therapy (Shenoy and Shenoy 2010) might confirm the endodontic origin

of the defect without any further concomitant causes, such as vertical root fracture or periodontal involvement. On the contrary, a persisting sinus track might imply periodontal involvement or unsolved endodontic infection (Harrington and Steiner 2002; Walton and Torabinejad 2002; Rotstein and Simon 2004).

4.5.2.10 Pulp Vitality Tests

Pulp vitality tests are very important to evaluate whether the lesion has an endodontic or periodontal origin (Walton and Torabinejad 2002). The *sensitivity* rather than the *vitality* of the pulp is assessed through sensory nerve stimulation. Two different stimuli, electric and/or thermal (cold or hot), can be applied, and complaints and painful sensations are recorded. Figure 4.13 summarizes the diagnostic tests for pulp health assessment, and

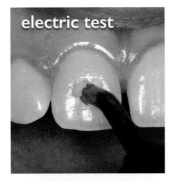
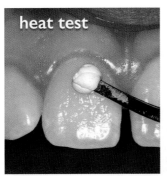
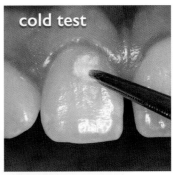
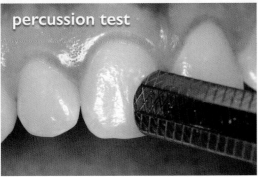
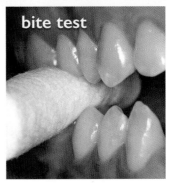

Figure 4.13 Diagnostic tests for pulp health assessment. *Source*: AIE—Collana di Monografie Piccin Nuova Libraria S.p.A 2014, pp. 266–268, 271.

Box 4.6 considers how sensitivity tests might be misinterpreted.

Vital teeth react to cold and hot stimuli by exhibiting short-lasting sharp pain or mild heat sensation, respectively. Intense and long-lasting painful reactions might indicate irreversible pulp changes. In molars, tissue degeneration might be limited to part of the pulp only (see Figure 4.14) and the reliability of the tests might be questioned, as false

> **Box 4.6 Clinical situations where pulp response to sensitivity tests might be misinterpreted.**
>
> - Teeth with calcified root canals.
> - Multi-rooted teeth with partially affected pulp.
> - Teeth with partial- or full-coverage restorations.
> - Traumatized teeth.
> - Endodontically treated teeth with untreated canals.

negatives can be wrongly recorded (Abou-Rass 1982; Mejàre et al. 2012; Levin 2013). A lack of response is often associated with pulp necrosis (Rowe and Pitt Ford 1990; Peters et al. 1994).

Vital teeth react to an electric test by exhibiting tingling, slight discomfort, or a burning sensation. Scored values per se do not mean the presence or absence of pathology, since no general threshold for pulpal disease has been established so far. As a general rule, the higher the scored values, the higher the probability of irreversible pulpal alterations. To better assess the response, healthy teeth should be taken as controls. By comparing the values obtained at different follow-up stages, more clinical information is provided for the diagnosis. However, false negatives and positives might make clinical evaluation somewhat challenging (Rotstein and Simon 2004; Gopikrishna et al. 2007; Chen and Abbott 2009; Jafarzadeh and Abbott 2010; Mejàre et al. 2012; Alghaithy and Qualtrough 2017).

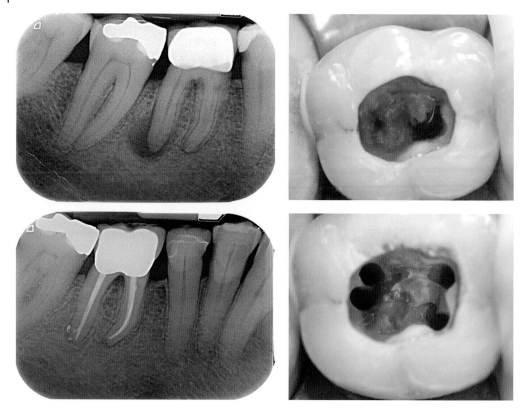

Figure 4.14 Pulp necrosis limited to the distal root on 4.6 (LR6) and result after root canal therapy.

While a lack of response can be associated with pulp necrosis, exaggerated or misleading responses following cold or electric tests can be the result of pulpitis, patient anxiety, dentinal hypersensitivity, trauma, or enamel-to-dentine cracks (Abou-Rass 1982; Eli 1993; Peters et al. 1994; Bastos et al. 2014). Cold and hot stimuli can respectively mitigate or exacerbate the symptoms in partially necrotic teeth.

Vital teeth with a history of deep caries, periodontitis, bruxism, or trauma may not respond to thermal or electrical stimuli because of the reparative changes in the pulp tissues (Bastos et al. 2014). Partial- or full-coverage restorations can also act as a barrier to thermal and, to a lesser degree, electrical stimuli, preventing the pulp from being properly evaluated (Rowe and Pitt Ford 1990; Peters et al. 1994; Myers 1998; Petersson et al. 1999).

The vitality rather than the sensitivity of the pulp can be assessed by measuring the pulp blood flow through laser doppler flow-metry or similar procedures. Many investigations have been conducted to validate the efficacy of these tests. However, their clinical applicability is still questioned (Gopikrishna et al. 2007; Mejàre et al. 2012; Alghaithy and Qualtrough 2017).

4.5.2.11 Cavity Test

By drilling the cavity without anaesthetic, the pulp status can be objectively evaluated through patient-referred symptoms. The so-called cavity test can be performed when all the aforementioned tests have failed to give comprehensive information about the vitality of the pulp. Positive and negative responses indicate vital and necrotic pulp, respectively. If no symptoms are reported by extending the cavity towards the pulp chamber, partial or complete pulp necrosis is confirmed and the endodontic treatment can be started (Kerns and Glickman 2011).

4.5.2.12 Selective Anaesthesia Test

To determine the origin of pain, teeth might be selectively anaesthetized by carefully injecting the anaesthetic through the periodontal ligament. Periodontal intraligament injection is limited to a single tooth without involving the adjacent teeth. The test is useful to identify the origin of pulpitis-related radiating pain (D'Souza et al. 1987; Rotstein and Simon 2004).

4.5.3 Management of Endodontic-periodontal Disease

To properly manage endodontic-periodontal pathology (Box 4.7; Berner and Graber 2008), prognosis and treatment decision-making should be based on scrupulous diagnosis. The pulp should be assessed for sensitivity, whereas bone defects should be assessed for severity, extension, and shape.

Primary endodontic disease is characterized by necrotic pulp and narrower calculus-free defect, thus the prognosis would mainly depend on the outcome of root canal therapy. Once calculus-related pockets are excluded and root canal treatment is properly performed, the diagnosis of primary endodontic lesions is confirmed by the disappearance of symptoms, physiological values on soft tissue probing, and bony remineralization on recall radiographs.

Primary periodontal lesions show vital pulp and a wide calculus-associated pocket. In this case, the prognosis depends on periodontal disease severity, treatment execution, and patient response, motivation, and compliance.

Box 4.7 Proper management of endodontic-periodontal pathology.

- Collect all the information referred to by the patient (i.e. previous trauma, pulp capping).
- Perform all the tests mentioned.
- Match and interpret the data collected.

Despite the similar clinical and radiographic findings, the presence of plaque and calculus is crucial for the diagnosis and prognosis of combined or true endodontic-periodontal lesions. From a treatment viewpoint, the calculus, if present, might be useful to detect the limit between the periodontal (rough surfaces due to calculus) and endodontic component of the defect (smooth surfaces without calculus). When this differential diagnosis is not possible, deep and heavy debridement should be avoided before root canal therapy, since healthy cementum might be wrongly removed, and a second re-evaluation of the site should be made two to three months after the endodontic treatment (Zehnder 2001; Parolia et al. 2013; Paul and Hutter 1997). This time is required for the initial bone remineralization, thus the extent of the periodontal component can be more precisely assessed.

Tooth maintainability should be deeply questioned once the extent of the defect is seen to depend more on periodontal than endodontic disease. The prognosis depends on periodontal disease severity, overall treatment execution, and patient response, motivation, and compliance. Cases of true combined disease might have more a guarded prognosis than the combined endodontic-periodontal lesions (Paul and Hutter 1997; Rotstein and Simon 2004; Bergenholtz and Hasselgreen 2008; Kerns and Glickman 2011; Schmidt et al. 2014).

4.5.4 Endodontic-periodontal Disease in Endodontically Treated Teeth

Sensitivity tests cannot be used for diagnostic purposes in endodontically treated teeth. Improper root canal treatment (see Figure 4.15) or iatrogenic injuries (see Figure 4.16), such as stripping or perforation, should be radiographically detected to determine whether the origin of the lesion is endodontic, particularly if there are no signs of periodontal disease. The diagnostic dilemma can only be solved through proper endodontic retreatment. By controlling the infection, clinical and radiographic healing

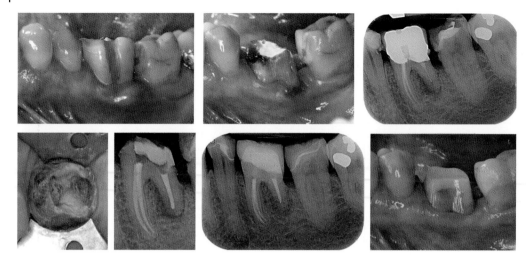

Figure 4.15 True combined lesion on 3.6 (LL6) with an incongruous root canal therapy. The endodontic infection led to the apical resorption of the distal root. Despite the inter-radicular radiolucency, furcation probing was negative. A periodontal defect was present on the distal aspect of the tooth. Two-year follow-up after non-surgical periodontal therapy, oral hygiene instructions, and root canal retreatment.

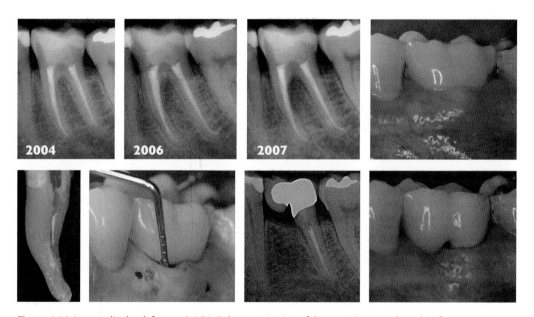

Figure 4.16 Inter-radicular defect on 3.6 (LL6) due to stripping of the mesial root and results after rizectomy.

can be expected within two to three months after the retreatment (European Society of Endodontology 2006; Shenoy and Shenoy 2010). If resolution does not occur, periodontal disease, vertical root fracture, or persisting endodontic infection can be individually considered as possible causes of the disease (Rotstein and Simon 2004).

4.6 Relationship Between Pulp and Periodontal Furcation Therapies

4.6.1 Non-surgical Periodontal Therapy

The previous chapter discussed how, since bacteria are the primary aetiological factor in periodontal disease, periodontal furcation therapy aims to subgingivally remove plaque and calculus from the contaminated root surfaces (Wennström et al. 2005; Tomasi and Wennström 2009). Despite the benefits for periodontal health (Löe et al. 1965), mechanical instrumentation might have some side effects on root integrity and, therefore, on the endodontium. Following root cementum and superficial dentine removal, bacteria can more easily penetrate into the tubules and induce a localized inflammatory response on the pulp (Adriaens et al. 1988; Bergenholtz and Ricucci 2008). Nevertheless, some authors have reported that cementum and dentine removal do not appear to have consequences for pulp health (Bergenholtz and Lindhe 1978), even when the exposed root is in contact with plaque (Nilvéus and Selvig 1983; Hattler and Listgarten 1984). In fact, the incidence of pulp lesions was seen to be similar between scaling and root planing–treated and untreated teeth (Bergenholtz and Lindhe 1978).

Among the instrumentation-related side effects, root dentine hypersensitivity is widely reported as a complaint by patients. In fact, half of cases usually report sensitivity after subgingival scaling and root planning (von Troil et al. 2002). Painful symptoms, which affect the upper premolars and first molars more than the rest of the teeth (Bartold 2006), are normally evoked by evaporative, tactile, thermal, or osmotic stimuli, and can prevent the patient from undertaking daily oral hygiene procedures. In accordance with the most accredited hydrodynamic theory, fluid shift across the exposed tubules can be responsible for the painful sensation (Pashley et al. 1996).

Generally, root dentine hypersensitivity disappears within a couple of weeks after subgingival debridement because of the natural occlusion of the tubules. Mineral crystal deposition on the tubular lumen inactivates the hydrodynamic mechanism for dentinal pain and limits the potential for an inward diffusion of bacterial elements towards the pulp (Yoshiyama et al. 1989; 1990).

Besides the patient's pain perception and threshold, eating habits, such as consumption of citrus fruit, fruit juice, yogurt, and wine, can promote the onset of root dentine hypersensitivity. Acid nourishment can act as conditioners for mineralized tissues, preventing the tubules from occluding (Bergenholtz and Ricucci 2008; Addy et al. 1987).

A wide number of treatment options seem to be effective in the management of dentinal hypersensitivity. Chemical or physical agents are professionally or domestically applied, to either desensitize the nerve or cover the exposed dentinal tubules (Gillam and Orchardson 2006). Sometimes, for stressed patients with poor eating habits and a low pain threshold, dentinal hypersensitivity can persist for months or years after mechanical instrumentation, and root canal treatment might be required to improve their daily oral hygiene and the related quality of life (Bartold 2006; Gillam and Orchardson 2006).

4.6.2 Regenerative Furcation Therapy

Chapters 6 and 7 will cover the regenerative options for periodontal furcation involvement (FI). Despite the effort to establish whether a negative effect of guided tissue regeneration (GTR) on the pulp exists, clear evidence is still lacking (Chen et al. 1997). According to Cortellini and Tonetti (2001), GTR of deep intrabony defects extended to the apical third of the root does not negatively influence the vitality of the tooth. This is particularly evident when the neuro-vascular bundle is not damaged by debridement. Clinical attachment level (CAL) gain following GTR appears to be quite similar between vital and endodontically treated teeth. In fact, the healing process does not seem to be influenced by root canal therapy successfully performed prior to the regeneration (Cortellini and Tonetti 2001).

As reported by other authors (Lasho et al. 1983; Polson et al. 1984; Gkranias et al. 2012; Garg et al. 2015), conditioners, such as citric acid and ethylenediaminetetraacetic acid

(EDTA), are effective in smear layer, endo-toxins, and anaerobic bacteria removal. Root conditioning improves the attractiveness of the surface as a substrate to which cells/blood components can adhere (Boyko et al. 1980), therefore the exposed collagen fibres can act as a matrix for a new connective tissue attachment to cementum (Pitaru and Melcher 1987). Conversely, smear layer dissolution can threaten pulp health. By removing this protective barrier, dentine permeability increases and the pulp might be more likely to be injured (Ryan et al. 1984; McInnes-Ledoux et al. 1985). As observed by Cotton and Siegel (1977), citric acid application on freshly cut dentine may have a detrimental toxic effect on human pulp. However, several studies do not endorse this finding (Nilvéus and Selvig 1983; Lambrianidis et al. 1988).

Without evidence-based operating proto-cols, the recommendations in Box 4.8 should be followed.

4.6.3 Resective Therapy

As discussed by Rotundo and Fonzar in Chapter 8, endodontic treatment is manda-tory before resective therapy whenever the tooth is vital or the previous endodontic treatment is incongruous (see Figures 4.17 and 4.18). Rubber dam is required for optimal working conditions (Ahmad 2009; Lin et al. 2014). During cleaning and shaping, root integrity has to be preserved as much as pos-sible by minimally removing the dentine along the canals. To avoid resection-related gutta-percha exposure, the canal space has to be filled 2–3 mm apical to the furcation (Marin et al. 1989). Prior to the resective therapy, resin composites can be used to adhesively build up the abutment. Endodontic posts or screws might be necessary whenever the retention for the build-up material is poor. When the endodontic and restorative protocols are properly followed, retention-related complications such as build-up debonding or breaking are generally avoided (Carnevale et al. 2008).

Occasionally, the FI might be preoperatively or intraoperatively underestimated and its resolution might not be obtained by barrelling only (Jameson and Malone 1982). The exposed root canal entrances have to be carefully sealed after the resective therapy, since the incidence of pulp failures increases over time (Smukler and Tagger 1976). In particular, 41%,

---

Box 4.8 Recommendations for regenerative furcation therapy.

- For deep periodontal defects, with or without furcation involvement, on impairment-free vital teeth, regenerative therapy may be performed without endodontic pre-treatment, since pulp vitality is likely to be preserved.
- For up-to-the-apex periodontal defects, scaling and root planing (SRP) procedures might dam-age the neuro-vascular bundle of the tooth. Since pulp necrosis might occur during periodon-tal healing, according to some authors root canal treatment could be preventively performed to avoid any interference with the regeneration process (Cortellini and Tonetti 2001).
- For deep periodontal defects on asymptomatic congruously root-filled teeth with periapical radiolucency, root canal retreatment should be delayed, since a periapical lesion might require up to five years for comprehensive radiographic healing (Molven et al. 2002; Zitzmann et al. 2009; Abbott 2011).
- For deep periodontal defects on symptomatic incongruously root-filled teeth with periapical radiolucency, root canal retreatment is mandatory before proceeding with guided tissue regeneration therapy.
- For deep periodontal defects on symptom-free incongruously root-filled teeth without peria-pical translucency, no evidence-based endodontic protocol has been defined so far, thus root canal retreatment may be performed or not, depending on restorative purposes.

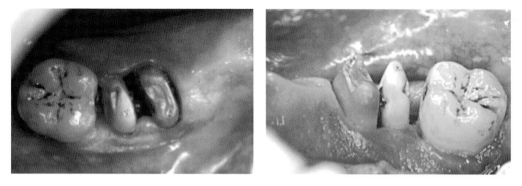

Figure 4.17 Pulp exposure after resective therapy on vital 4.6 (LR6). Root canal treatment was performed one week later.

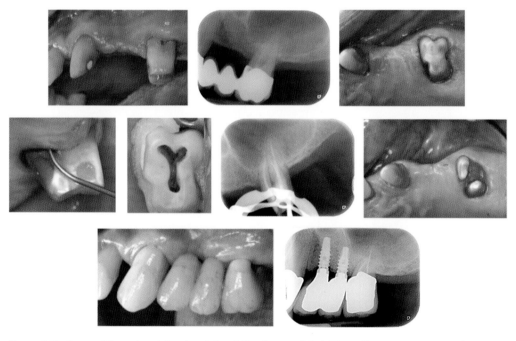

Figure 4.18 Degree II furcation defect (mesial and distal) on 2.6 (UL6). Minimally invasive access to the endodontic space was obtained after isolation with rubber dam. Canals were conservatively shaped and filled with gutta-percha apical to the furcation floor. Resin composite was used to fill the root canal entrances and to build up the cavity access. The rizotomy (root separation) of the mesio-buccal and palatal roots and the rizectomy (root amputation) of the disto-buccal root were performed after endodontic treatment. All the root canals were endodontically treated, since there was no pre-operative certainty of the extraction of the distal root.

62%, and 87% of resected teeth show pulp necrosis after six months, one year, and five years, respectively (Filipowicz et al. 1984). Because of the poor short-term endodontic prognosis, vital teeth should be devitalized before the resective therapy, or at least within two weeks afterwards (Smukler and Tagger 1976).

The operating recommendations in Box 4.9 should be followed.

Box 4.9 Recommendations for resective therapy.

- Cleaning and shaping should be conservatively performed, and residual dentine thickness should be preserved as much as possible to avoid root weakening.
- For canal filling, gutta-percha should be extended 2–3 mm apical to the furcation.
- For the build-up, resin composite should be used to adhesively restore the abutment.
- Endodontic posts or screws should be placed only in low-retention teeth.
- Vital resected teeth should be endodontically treated within two weeks after the resective therapy.

Summary of Evidence

- Endodontium and periodontium influence each other during health, function, and disease.
- The histological pulp changes induced by periodontal disease can be reparative or degenerative. Pulp necrosis generally occurs when the apical neuro-vascular bundle is involved.
- Accessory canals in the furcation region are frequent and might represent a communication pathway between endodontic and periodontal pathologies through the induction of inflammatory responses.
- Primary endodontic lesions might resemble a furcation class III periodontal defect, when the fistulous sinus tract drains through the periodontal ligament in the inter-radicular space of multi-rooted teeth.
- Pulp sensitivity tests and periodontal probing are essential for the differential diagnosis of endodontic and periodontal diseases.
- When combined endodontic and periodontal lesions merge, root canal therapy should be carried out a few months before any further surgical periodontal treatment, in order to evaluate the part of the defect originating from the endodontic disease.
- The vitality of the pulp seems to hinder bacteria migration from the periodontal pocket to the endodontium.
- Except for root resective therapy, non-surgical, surgical, and regenerative periodontal therapies for furcation lesions do not benefit from any preventive root canal treatment.

References

Abbott, P.V. (2011). Diagnosis and management planning for root-filled teeth with persisting or new apical pathosis. *Endodontic Topics* 19, 1–21.

Abbott, P.V., and Salgado, J.C. (2009). Strategies for the endodontic management of concurrent endodontic and periodontal diseases. *Australian Dental Journal* 54, 70–85.

Abou-Rass, M. (1982). The stressed pulp condition: An endodontic-restorative diagnostic concept. *Journal of Prosthetic Dentistry* 48, 264–267.

Addy, M., Mostafa, P., and Newcombe, R.G. (1987). Dentine hypersensitivity: The distribution of recession, sensitivity and plaque. *British Dental Journal* 162, 253–256.

Adriaens, P.A., De Boever, J.A., and Loesche, W.J. (1987). Bacterial invasion in root cementum and radicular dentin of periodontally diseased teeth in humans: A reservoir of periodontopathic bacteria. *Journal of Periodontology* 59, 222–230.

Adriaens, P.A., Edwards, C.A., De Boever, J.A., and Loesche, W.J. (1988). Ultrastructural observations on bacterial invasion in cementum and radicular dentin of periodontally diseased human teeth. *Journal of Periodontology* 59, 493–503.

Aguiar, T.R., Tristao, G.C., Mandarino, D. et al. (2014). Histopathologic changes in dental pulp of teeth with chronic periodontitis. *Compendium of Continuing Education in Dentistry* 35, 344–351.

Ahmad, I.A. (2009). Rubber dam usage for endodontic treatment: A review. *International Endodontic Journal* 42, 963–972.

AIE Accademia Italiana di Endodonzia (2014). Patologia da carico e sovraccarico dentale. In: *Elementi di anatomia, fisiologia e patologia del complesso pulpo-dentinale: La diagnosi* (ed. F. Fonzar and M. Venturi), 139. Padova: Piccin Nuova Libraria.

Aleo, J,J., De Renzis, F.A., Farber, P.A., and Varboncoeur, A.P. (1974), The presence and biologic activity of cementum-bound endotoxin. *Journal of Periodontology* 45, 672–675.

Alghaithy, R.A., and Qualtrough, A.J. (2017). Pulp sensibility and vitality tests for diagnosing pulpal health in permanent teeth: A critical review. *International Endodontic Journal* 50, 135–142.

American Association of Endodontists (2015). *Glossary of Endodontic Terms*, 9th edn. Chicago, IL: American Association of Endodontists.

Andreasen, F.M., and Andersson, L. (2007). *Textbook and Color Atlas of Traumatic Injuries to the Teeth*, 4th edn. Oxford: Blackwell.

Bartold, P.M. (2006). Dentinal hypersensitivity: A review. *Australian Dental Journal* 51, 212–218.

Bastos, J.V., Goulart, E.M., and de Souza Côrtes, M.I. (2014). Pulpal response to sensibility tests after traumatic dental injuries in permanent teeth. *Dental Traumatology* 30, 188–192.

Bender, I.B., and Seltzer, S. (1972). The effect of periodontal disease on the pulp. *Oral Surgery, Oral Medicine, Oral Pathology* 33, 458–474.

Bergenholtz, G. (1981). Inflammatory response of the dental pulp to bacterial irritation. *Journal of Endodontics* 7, 100–104.

Bergenholtz, G., and Hasselgreen, G. (2008). Endodontics and periodontics. In: *Clinical Periodontology and Implant Dentistry*, 5th edn (ed. J. Lindhe, N.P. Lang, and T. Karring), 848–874. Oxford: Blackwell Munksgaard.

Bergenholtz, G., and Lindhe, J. (1978). Effect of experimentally induced marginal periodontitis and periodontal scaling on the dental pulp. *Journal of Clinical Periodontology* 5, 59–73.

Bergenholtz, G., and Ricucci, D. (2008). Lesions of endodontic origin. In: *Clinical Periodontology and Implant Dentistry*, 5th edn (ed. J. Lindhe, N.P. Lang, and T. Karring), 518–519. Oxford: Blackwell Munksgaard.

Berner, E.S., and Graber, M.L. (2008). Overconfidence as a cause of diagnostic error in medicine. *American Journal of Medicine* 121, 2–23.

Biancu, S., Ericsson, I., and Lindhe, J. (1995). Periodontal ligament tissue reactions to trauma and gingival inflammation: An experimental study in the beagle dog. *Journal of Clinical Periodontology* 22, 772–779.

Boyko, G.A., Brunette, D.M., and Melcher, A.H. (1980). Cell attachment to demineralized root surfaces in vitro. *Journal of Periodontal Research* 15, 297–303.

Burch, J.G., and Hulen, S. (1974). A study of the presence of accessory foramina and the topography of molar furcations. *Oral Surgery, Oral Medicine, Oral Pathology* 38, 451–455.

Cameron, C.E. (1964). Cracked-tooth syndrome. *Journal of the American Dental Association* 68, 405–411.

Carnevale, G., Pontoriero, R., and Lindhe, J. (2008). Treatment of furcation-involved teeth. In: *Clinical Periodontology and Implant Dentistry*, 5th edn (ed. J. Lindhe, N.P. Lang, and T. Karring), 349–374. Oxford: Blackwell Munksgaard.

Chan, C.P., Lin, C.P., Tseng, S.C., and Jeng, J.H. (1999). Vertical root fracture in endodontically versus non endodontically treated teeth: A survey of 315 cases in Chinese patients. *Oral Surgery, Oral Medicine, Oral Pathology, Oral Radiology, Endodontics* 87, 504–507.

Chen, E., and Abbott, P.V. (2009). Dental pulp testing: A review. *International Journal of Dentistry* 2009, 1–12.

Chen, S.Y., Wang, H.L., and Glickman, G.N. (1997). The influence of endodontic treatment upon periodontal wound healing. *Journal of Clinical Periodontology* 24, 449–456.

Cheron, R.A., Marshall, S.J., Goodis, H.E., and Peters, O.A. (2011). Nanomechanical properties of endodontically treated teeth. *Journal of Endodontics* 37, 1562–1565.

Cortellini, P., and Tonetti, M.S. (2001). Evaluation of the effect of tooth vitality on regenerative outcomes in infrabony defects. *Journal of Clinical Periodontology* 28, 672–679.

Cotton, W.R., and Siegel, R.L. (1977). Pulp response to citric acid cavity cleanser. *US Navy Medicine* 68, 27–29.

Czarnecki, R.T., and Schilder, H. (1979). A histological evaluation of the human pulp in teeth with varying degrees of periodontal disease. *Journal of Endodontics* 5, 242–253.

Daly, C.G., Seymour, G.J., Kieser, J.B., and Corbet, E.F. (1982). Histological assessment of periodontally involved cementum. *Journal of Clinical Periodontology* 9, 266–274.

De Deus, Q.D. (1975). Frequency, location, and direction of the lateral, secondary, and accessory canals. *Journal of Endodontics* 1, 361–366.

D'Souza, J.E., Walton, R.E., and Peterson, L.C. (1987). Periodontal ligament injection: An evaluation of the extent of anaesthesia and postinjection discomfort. *Journal of the American Dental Association* 114, 341–344.

Eli, I. (1993). Dental anxiety: A cause for possible misdiagnosis of tooth vitality. *International Endodontic Journal* 26, 251–253.

European Society of Endodontology (2006). Quality guidelines for endodontic treatment:

Consensus report of the European Society of Endodontology. *International Endodontic Journal* 39, 921–930.

Faria, A.C., Rodrigues, R.C., de Almeida Antunes, R.P. et al. (2011). Endodontically treated teeth: Characteristics and considerations to restore them. *Journal of Prosthodontic Research* 55, 69–74.

Filipowicz, F., Umstott, P., and England, M. (1984). Vital root resection in maxillary molar teeth: A longitudinal study. *Journal of Endodontics* 10, 264–268.

Garg, J., Maurya, R., Gupta, A. et al. (2015). An in vitro scanning electron microscope study to evaluate the efficacy of various root conditioning agents. *Journal of Indian Society of Periodontology* 19, 520–524.

Gargiulo, A.V., Jr (1984). Endodontic-periodontic interrelationships: Diagnosis and treatment. *Dental Clinics of North America* 28, 767–781.

Ghazali, F.B. (2003). Permeability of dentine. *Malaysian Journal of Medical Sciences* 10, 27–36.

Gillam, D.G., and Orchardson, R. (2006). Advances in the treatment of root dentine sensitivity: Mechanisms and treatment principles. *Endodontic Topics* 13, 13–33.

Giuliana, G., Ammatuna, P., Pizzo, G. et al. (1997). Occurrence of invading bacteria in radicular dentin of periodontally diseased teeth: Microbiological findings. *Journal of Clinical Periodontology* 24, 478–485.

Gkranias, N.D., Graziani, F., Sculean, A., and Donos, N. (2012). Wound healing following regenerative procedures in furcation degree III defects: Histomorphometric outcomes. *Clinical Oral Investigation* 16, 239–249.

Goldberg, F., Massone, E.J., Soares, I., and Bittencourt, A.Z. (1987). Accessory orifices: Anatomical relationship between the pulp chamber floor and the furcation. *Journal of Endodontics* 13, 176–181.

Gopikrishna, V., Tinagupta, K., and Kandaswamy, D. (2007). Comparison of electrical, thermal, and pulse oximetry methods for assessing pulp vitality in recently traumatized teeth. *Journal of Endodontics* 33, 531–535.

Gorni, F.G., Andreano, A., Ambrogi, F. et al. (2016). Patient and clinical characteristics associated with primary healing of iatrogenic perforations after root canal treatment: Results of a long-term Italian study. *Journal of Endodontics* 42, 211–215.

Guldener, P.H. (1985). The relationship between periodontal and pulpal disease. *International Endodontic Journal* 18, 41–54.

Gutmann, J.L. (1978). Prevalence, location, and patency of accessory canals in the furcation region of permanent molars. *Journal of Periodontology* 49, 21–26.

Haapasalo, M., Parhar, M., Huang, X. et al. (2015). Clinical use of bioceramic materials. *Endodontic Topics* 32, 97–117.

Hahn, C.L., and Overton, B. (1997). The effects of immunoglobulins on the convective permeability of human dentine in vitro. *Archives of Oral Biology* 42, 835–843.

Harrington, G.W., and Steiner, D.R. (2002). Periodontal-endodontic considerations. In: *Principles and Practice of Endodontics*, 3rd edn (ed. R.E. Walton and M. Torabinejad), 466–484. Philadelphia, PA: W.B. Saunders.

Harrington, G.W., Steiner, D.R., and Ammons, W.F. (2002). The periodontal-endodontic controversy. *Periodontology 2000* 30, 123–130.

Hattler, A.B., and Listgarten, M.A. (1984). Pulpal response to root planing in a rat model. *Journal of Endodontics* 10, 471–476.

Hoffman, I.D., and Gold, W. (1971). Distances between plaque and remnants of attached periodontal tissues on extracted teeth. *Journal of Periodontology* 42, 29–30.

Huang, T.J., Schilder, H., and Nathanson, D. (1992). Effects of moisture content and endodontic treatment on some mechanical properties of human dentin. *Journal of Endodontics* 18, 209–215.

Jafarzadeh, H., and Abbott, P.V. (2010). Review of pulp sensibility tests. Part II: Electric pulp tests and test cavities. *International Endodontic Journal* 43, 945–958.

Jameson, L.M., and Malone, W.F. (1982). Crown contours and gingival response. *Journal of Prosthetic Dentistry* 47, 620–624.

Kerns, D.G., and Glickman G.N. (2011). Endodontic and periodontal interrelationships. In: *Cohen's Pathways of the Pulp*, 10th edn (ed. K.M. Hargraves and S. Cohen), 655–670. St Louis, MO: Elsevier.

Kirkham, D.B. (1975). The location and incidence of accessory pulpal canals in periodontal pockets. *Journal of the American Dental Association* 91, 353–356.

Kobayashi, T., Hayashi, A., Yoshikawa, R. et al. (1990). The microbial flora from root canals and periodontal pockets of non-vital teeth associated with advanced periodontitis. *International Endodontic Journal* 23, 100–106.

Kurihara, H., Kobayashi, Y., Francisco, I.A. et al. (1995). A microbiological and immunological study of endodontic-periodontic lesions. *Journal of Endodontics* 21, 617–621.

Lambrianidis, T., Tziafas, D., and Kolokuris, I. (1988). Pulpal response to topical application of citric acid to root dentin. *Endodontics and Dental Traumatology* 4, 12–15.

Langeland, K., Rodrigues, H., and Dowden, W. (1974). Periodontal disease, bacteria, and pulpal histopathology. *Oral Surgery, Oral Medicine, Oral Pathology* 37, 257–270.

Lantelme, R.L., Handelman, S.L., and Herbison, R.J. (1976). Dentin formation in periodontally diseased teeth. *Journal of Dental Research* 55, 48–51.

Lasho, D.J., O'Leary, T.J., and Kafrawy, A.H. (1983). A scanning electron microscope study of the effects of various agents on instrumented periodontally involved root surfaces. *Journal of Periodontology* 54, 210–220.

Levin, L.G. (2013). Pulp and periradicular testing. *Journal of Endodontics* 39, 13–19.

Lewinstein, I., and Grajower, R. (1981). Root dentin hardness of endodontically treated teeth. *Journal of Endodontics* 7, 421–422.

Liewehr, F.R. (2001). An inexpensive device for transillumination. *Journal of Endodontics* 27, 130–131.

Lin, P.Y., Huang, S.H., Chang, H.J., and Chi, L.Y. (2014). The effect of rubber dam usage on the survival rate of teeth receiving initial root canal treatment: A nationwide population-based study. *Journal of Endodontics* 40, 1733–1737.

Lindhe, J., Nyman S., and Ericsson I. (2008). Trauma from occlusion: Periodontal tissues. In: *Clinical Periodontology and Implant Dentistry*, 5th edn (ed. J. Lindhe, N.P. Lang, and T. Karring), 349–374. Oxford: Blackwell Munksgaard.

Löe H., Theilade, E., and Jensen, S.B. (1965). Experimental gingivitis in man. *Journal of Periodontology* 36, 177–187.

Love, R.M., and Jenkinson, H.F. (2002). Invasion of dentinal tubules by oral bacteria. *Critical Reviews in Oral Biology and Medicine* 13, 171–183.

Lowman, J.V., Burke, R.S., and Pelleu, G.B. (1973). Patent accessory canals: Incidence in molar furcation region. *Oral Surgery, Oral Medicine, Oral Pathology* 36, 580–584.

Lubisich, E.B., Hilton, T.J., and Ferracane, J. (2010). Cracked teeth: A review of the literature. *Journal of Esthetic and Restorative Dentistry* 22, 158–167.

Marin, C., Carnevale, G., Di Febo, G., and Fuzzi, M. (1989). Restoration of endodontically treated teeth with interradicular lesions before root removal and/or root separation. *International Journal of Periodontics and Restorative Dentistry* 9, 42–57.

Marroquin, B.B., El-Sayed, M.A., and Willershausen-Zönnchen, B. (2004). Morphology of the physiological foramen: I. *Maxillary and mandibular molars. Journal of Endodontics* 30, 321–328.

Mazur, B., and Massler, M. (1964). Influence of periodontal disease on the dental pulp. *Oral Surgery, Oral Medicine, Oral Pathology* 17, 592–603.

McInnes-Ledoux, P., Cleaton-Jones, P.E., and Austin, J.C. (1985). The pulpal response to dilute citric acid smear removers. *Journal of Oral Rehabilitation* 12, 215–228.

Mejàre, I.A., Axelsson, S., Davidson, T. et al. (2012). Diagnosis of the condition of the dental pulp: A systematic review. *International Endodontic Journal* 45, 597–613.

Mjör, I.A., Smith, M.R., Ferrari, M., and Mannocci, F. (2001). The structure of dentin in the apical region of human teeth. *International Endodontic Journal* 34, 346–353.

Mohammadi, Z., Palazzi, F., Giardino, L., and Shalavi, S. (2013). Microbial biofilms in endodontic infections: An update review. *Biomedical Journal* 36, 59–70.

Molven, O., Halse, A., Fristad, I., and MacDonald-Jankowski, D. (2002). Periapical changes following root-canal treatment observed 20–27 years postoperatively. *International Endodontic Journal* 35, 784–790.

Myers, J.W. (1998). Demonstration of a possible source of error with an electric pulp tester. *Journal of Endodontics* 24, 199–200.

Nagaoka, S., Miyazaki, Y., Liu, H.J. et al. (1995). Bacterial invasion into dentinal tubules of human vital and nonvital teeth. *Journal of Endodontics* 21, 70–73.

Ng, Y.L., Mann, V., Rahbaran, S. et al. (2007). Outcome of primary root canal treatment: Systematic review of the literature. Part 1: Effects of study characteristics on probability of success. *International Endodontic Journal* 40, 921–939.

Nibali, L., Pometti, D., Chen, T.T., and Tu, Y.K. (2015). Minimally invasive non-surgical approach for the treatment of periodontal intrabony defects: A retrospective analysis. *Journal of Clinical Periodontology* 42, 853–859.

Nilvéus, R., and Selvig, K.A. (1983). Pulpal reactions to the application of citric acid to root-planed dentin in beagles. *Journal of Periodontal Research* 18, 420–428.

Page, R.C. (1999). Milestones in periodontal research and the remaining critical issues. *Journal of Periodontal Research* 34, 331–339.

Parirokh, M., and Torabinejad, M. (2010). Mineral trioxide aggregate: A comprehensive literature review. Part III: Clinical applications, drawbacks, and mechanism of action. *Journal of Endodontics* 36, 400–413.

Parolia, A., Gait, T.C., Porto, I.C.C.M., and Mala, K. (2013). Endo-perio lesion: A dilemma from 19th until 21st century. *Journal of Interdisciplinary Dentistry* 3, 2–11.

Pashley, D.H. (1990). Mechanisms of dentin sensitivity. *Dental Clinics of North America* 34, 449–473.

Pashley, D.H., Matthews, W.G., Zhang Y., and Johnson, M. (1996). Fluid shifts across human dentine in vitro in response to hydrodynamic stimuli. *Archives of Oral Biology* 41, 1065–1072.

Pashley, D.H., Pashley, E.I., Carvalho, R.M., and Tay, F.R. (2002). The effects of dentin permeability on restorative dentistry. *Dental Clinics of North America* 46, 211–245.

Patel, S., Ricucci, D., Durak, C., and Tay, F. (2010). Internal root resorption: A review. *Journal of Endodontics* 36, 1107–1121.

Paul, B.F., and Hutter, J.W. (1997). The endodontic-periodontal continuum revisited: New insights into aetiology, diagnosis and treatment. *Journal of the American Dental Association* 128, 1541–1548.

Peters, D.D., Baumgartner, J.C., and Lorton, L. (1994). Adult pulpal diagnosis. I: Evaluation of the positive and negative responses to cold and electrical pulp tests. *Journal of Endodontics* 20, 506–511.

Petersson, K., Söderström, C., Kiani-Anaraki, M., and Lévy, G. (1999). Evaluation of the ability of thermal and electrical tests to register pulp vitality. *Endodontics and Dental Traumatology* 15, 127–131.

Pinheiro, E.T., Gomes, B.P., Ferraz, C.C. et al. (2003). Microorganisms from canals of root-filled teeth with periapical lesions. *International Endodontic Journal* 36, 1–11.

Pitaru, S., and Melcher, A.H. (1987). Organization of an oriented fiber system in vitro by human gingival fibroblasts attached to dental tissue: Relationship between cells and mineralized and demineralized tissue. *Journal of Periodontal Research* 22, 6–13.

Polson, A.M., Frederick, G.T., Ladenheim, S., and Hanes, P.J. (1984). The production of a root surface smear layer by instrumentation and its removal by citric acid. *Journal of Periodontology* 55, 443–446.

Rapp, R., Matthews, G., Simpson, M., and Pashley, D.H. (1992). In vitro permeability of furcation dentin in permanent teeth. *Journal of Endodontics* 18, 444–447.

Rathod, S.R., Fande P., and Sarda, T.S. (2014). The effect of chronic periodontitis on dental pulp: A clinical and histopathological study. *Journal of the International Clinical Dental Research Organization* 6, 107–111.

Rôças, I.N., Siqueira, J.F., Jr, and Santos, K.R. (2004). Association of *Enterococcus faecalis* with different forms of periradicular diseases. *Journal of Endodontics* 30, 315–320.

Ross, I.F., and Thompson, R.H. (1978). A long term study of root retention in the treatment of maxillary molars with furcation involvement. *Journal of Periodontology* 49, 238–244.

Rotstein, I., and Simon, J.H.S. (2004). Diagnosis, prognosis and decision-making in the treatment of combined periodontal-endodontic lesions. *Periodontology 2000* 34, 165–203.

Rowe, A.H., and Pitt Ford, T.R. (1990). The assessment of pulpal vitality. *International Endodontic Journal* 23, 77–83.

Rubach, W.C., and Mitchell, D.F. (1965). Periodontal disease, age, and pulp status. *Oral Surgery, Oral Medicine, Oral Pathology* 19, 482–493.

Ryan, P.C., Newcomb, G.M., Seymour, G.J., and Powell, R.N. (1984). The pulpal response to citric acid in cats. *Journal of Clinical Periodontology* 11, 633–643.

Sakamoto, M., Siqueira, J.F., Jr, Rôças, I.N., and Benno, Y. (2008). Molecular analysis of the root canal microbiota associated with endodontic treatment failures. *Oral Microbiology and Immunology* 23, 275–281.

Schmidt, J.C., Walter, C., Amato, M., and Weiger, R. (2014). Treatment of periodontal-endodontic lesions: A systematic review. *Journal of Clinical Periodontology* 41, 779–790.

Séguier, S., Godeau, G., and Brousse, N. (2000). Collagen fibers and inflammatory cells in healthy and diseased human gingival tissues: A comparative and quantitative study by immunohistochemistry and automated image analysis. *Journal of Periodontology* 71, 1079–1085.

Seltzer, S., Bender, I.B., and Ziontz, M. (1963). The interrelationship of pulp and periodontal disease. *Oral Surgery, Oral Medicine, Oral Pathology* 16, 1474–1490.

Shenoy, N., and Shenoy, A. (2010). Endo-perio lesions: Diagnosis and clinical considerations. *Indian Journal of Dental Research* 21, 579–585.

Sheykhrezaee, M.S., Eshghyar, N., Khoshkhounejad, A.A., and Khoshkhounejad, M. (2007). Evaluation of histopathologic changes of dental pulp in advanced periodontal diseases. *Acta Medica Iranica* 45, 51–57.

Simon, J.H., Glick, D.H., and Frank, A.L. (1972). The relationship of endodontic-periodontic lesions. *Journal of Periodontology* 43, 202–208.

Simring, M., and Goldberg, M. (1964). The pulpal pocket approach: Retrograde periodontitis. *Journal of Periodontology* 35, 22–48.

Smukler, H., and Tagger, M. (1976). Vital root amputation: A clinical and histological study. *Journal of Periodontology* 47, 324–330.

Sugaya, T., Nakatsuka, M., Inoue, K. et al. (2015). Comparison of fracture sites and post lengths in longitudinal root fractures. *Journal of Endodontics* 41, 159–163.

Sundqvist, G. (1994). Taxonomy, ecology, and pathogenicity of the root canal flora. *Oral Surgery, Oral Medicine, Oral Pathology* 78, 522–530.

Sundqvist, G., Figdor, D., Persson, S., and Sjögren, U. (1998). Microbiologic analysis of teeth with failed endodontic treatment and the outcome of conservative re-treatment. *Oral Surgery, Oral Medicine, Oral Pathology, Oral Radiology, Endodontics* 85, 86–93.

Sunitha, V.R., Emmadi, P., Namasivayam, A. et al. (2008). The periodontal-endodontic continuum: A review. *Journal of Conservative Dentistry* 11, 54–62.

Tomasi, C., and Wennström, J.L. (2009). Full-mouth treatment vs. the conventional staged approach for periodontal infection control. *Periodontology 2000* 51, 45–62.

Torabinejad, M., and Kiger, R.D. (1985). A histologic evaluation of dental pulp tissue of a patient with periodontal disease. *Oral Surgery, Oral Medicine, Oral Pathology* 59, 198–200.

Toto, P.D., and Gargiulo, A.W. (1970). Epithelial and connective tissue changes in periodontitis. *Journal of Periodontology* 41, 587–590.

Tronstad, L. (1988). Root resorption: Aetiology, terminology and clinical manifestations. *Endodontics and Dental Traumatology* 4, 241–252.

Trope, M. (1998). Subattachment inflammatory root resorption: Treatment strategies. *Practical Periodontics and Aesthetic Dentistry* 10, 1005–1010.

Trope, M., Tronstad, L., Rosenberg, E.S., and Listgarten, M. (1988). Darkfield microscopy as a diagnostic aid in differentiating exudates from endodontic and periodontal abscesses. *Journal of Endodontics* 14, 35–38.

Tsesis, I., Rosenberg, E., Faivishevsky, V. et al. (2010). Prevalence and associated periodontal status of teeth with root perforation: A retrospective study of 2,002 patients' medical records. *Journal of Endodontics* 36, 797–800.

Vertucci, F.J. (2005). Root canal morphology and its relationship to endodontic procedures. *Endodontic Topics* 10, 3–29.

von Troil, B., Needleman, I., and Sanz, M. (2002). A systematic review of the prevalence of root sensitivity following periodontal therapy. *Journal of Clinical Periodontology* 29, 173–177.

Vongsavan, N., and Matthews, B. (1991). The permeability of cat dentine in vivo and in vitro. *Archives of Oral Biology* 36, 641–646.

Vongsavan, N., and Matthews, B. (1992). Fluid flow through cat dentine in vivo. *Archives of Oral Biology* 37, 175–185.

Walton, R.E., and Torabinejad, M. (2002). Diagnosis and treatment planning. In:

Principles and Practice of Endodontics, 3rd edn (ed. R.E. Walton and M. Torabinejad), 49–70. Philadelphia, PA: W.B. Saunders.

Weldon, J.K., Jr, Pashley, D.H., Loushine, R.J. et al. (2002). Sealing ability of mineral trioxide aggregate and super-EBA when used as furcation repair materials: A longitudinal study. *Journal of Endodontics* 28, 467–470.

Wennström, J.L., Tomasi, C., Bertelle, A., and Dellasega, E. (2005). Full-mouth ultrasonic debridement versus quadrant scaling and root planing as an initial approach in the treatment of chronic periodontitis. *Journal of Clinical Periodontology* 32, 851–859.

Yoshiyama, M., Masada, J., Uchida, A., and Ishida, H. (1989). Scanning electron microscopic characterization of sensitive vs. insensitive human radicular dentin. *Journal of Dental Research* 68, 1498–1502.

Yoshiyama, M., Noiri, Y., Ozaki, K. et al. (1990). Transmission electron microscopic characterization of hypersensitive human radicular dentin. *Journal of Dental Research* 69, 1293–1297.

Zehnder, M. (2001). Endodontic infection caused by localized aggressive periodontitis: A case report and bacteriologic evaluation. *Oral Surgery, Oral Medicine, Oral Pathology, Oral Radiology, Endodontics* 92, 440–445.

Zehnder, M., Gold, S.I., and Hasselgren, G. (2002). Pathologic interactions in pulpal and periodontal tissues. *Journal of Clinical Periodontology* 29, 663–671.

Zitzmann, N.U., Krastl, G., Hecker, H. et al. (2009). Endodontics or implants? A review of decisive criteria and guidelines for single tooth restorations and full arch reconstructions. *International Endodontic Journal* 42, 757–774.

Zuza, E.P., Carrareto, A.L., Lia, R.C. et al. (2012). Histopathological features of dental pulp in teeth with different levels of chronic periodontitis severity. *International Scholarly Research Notices Dentistry* 2012, 1–6.

Chapter 5

Why do We Really Care About Furcations? Long-term Tooth Loss Data

Luigi Nibali

Centre for Immunobiology and Regenerative Medicine, Centre for Oral Clinical Research, Institute of Dentistry, Barts and the London School of Medicine and Dentistry, Queen Mary University of London (QMUL), London, UK

5.1   Introduction

Chapter 1 highlighted how the anatomy of multi-rooted teeth favours microbial accumulation, leading to periodontal breakdown inside the root separation area. Furthermore, we have now learned (see Chapter 3) that plaque removal inside the furcation area is a rather daunting and difficult task, both for the clinician and for patients themselves. It is therefore natural to assume that teeth affected by furcation involvement (FI), being more exposed to the microbial challenge, will develop periodontal progression more rapidly and will have a higher risk of tooth loss. This chapter reviews the evidence for this and aims to provide long-term data on tooth loss in teeth with FI. This answers the question 'Why do really we care about furcations?' and perhaps provides the rationale for the whole book, justifying the interest in furcations as a therapeutic challenge for periodontists, general dentists, and hygienists.

5.2   Measures of Disease Progression

The reader of this book will be well aware that periodontitis causes inflammatory resorption of the attachment apparatus of the tooth, which results in gingival bleeding, discomfort, and eventually tooth mobility and exfoliation. This is also potentially associated with onset of systemic diseases like diabetes mellitus, rheumatoid arthritis, and cardiovascular disease (EFP 2014). Therefore, the 'effects' or end-points of periodontitis could be measured as tooth loss, decreased patient quality of life (QOL), and perhaps systemic effects of the periodontal inflammatory reaction. It is logical to assume that these would be the outcomes measured by any study assessing the impact of periodontitis. However, reality tells us that, since periodontitis is a chronic disease that usually occurs over a long time span, most periodontal studies focus on other, shorter-term measures of disease as main outcomes, such as probing pocket depth (PPD), clinical attachment levels (CAL), and bleeding on probing (BOP). This is done with the understanding that these are surrogate markers of the really relevant outcomes just described.

Recent systematic reviews on furcations followed this approach and focused on short-term outcomes after regenerative surgery (Graziani et al. 2015; Reddy et al. 2015; see Chapters 6 and 7). This clearly represents a limitation as, although an association exists between these clinical parameters and disease progression and tooth loss (Claffey and Egelberg 1995; Chambrone et al. 2010), it is a far from ideal approach. On the other end, the outcome 'tooth loss' is severely influenced by the treating clinician, and by their treatment philosophy and inclination to be more or less conservative. With this in mind, in the view of this author studies on FI should ideally measure 'tooth loss', QOL measures, and measures of systemic burden of periodontitis as outcomes. In reality, what emerges from the periodontal literature is that only the outcome 'tooth loss' has been assessed by a large enough number of studies to allow for making conclusions on how it can be influenced by FI.

5.3 Tooth Loss

Although natural tooth exfoliation can still occur in the general population, it is assumed that 'tooth loss' usually occurs as tooth extraction performed by a dentist, at least in industrialized countries. Severe periodontitis is estimated to be the sixth most prevalent chronic disease in humans (Kassebaum et al. 2014) and it is considered one of the main causes of tooth loss (Hull et al. 1997; Al-Shammari et al. 2005; Akhter et al. 2008). Periodontal treatment classically consists of oral hygiene instructions, supra- and subgingival tooth debridement (with or without adjunctive therapy such as antimicrobials), followed by a re-evaluation. At this stage,

cases deemed to have reached stability will enter a phase named 'maintenance care' or 'supportive periodontal therapy' (SPT) directly or after the provision of surgical therapy, depending on the case (see Figure 5.1).

Provision of regular SPT, consisting of oral hygiene reinforcement and motivation, periodontal charting, and supra- and subgingival debridement, is associated with a reduced risk of tooth loss (Lee et al. 2015). Long-term longitudinal studies in unspecified periodontitis cohorts or chronic periodontitis in SPT reported tooth loss of approximately 0.10 (Hirschfeld and Wasserman 1978), 0.13 (McGuire and Nunn 1996), 0.15 (Eickholz et al. 2008), 0.18 (McFall 1982), and up to 0.30 teeth per patient per year (Tsami et al. 2009). A systematic review of studies including periodontal maintenance care following comprehensive periodontal treatment showed that in the studies included, 3919 teeth from a total of 41 404 were lost during the maintenance period. From 36 to 88.5% of patients did not experience tooth loss during the follow-up period in the different studies. The percentages of tooth loss due to periodontal reasons varied from 1.5 to 9.8%. Patient-related factors (i.e. age and smoking) and tooth-related factors (tooth type and location, and the initial tooth prognosis) were associated with tooth loss (Chambrone et al. 2010). In a more recent systematic review, Trombelli and co-workers

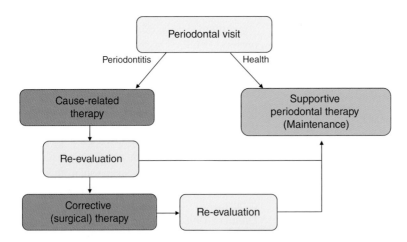

Figure 5.1 The different steps of periodontal therapy.

observed a weighted mean yearly tooth loss rate during SPT of 0.15 and 0.09 teeth/patient/year for follow-up of 5 years and 12–14 years, respectively (Trombelli et al. 2015). Another systematic review in aggressive periodontitis (AgP) cases, including 16 longitudinal studies, revealed that the average tooth loss for all AgP cases was 0.09 teeth/patient/year (95% confidence interval [CI] = 0.06–0.16), therefore in line with chronic periodontitis (CP) studies (Nibali et al. 2013).

But what is the relative contribution of FI to the tooth loss outcome? The following paragraphs will review the evidence from the periodontal literature for tooth loss in molars with FI.

5.4 Tooth Loss for Untreated Furcation-involved Teeth

Although it seems almost obvious from what has been discussed so far that molars with FI have a greater risk of being extracted compared with molars with no FI, very few studies have systematically assessed this question and the magnitude of such a risk, especially in untreated populations. Bjorn and Hjort (1982) published the results of a longitudinal study on a sample of 221 staff members of a Swedish industrial company, originally examined in 1965 and then re-examined in 1978. These subjects were not receiving a specific treatment protocol. Radiographic mandibular molar inter-radicular bone destruction was used for furcation diagnosis, in the absence of clinical data. Only 1.1–2.7% of the molars had bone loss affecting more than 50% of the distance vertex to apex, and bone loss in furcation increased from 18 to 32% in the 13-year follow-up period. During this time, 9% of furcated molars were lost, but only 2.5% were estimated to have been lost due to progressive FI. Although these percentages are relatively low, we should highlight that this was a general population (not specifically subjects selected for having periodontitis) and it is not clear what

treatment if any they received during the follow-up period.

Similarly, data were recently published on a total of 3267 molars of 1897 subjects participating in the 11-year follow-up of the Study of Health in Pomerania (SHIP; Nibali et al. 2017). All subjects had half-mouth periodontal examinations, including FI measurements with a straight probe in one upper and one lower molar at baseline. Only 28% of subjects reported having had some form of unspecified 'gum treatment' throughout the course of the observational period. In total, 375 subjects (19.8%) lost molars during the follow-up period. Respectively 5.6%, 12.7%, 34.0%, and 55.6% of molars without FI, degree I FI, degree II FI, and degree III FI were lost. As well as initial PPD and CAL and diagnosis of periodontitis ($p < 0.001$), FI was associated with molar loss in the 11-year follow-up. The calculated incidence rate ratios (IRR) for molar loss were 1.73 (95% CI = 1.34–2.23, $p < 0.001$) for degree I FI and 3.88 (95% CI = 2.94–5.11, $p < 0.001$) for degree II–III, compared with without FI at baseline. These results were confirmed in subanalysis of the 72% of subjects who had no periodontal treatment during the course of the study (who could more genuinely be considered 'untreated'; Nibali et al. 2017).

5.5 Tooth Loss for Treated Furcation-involved Teeth

Fu and Wang summarized in Table 3.1 some longitudinal studies reporting tooth loss by FI by research groups in the USA and Europe. The classic study by Hirschfeld and Wasserman (1978) was perhaps the first large published study assessing long-term tooth prognosis in patients with periodontitis. Following up 600 patients during SPT for at least 15 years retrospectively (average 22 years), the authors observed that 300 patients had lost no teeth from periodontal disease, 199 had lost 1–3 teeth, 76 had lost 4–9 teeth, and 25 had lost 10–23 teeth. These figures helped identify three different groups of patients based on progression pattern: 'well-maintained' (the great majority), 'down-hill', and 'extreme downhill'. Of 1464 teeth which originally had FI, 460 were lost after the average 22 years follow-up, 240 of them by one-sixth of the patients who deteriorated the most.

A systematic review on long-term tooth loss related to FI revealed that the survival rate of molars treated non-surgically was more than 90% after 5–9 years, with different breakdowns according to treatment protocols and varying degrees of disease severity (Huynh-Ba et al. 2009). Although no meta-analysis could be produced, the authors concluded that initial FI (degree I) could be successfully managed by non-surgical mechanical debridement, and that vertical root fractures and endodontic failures were the most frequent complications observed following resective procedures of molars with FI.

A more recent systematic review tried to answer the focused question: 'What is the risk of tooth loss in teeth with furcation involvement and which factors affect the outcome?' (Nibali et al. 2016). Longitudinal human studies in patients with CP presenting data on furcation diagnosis and tooth loss were considered eligible. In order to be included, studies had to have 'secure' furcation diagnosis (clinical with Nabers probe or equivalent), treatment of FI provided, a follow-up of at least three years, and had to report tooth loss data by furcation diagnosis. The literature search was conducted at Ovid Medline, Embase, LILACS, and Cochrane Library and complemented by a hand search. Studies were selected in two-stage screening carried out by two independent reviewers. Following an initial screening of 1207 articles, full-text review resulted in 21 articles which met the defined inclusion criteria.

Table 5.1 reports the characteristics of the sample included in the reviewed studies, which had been carried out in the USA (n = 11), Germany (n = 6), Sweden (n = 2), Switzerland (n = 1), and Italy (n = 1) across five decades from the 1970s to the 2010s, and the interventions of these studies (divided into active and supportive periodontal therapy). Five of the included papers focused on specific treatment for a specific group of furcation-involved teeth (Haney et al. 1997; Yukna and Yukna 1997; Eickholz and Hausmann 2002; Little et al. 1995; Zafiropoulos et al. 2009), while fourteen papers assessed long-term tooth loss in cohorts of periodontitis patients during maintenance care and were suitable for meta-analysis. SPT protocols (when specified) generally included periodic (3- to 6- to 12-monthly) periodontal clinical measurements, oral hygiene instructions, and subgingival debridement and a range of different periodontal surgeries if considered necessary. The risk of bias analyses performed using the Newcastle Ottawa scale showed that study quality scores ranged from a total of 3 to a total of 5 (out of a maximum total of 9 stars). The asymmetrical results of funnel plots of meta-analysis of relative risk for tooth loss based on follow-up periods revealed potential publication bias (see Nibali et al. 2016).

Data on tooth loss by furcation diagnosis was obtained, when possible with a breakdown on first, second, and third molars. Although studies focusing only on AgP had been excluded, some of the included studies incorporated a small subset of AgP cases (Dannewitz et al. 2006; Pretzl et al. 2008; Salvi et al. 2014; Graetz et al. 2015) and only in one of these papers was it possible to obtain separate data on CP from the authors (Dannewitz et al. 2006). Only data on tooth loss following initial therapy (during maintenance care) were analysed.

5.5.1 Tooth Loss for FI vs No FI

Grouping studies reporting data on tooth loss for molars with and without FI, a total of 8143 molars without FI and a total of 5772 molars with FI were included. Tooth survival ranged from 94 to 100% after 4–7.5 years in regeneration studies (Haney et al. 1997; Yukna and

Table 5.1 Summary of study procedures for all included studies.

Author/Year	Sample no.	Follow-up years (range)	Inclusion/disease classification	Active periodontal therapy (APT)	Supportive periodontal therapy (SPT)
Lindhe and Nyman 1975	75	5	≥50% loss of periodontal support and optimal oral hygiene	OHI, SRP, restorative therapy if needed, periodontal surgery in PPDs >4 mm (gingivectomy, Widman flaps, bone recontouring, furcation plasty, tunnelling, root resection as indicated)	3–6 monthly OHI and prophylaxis by hygienist, yearly periodontal examinations and radiographs
Hirschfeld and Wasserman 1978	600	22 (15–53)	'Early': PPD of 4 mm or less, with gingival inflammation and subgingival calculus; 'intermediate': PPD of 4–7 mm; 'advanced': PPD >7 mm, furcation involvement	Subgingival scaling with or without surgery (additional surgical procedure or non-surgical procedure performed depending on tooth diagnosis)	Deep scaling + 'problem areas' retreated when necessary, occlusion checked and adjusted as indicated, OHI
McFall 1982	100	19 (15–29)	'Early': PPD ≤4 mm (n = 11); 'intermediate': PPD 4–7 mm (n = 53); 'advanced' PPD >7 mm (n = 36)	Supragingival and subgingival scaling, polishing, OHI, occlusal adjustment and biteguards if needed, gingival curettage, gingivectomy, gingivoplasty, ostectomy, osteoplasty	Generally every 3–4 to 6 months (including curettage, muco-periosteal flaps, osseous surgery, root resection if needed)
Goldman et al. 1986	211	22.2 (15–34)	CP	Oral physiotherapy, supragingival and subgingival scaling, OHI	3–6-month recalls (selective grinding and coronal reshaping, adjunct restorative treatment if needed)
Wood et al. 1989	63	13.6 (10–34)	Patients with moderate periodontitis treated and maintained by SRP for 10 years or longer	OHI, non-surgical (SRP, curettage, occlusal adjustment) and surgical treatment (gingivectomy, flap surgery, flap curettage, osseous contouring, osseous grafting, root amputation)	Not reported
Kuhrau et al. 1990	59	5.8 (4–8)	Patients with periodontitis with furcation-involved teeth treated surgically	Surgical therapy (modified Widman flap, root resection, tunnelling)	'Regular'
Wang et al. 1994	24	8	Patients with CP who had completed an 8-year clinical trial and had no more than 2 first or second molars missing at baseline	SRP followed by one of three procedures: pocket elimination surgery, modified Widman flap surgery, or gingival curettage	3-month recall interval for maintenance prophylaxis and yearly examinations

(*Continued*)

Table 5.1 (Continued)

Author/Year	Sample no.	Follow-up years (range)	Inclusion/disease classification	Active periodontal therapy (APT)	Supportive periodontal therapy (SPT)
Little et al. 1995	18	4.6	Patient with periodontal disease with deep class II or III molar furcation invasion	Surgical therapy consisting of osseous resectioning and/or recontouring to the adjacent mesial tooth and tunnelling	3-monthly following surgery to control plaque and potential bacterial pathogens
McGuire and Nunn 1996	100	10	Chronic generalized moderate to severe adult periodontitis	SRP, OHI, removal of fremitus, surgery if indicated (osseous surgery, open SRP, rarely bone grafts)	2- or 3-month intervals (majority under a 3-month interval) – SRP, polishing, minor occlusal adjustments
Haney et al. 1997	13	4–5	CP	Coronally advanced flap procedures and citric acid root treatment with or without adjunctive implantation of freeze-dried. demineralized, allogeneic bone	6-monthly for 5 years
Yukna and Yukna 1997	13	6.7 (6–7.5)	Grade II molar furcation defects, with adjacent bone crest height >75% of the root length and coronal to the furcation bone level	Regenerative surgery with bone grafts and coronally advanced flaps	Weekly, then monthly deplaquing until surgical re-entry at 6–12 months, then 3-month recalls
McLeod et al. 1998	114	12.5 (5–29)	Moderate to advanced periodontitis with 4–7 mm or greater AL	Non-surgical therapy (OHI, SRP, occlusal adjustment, occasional use of systemic AB) followed by surgical treatment (pocket reduction, pocket elimination, occasional regeneration)	6-monthly
Eickholz and Hausmann 2002	9	5	Advanced periodontal disease	Guided tissue regeneration	3-monthly for the first 2 years (OHI and professional tooth cleaning), then 3–6-monthly according to individual risk
Checchi et al. 2002	92	6.7 (3–12)	Chronic adult periodontitis who completed APT and have been on a recall SPT schedule	OHI, SRP, re-evaluation, and periodontal surgery	3–4-monthly hygienist appointment recall

Dannewitz et al. 2006	71	5	CP or AgP (≥50% bone loss in at least 2 permanent teeth)	OHI, professional tooth cleaning, SRP, surgical intervention included access flap surgery, GTR, tunnelling, resective procedures, or tooth extraction	3–6- or 12-monthly (clinical measurements, plaque score, and if needed re-instrumentation of PPD ≥4 mm and BOP, or ≥5 mm)
Pretzl. et al. 2008	100	10	Generalized moderate CP and generalized severe or aggressive periodontitis	Subgingival debridement under local anaesthesia and periodontal surgery if required	Patients with and without SPT (3–6-monthly including OHI, professional tooth cleaning, polishing, application of a fluoride gel)
Zafiropoulos et al. 2009	60	Min. 4	CP with a minimum of 4 sites with CAL loss <4 mm, radiographic evidence of bone loss, and BOP in 4 sites	56 mandibular first and second molars treated by hemisection (Group H, n = 32); 36 implants in the mandible to replace periodontally involved first and second molars (Group I, n = 28).	6-monthly (OHI, supra- and subgingival debridement, polishing)
Johansson et al. 2013	64	14.8 (13–16)	Patients referred to the Department of Periodontology	OH, supra- and subgingival scaling, selective periodontal surgeries (occasionally regenerative)	3–4-monthly for 2 years by dental hygienists (then referred back to general dentist/hygienist for supportive care)
Miller et al. 2014	106	15	Moderate to severe CP	Non-surgical and surgical periodontal treatment	Lasted for as long as the patient continued to be seen (periodontal health and oral hygiene assessment, retreatment and surgery when necessary)
Salvi et al. 2014	199	11.5	CP or AgP (Level 1: proximal AL ≥3 mm at ≥2 non-adjacent teeth; level 2: proximal AL ≥5 mm in ≥30% of teeth)	OHI, SRP, surgery if needed (OFD, regeneration, tunnelling, or resective surgery)	SPT at Department of Periodontology or private practice according to needs (some 'non-compliers')
Graetz et al. 2015	379	18.3	Chronic or aggressive periodontitis with at least one first or second molar present, regular SPT, and complete radiological documentation at baseline and last visit	SRP, OFD in case of PPD ≥5 mm with BOP, or PPD ≥6 mm (tunnelling or root resection when needed)	3–12-monthly (non-surgical or surgical subgingival debridement with or without AB)

AB = antibiotic; AgP = aggressive periodontitis); AL = attachment loss: APT = active periodontal treatment; BOP = bleeding on probing; CP = chronic periodontitis; OFD = Open flap debridement; OHI = oral hygiene instructions; PPD = probing pocket depth; SPT = supportive periodontal therapy; SRP = scaling and root planing.
Source: Adapted from Nibali et al. (2016).

Yukna 1997; Eickholz and Hausmann 2002), 89% after 5.8 years in a tunnelling study (Little et al. 1995), 79% after a minimum of 4 years in a root resection study (Zafiropoulos et al. 2009), and 43–100% after 5–53 years for studies including combined therapies (Hirschfeld and Wasserman 1978; McFall 1982; Goldman et al. 1986; Wood et al. 1989; Kuhrau et al. 1990; Wang et al. 1994; McGuire and Nunn 1996; Checchi et al. 2002; Dannewitz et al. 2006; Pretzl et al. 2008; Johansson et al. 2013; Miller et al. 2014; Salvi et al. 2014; Graetz et al. 2015). Among teeth reported in these studies, the average tooth loss/patient/year was 0.01 and 0.02 for molars without and with FI, respectively. Periodontal progression, endodontic complications, caries, and fractures were reported as main causes of tooth loss (Kuhrau et al. 1990; McLeod et al. 1998; Haney et al. 1997; Yukna and Yukna 1997; Dannewitz et al. 2006).

In studies reporting data for only first and second molars (Hirschfeld and Wasserman 1978; McFall 1982; Goldman et al. 1986; Wood et al. 1989; Dannewitz et al. 2006; Pretzl et al. 2008; Johansson et al. 2013; Miller et al. 2014; Graetz et al. 2015), the following relative risks (RR) of tooth loss were detected (see Figure 5.2):

- RR = 2.90 (95% CI = 2.01–4.18) for molars with FI vs no FI ($p < 0.0001$; various lengths of follow-up).
- RR = 1.46 (95% CI = 0.99–2.15, $p = 0.06$) for molars with FI vs no FI ($p < 0.0001$; 5–10 years follow-up).

	With FI		No FI			Risk Ratio	
Study or Subgroup	Events	Total	Events	Total	Weight	IV. Random, 95% CI	Year
5–10 years							
Dannewitz et al. 2006	23	240	5	111	6.9%	2.13 [0.83, 5.45]	2006
Pretzl et al. 2008	51	390	30	309	11.0%	1.35 [0.88, 2.06]	2008
Subtotal (95% CI)		**630**		**420**	**17.9%**	**1.67 [1.14, 2.43]**	
Total events	74		35				
Heterogeneity: $Tau^2 = 0.00$; $Chi^2 = 0.75$, df = 1 (P = 0.39); $I^2 = 0\%$							
Test for overall effect: Z = 1.90 (P = 0.06)							
10–15 years							
Wood et al. 1989	35	151	27	215	10.7%	1.86 [1.17, 2.91]	1989
Johansson et al. 2013	30	94	37	267	11.1%	2.18 [1.44, 3.31]	2013
Miller et al. 2014	127	419	50	397	11.9%	2.41 [1.79, 3.24]	2014
Subtotal (95% CI)		**664**		**879**	**33.7%**	**2.21 [1.79, 2.74]**	
Total events	192		116				
Heterogeneity: $Tau^2 = 0.00$; $Chi^2 = 0.92$, df = 2 (P = 0.63); $I^2 = 0\%$							
Test for overall effect: Z = 7.30 (P < 0.0001)							
>15 years							
Hirchfeld & Wasserman 1978	384	1285	124	2250	12.5%	5.42 [4.48, 6.56]	1978
McFall 1982	82	147	25	492	11.1%	10.98 [7.30, 16.51]	1982
Goldman et al. 1986	235	562	110	835	12.4%	3.17 [2.60, 3.88]	1986
Graetz et al. 2015	315	1183	118	1022	12.4%	2.31 [1.90, 2.80]	2015
Subtotal (95% CI)		**3177**		**4599**	**38.4%**	**4.46 [2.62, 7.62]**	
Total events	192		116				
Heterogeneity: $Tau^2 = 0.28$; $Chi^2 = 67.73$, df = 3 (P = 0.00001); $I^2 = 96\%$							
Test for overall effect: Z = 5.49 (P < 0.0001)							
Total (95% CI)		**4471**		**5898**	**100.0%**	**2.90 [2.01, 4.18]**	
Total events	1282		528				
Heterogeneity: $Tau^2 = 0.27$; $Chi^2 = 104.40$, df = 8 (P < 0.00001); $I^2 = 92\%$							
Test for overall effect: Z = 5.72 (P < 0.0001)							

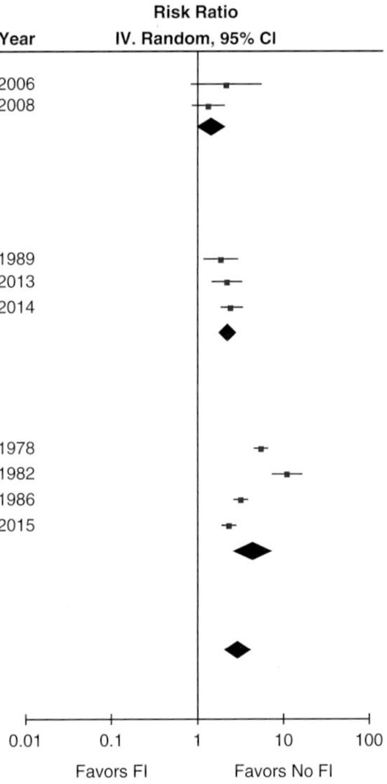

Figure 5.2 Forest plot presenting relative risk (RR) of tooth loss based on follow-up periods (excluding third molars). Meta-analysis for the comparison of tooth loss among selected studies presented an overall odds ratio of 2.90 (95% confidence interval [CI] = 2.01–4.18, $p < 0.0001$). For studies with a follow-up period of 5–10 years, 10–15 years, and > 15 years, the RR of tooth loss between teeth with and without furcation involvement was 1.46 (95% CI = 0.99–2.15, $p = 0.06$), 2.21 (95% CI = 1.79–2.74, $p < 0.0001$), and 4.46 (95% CI = 2.62–7.62, $p < 0.0001$), respectively. *Source*: Nibali et al. (2016).

- RR = 2.21 (95% CI = 1.79–2.74, p < 0.0001) for molars with FI vs no FI (p < 0.0001; 10–15 years follow-up).
- RR = 4.46 (95% CI = 2.62–7.62, p < 0.0001) for molars with FI vs no FI (p < 0.0001; > 15 years follow-up).

Only the comparison for studies over more than 15 years had a high degree of heterogeneity (p value for chi-square test < 0.0001 and I^2 test = 96%), hence it needs to be interpreted cautiously. When third molars were included, only small changes to the summary estimate for risk of tooth loss by FI were detected (see Nibali et al. 2016 for details).

5.5.2 Tooth loss by Different Furcation Degree

An important question with clinical relevance is whether the degree of FI affects the risk of tooth loss. We previously (Section 5.4) discussed an increased risk of tooth loss by increased degree of FI in a largely untreated population participating in the SHIP in Pomerania (Nibali et al. 2017). When studies included in Nibali et al.'s (2016) systematic review of treated patients reporting tooth loss by degree of FI were considered (McGuire and Nunn 1996; Dannewitz et al. 2006; Johansson et al. 2013; Salvi et al. 2014, Graetz et al. 2015), 8%, 18%, and 30% of the total of teeth with furcation degrees I, II, and III, respectively, were lost in the follow-up period (0.01, 0.02, and 0.03 teeth/patient/year). Meta-analysis for tooth loss among the included studies (see Figure 5.3) presented a relative risk of tooth loss of:

- RR = 1.67 (95% CI = 1.14–2.43, p = 0.008) for FI degree II vs I.
- RR = 1.83 (95% CI = 1.37–2.45, p < 0.0001) for FI degree III vs II.
- RR = 3.13 (95% CI = 2.30–4.24, p < 0.0001) for FI degree III vs I.

The comparisons presented a low to moderate degree of heterogeneity among the selected studies (p value for chi-square test = 0.04, 0.20, and 0.26, and I^2 test = 61%, 33%, and 25%, for degree II vs I, III vs II, and III vs I comparisons, respectively).

5.5.3 Tooth Loss by Vertical Furcation Component

The previous discussion points to the fact that the great majority of long-term follow-up studies of molars with FI have focused on the horizontal component, as measured by the Hamp classification (Hamp et al. 1975). Chapter 2 also introduced the concept of 'vertical' FI and its relative subclassification into A, B, and C (Tarnow and Fletcher 1984), which could be associated with the measure of horizontal involvement. A recent paper hypothesized that different levels of vertical FI may have a bearing on the risk of tooth loss of horizontal degree II FI (Tonetti et al. 2017). The authors retrospectively assessed 200 molars followed up for 10 years of supportive therapy after conservative periodontal surgery with limited osseous surgery. Vertical furcation subclassification was established according to a modification of the classification proposed by Tarnow and Fletcher (1984) using bone loss observed in a periapical radiograph and clinical probing depths/CAL. A gradually higher incidence of tooth loss was observed for degree II FI with bone loss up to the apical third, middle third, or coronal third of the root (respectively 77%, 33%, and 9% tooth loss at 10 years). The authors advocated that the vertical component might be an important predictor of tooth loss in molars with degree II horizontal FI. They also suggested that vertical involvement of the apical third is often associated with the presence of an intrabony defect within the furcation defect. Treating such intrabony defects may reduce the level of vertical FI, thus potentially reducing the future risk of molar loss (Tonetti et al. 2017).

5.6 Conclusions on Risk of Tooth Loss by Furcation Involvement

Based on the review presented here (Nibali et al. 2016), FI approximately doubles the risk of tooth loss for molars in supportive periodontal therapy for up to 10–15 years. In

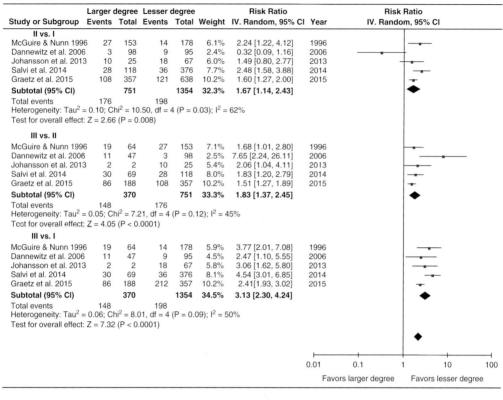

Figure 5.3 Forest plot presenting relative risk (RR) of tooth loss based on degrees of furcation involvement (excluding third molars). Meta-analysis for the comparison of tooth loss among selected studies presented an RR of 1.67 (95% confidence interval [CI] = 1.14–2.43, p = 0.008), 1.83 (95% CI = 1.37–2.45, p < 0.0001), and 3.13 (95% CI = 2.30–4.24, p < 0.0001) when comparing degree II to I, degree III to II, and degree III to I furcation involvement, respectively. *Source*: Nibali et al. (2016).

particular, first and second molars with FI had an RR of tooth loss of 1.46 (p = 0.06) up to 10 years and of 2.21 from 10 to 15 years (p < 0.0001), compared with molars with no FI (RR 1.69 and 2.06, respectively, including third molars). Studies up to 15 years of follow-up had consistent results and reported similar relative risk for tooth loss. This may be attributable to the similar designs of these studies, consisting of initial periodontal therapy, surgical therapy when needed (including access flaps, osseous resective surgery, root resection, tunnelling, or occasionally regenerative surgery), and then supportive periodontal therapy (at regular intervals for most studies, generally every 3, 4, 6, or up to 12 months). A three to four times higher risk of tooth loss was observed for studies with longer follow-ups (>15 years, up to 53 years), although data relative to this outcome have to be interpreted cautiously due to high heterogeneity. A similar

and perhaps higher risk of tooth loss could be attributed to molars with furcation not undergoing regular periodontal treatment (Nibali et al. 2017). Furthermore, there is enough evidence that the degree of FI (Hamp et al. 1975) is significantly associated with risk of tooth loss during supportive periodontal therapy, increasing from furcation degree I to II to III (Nibali et al. 2016, 2017). The vertical furcation subclassification and potential intrabony defects associated with one or multiple roots within the furcation may also affect the long-term tooth loss risk (Tonetti et al. 2017).

Based on the available evidence, it is worth mentioning that it is not possible to discriminate the relative contribution of FI and PPD on molar loss. In other words, we cannot be certain that the higher risk of tooth loss in molars with FI is due to them having FI rather than to them having a deep pocket. The relative contribution of FI to

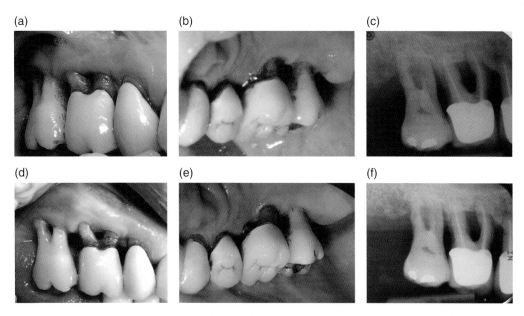

Figure 5.4 (a, b) Clinical photographs of 55-year-old male patient affected by chronic periodontitis; (c) periapical radiographs of upper right molars showing triple degree III furcation involvement on UR6 and 7; (d, e) clinical photographs taken 10 years after tunnelling surgery; (f) Periapical photographs at 10-year follow-up.

molar loss could be tested by assessing risk of tooth loss prospectively in molars with similar pocket depth differing only by FI (for example, a 6 mm vertical PPD in a buccal surface of a lower molar with no FI vs a 6 mm vertical PPD of a lower molar with degree II FI). However, we are not aware of any studies testing this hypothesis. An indirect comparison of the risk of tooth loss attributable only to residual PPD is difficult, as limited data are available and merely on single-rooted teeth, since most studies present short-term disease progression data only (Badersten et al. 1984) or tooth loss data for all teeth combined (Matuliene et al. 2008).

In conclusion, in patients undergoing comprehensive periodontal treatment (cause-related, surgical therapy if needed, and SPT),

most molars affected by FI respond well to periodontal treatment, judging by the fact that even in the presence of degree III FI, only 30% of molars were lost with up to 15 years of follow-up (see Figure 5.4).

The risk of tooth loss (for FI vs non-FI molars) is in the region of 1.5–2.2 up to 15 years in maintenance. Such risk seems to increase sharply after the 15-year time point, although study heterogeneity does not allow clear conclusions on this. Similarly, an increased risk of tooth loss by FI exists for cases not undergoing periodontal maintenance. Among the relevant long-term outcomes introduced in Section 5.2, we are not aware of any studies specifically assessing the effect of FI on the systemic inflammatory burden, while patient-reported outcomes are covered in Chapter 13.

Summary of Evidence

- Periodontal treatment and maintenance care lead to low tooth loss rates of molars with furcation involvement (FI).
- The tooth loss of molars with FI is approximately double that of molars without FI up to 15 years of follow-up.
- Degree of horizontal FI affects risk of tooth loss (increasing from degree I to II to III).
- Degree of vertical FI may also affect the risk of tooth loss (increasing from subclassification A to B to C).

References

Akhter, R., Hassan, N.M., Aida, J. et al. (2008). Risk indicators for tooth loss due to caries and periodontal disease in recipients of free dental treatment in an adult population in Bangladesh. *Oral Health & Preventive Dentistry* 6, 199–207.

Al-Shammari, K.F., Al-Khabbaz, A.K., Al-Ansari, J.M. et al. (2005). Risk indicators for tooth loss due to periodontal disease. *Journal of Periodontology* 76, 1910–1918.

Badersten, A., Nilveus, R., and Egelberg, J. (1984). Effect of nonsurgical periodontal therapy. *II. Severely advanced periodontitis. Journal of Clinical Periodontology* 11, 63–76.

Bjorn, A.L., and Hjort, P. (1982). Bone loss of furcated mandibular molars: A longitudinal study. *Journal of Clinical Periodontology* 9, 402–408.

Chambrone, L., Chambrone, D., Lima, L.A., and Chambrone, L.A. (2010). Predictors of tooth loss during long-term periodontal maintenance: A systematic review of observational studies. *Journal of Clinical Periodontology* 37, 675–684.

Checchi, L., Montevecchi, M., Gatto, M.R., and Trombelli, L. (2002). Retrospective study of tooth loss in 92 treated periodontal patients. *Journal of Clinical Periodontology* 29, 651–656.

Claffey, N., and Egelberg, J. (1995). Clinical indicators of probing attachment loss following initial periodontal treatment in advanced periodontitis patients. *Journal of Clinical Periodontology* 22, 690–696.

Dannewitz, B., Krieger, J.K., Husing, J., and Eickholz, P. (2006). Loss of molars in periodontally treated patients: A retrospective analysis five years or more after active periodontal treatment. *Journal of Clinical Periodontology* 33, 53–61.

Eickholz, P., and Hausmann, E. (2002). Evidence for healing of periodontal defects 5 years after conventional and regenerative therapy: Digital subtraction and bone level measurements. *Journal of Clinical Periodontology* 29, 922–928.

Eickholz, P., Kaltschmitt, J., Berbig, J. et al. (2008). Tooth loss after active periodontal therapy. 1: Patient-related factors for risk, prognosis, and quality of outcome. *Journal of Clinical Periodontology* 35, 165–174.

EFP European Federation of Periodontology (2004). EFP Manifesto: Perio and General Health. http://www.efp.org/efp-manifesto/index.html (accessed 6 February 2018).

Goldman, M.J., Ross, I.F., and Goteiner, D. (1986). Effect of periodontal therapy on patients maintained for 15 years or longer: A retrospective study. *Journal of Periodontology* 57, 347–353.

Graetz, C., Schutzhold, S., Plaumann, A. et al. (2015). Prognostic factors for the loss of molars: An 18-years retrospective cohort study. *Journal of Clinical Periodontology* 42, 943–950.

Graziani, F., Gennai, S., Karapetsa, D. et al. (2015). Clinical performance of access flap in the treatment of class II furcation defects: A systematic review and meta-analysis of randomized clinical trials. *Journal of Clinical Periodontology* 42, 169–181.

Hamp, S.E., Nyman, S., and Lindhe, J. (1975). Periodontal treatment of multirooted teeth: Results after 5 years. *Journal of Clinical Periodontology* 2, 126–135.

Haney, J.M., Leknes, K.N., and Wikesjo, U.M. (1997). Recurrence of mandibular molar furcation defects following citric acid root treatment and coronally advanced flap procedures. *International Journal of Periodontics and Restorative Dentistry* 17, 528–535.

Hirschfeld, L., and Wasserman, B. (1978). A long-term survey of tooth loss in 600 treated periodontal patients. *Journal of Periodontology* 49, 225–237.

Hull, P.S., Worthington, H.V., Clerehugh, V. et al. (1997). The reasons for tooth extractions in adults and their validation. *Journal of Dentistry* 25, 233–237.

Huynh-Ba, G., Kuonen, P., Hofer, D. et al. (2009). The effect of periodontal therapy on the survival rate and incidence of complications of multirooted teeth with furcation involvement after an observation period of at least 5 years: A systematic review. *Journal of Clinical Periodontology* 36, 164–176.

Johansson, K.J., Johansson, C.S., and Ravald, N. (2013). The prevalence and alterations of furcation involvements 13 to 16 years after periodontal treatment. *Swedish Dental Journal* 37, 87–95.

Kassebaum, N.J., Bernabe, E., Dahiya, M. et al. (2014). Global burden of severe periodontitis in 1990–2010: A systematic review and meta-regression. *Journal of Dental Research* 93, 1045–1053.

Kuhrau, N., Kocher, T., and Plagmann, H.C. (1990). [Periodontal treatment of furcally involved teeth: With or without root resection?] *Deutsche Zahnarztliche Zeitschrift* 45, 455–457.

Lee, C.T., Huang, H.Y., Sun, T.C., and Karimbux, N. (2015). Impact of patient compliance on tooth loss during supportive periodontal therapy: A systematic review and meta-analysis. *Dental Research* 94, 777–786.

Lindhe, J., and Nyman, S. (1975). The effect of plaque control and surgical pocket elimination on the establishment and maintnance of periodontal health: A longitudinal study of periodontal therapy in cases of advanced disease. *Journal of Clinical Periodontology* 2, 67–79.

Little, L.A., Beck, F.M., Bagci, B., and Horton, J.E. (1995). Lack of furcal bone loss following the tunnelling procedure. *Journal of Clinical Periodontology* 22, 637–641.

Matuliene, G., Pjetursson, B.E., Salvi, G.E. et al. (2008). Influence of residual pockets on progression of periodontitis and tooth loss: Results after 11 years of maintenance. *Journal of Clinical Periodontology* 35, 685–695.

McFall, W.T., Jr (1982). Tooth loss in 100 treated patients with periodontal disease: A long-term study. *Journal of Periodotology* 53, 539–549.

McGuire, M.K., and Nunn, M.E. (1996). Prognosis versus actual outcome. *III: The effectiveness of clinical parameters in accurately predicting tooth survival. Journal of Periodontology* 67, 666–674.

McLeod, D.E., Lainson, P.A., and Spivey, J.D. (1998). The predictability of periodontal treatment as measured by tooth loss: A retrospective study. *Quintessence International* 29, 631–635.

Miller, P.D., Jr, McEntire, M.L., Marlow, N.M., and Gellin, R.G. (2014). An evidenced-based scoring index to determine the periodontal prognosis on molars. *Journal of Periodontology* 85, 214–225.

Nibali, L., Farias, B.C., Vajgel, A. et al. (2013). Tooth loss in aggressive periodontitis: A systematic review. *Journal of Dental Research* 92, 868–875.

Nibali, L., Krajewski, A. Donos, N. et al. (2017). The effect of furcation involvement on tooth loss in a population without regular periodontal therapy. *Journal of Clinical Periodontology* 44, 813–821.

Nibali, L., Zavattini, A., Nagata, K. et al. (2016). Tooth loss in molars with and without furcation involvement: A systematic review and meta-analysis. *Journal of Clinical Periodontology* 43, 156–166.

Pretzl, B., Kaltschmitt, J., Kim, T.S. et al. (2008). Tooth loss after active periodontal therapy. 2: Tooth-related factors. *Journal of Clinical Periodontology* 35, 175–182.

Reddy, M.S., Aichelmann-Reidy, M.E., Avila-Ortiz, G. et al. (2015). Periodontal regeneration – furcation defects: A consensus report from the AAP Regeneration Workshop. *Journal of Periodontology* 86, S131–S133.

Salvi, G.E., Mischler, D.C., Schmidlin, K. et al. (2014). Risk factors associated with the longevity of multi-rooted teeth: Long-term outcomes after active and supportive periodontal therapy. *Journal of Clinical Periodontology* 41, 701–707.

Tarnow, D., and Fletcher, P. (1984). Classification of the vertical component of furcation involvement. *Journal of Periodontology* 55, 283–284.

Tonetti, M., Christianes, A., and Cortellini, P. (2017). Vertical sub-classification predicts survival of molars with class II furcation involvement during supportive periodontal care. *Journal of Clinical Periodontology* 44, 1140–1144.

Trombelli, L., Franceschetti, G., and Farina, R. (2015). Effect of professional mechanical plaque removal performed on a long-term, routine basis in the secondary prevention of periodontitis: A systematic review. *Journal of Clinical Periodontology* 42 (Suppl. 16), S221–S236.

Tsami, A., Pepelassi, E., Kodovazenitis, G., and Komboli, M. (2009). Parameters affecting tooth loss during periodontal maintenance in a Greek population. *Journal of the American Dental Association* 140, 1100–1107.

Wang, H.L., Burgett, F.G., Shyr, Y., and Ramfjord, S. (1994). The influence of molar furcation involvement and mobility on future clinical periodontal attachment loss. *Journal of Periodontology* 65, 25–29.

Wood, W.R., Greco, G.W., and McFall, W.T., Jr (1989). Tooth loss in patients with moderate periodontitis after treatment and long-term maintenance care. *Journal of Periodontology* 60, 516–520.

Yukna, R.A., and Yukna, C.N. (1997). Six-year clinical evaluation of HTR synthetic bone grafts in human grade II molar furcations. *Journal of Periodontal Research* 32, 627–633.

Zafiropoulos, G.G., Hoffmann, O., Kasaj, A. et al. (2009). Mandibular molar root resection versus implant therapy: A retrospective nonrandomized study. *Journal of Oral Implantology* 35, 52–62.

Chapter 6

Regenerative Therapy of Furcation Involvements in Preclinical Models: What is Feasible?

Nikolaos Donos[1], Iro Palaska[1], Elena Calciolari[1], Yoshinori Shirakata[2], and Anton Sculean[3]

[1] Centre for Immunobiology and Regenerative Medicine, Centre for Oral Clinical Research, Institute of Dentistry, Barts and the London School of Medicine and Dentistry, Queen Mary University of London (QMUL), London, UK
[2] Department of Periodontology, Kagoshima University Graduate School of Medical and Dental Sciences, Kagoshima, Japan
[3] Department of Periodontology, School of Dental Medicine, University of Bern, Bern, Switzerland

6.1 Introduction

In everyday clinical practice, the presence of furcation involvement constitutes a significant challenge (de Santana et al. 1999; Avila-Ortiz et al. 2015). Regeneration of the furcation defect with *restitution ad integrum* is a highly desirable outcome in these cases. This chapter and the next will review the current evidence on pre-clinical and clinical human studies on the potential to regenerate furcation defects.

The regeneration of furcation involvements following the use of various biological materials, extracellular matrix proteins, growth factors, and cell therapy is a complex biological process involving various tissue components, including epithelium, connective tissue, cementum, and alveolar bone (Ivanovic et al. 2014). Historically, animal models have been used as proof-of-principle models and for providing first-level in vivo evidence in potential translation of different regenerative materials to the clinical setting.

6.2 Available Preclinical Models

Different animal species have been used to evaluate the regeneration of furcation defects, with non-human primates, dogs, rabbits, and pigs being the most commonly employed (Struillou et al. 2010; Kantarci et al. 2015). Variations between species include anatomy, dimensions of teeth and alveolar process, gingival biotype, local physiological environment, animal behaviour, and healing rate (Caton et al. 1994).

Small animals (especially mice and rats) have generated substantial data on the pathogenetic mechanisms of systemic inflammation and their correlation with periodontal disease in transgenic and knockout animal models (Graves et al. 2008). The major drawback of small animals is the limited similarity of their dentition to the human dentition, which limits the possibility of translating the results to the clinical situation. Conversely, the dental anatomy of large animals (mainly non-human primates and dogs) may resemble better the human dento-alveolar architecture. In these animals, it has been suggested that it is feasible to study wound healing/regeneration in periodontal defects of clinically relevant size and configuration (Selvig 1994).

6.2.1 Non-human Primates

Non-human primates have naturally occurring dental plaque, calculus, oral microbial pathogens, and periodontal disease, although this occurs late in life and the lesions tend to be asymmetrical (Schou et al. 1993; Oz and Puleo 2011). Therefore, if osseous lesions are investigated, they are usually experimentally induced. Similar dental anatomy and periodontal wound healing (Caton and Kowalski 1976), suitability of furcation sites (Giannobile et al. 1994), and experimentally induced defects that do not spontaneously regenerate indicated that mature, adult, *Macaca mulatta* and *Macaca fascicularis* species could be used as models for evaluating periodontal regenerative procedures (Schou et al. 1993). However, it should be emphasized that their use is controversial, as this model shares some structural and functional features with humans, thus raising significant ethical concerns. Besides the ethical issues related to the close phylogenetic relationship with humans, primate research also requires expensive facilities, with dedicated and trained personnel and environmental enrichment.

6.2.2 Dog Model

Dogs are among the most widely used experimental animals for studying naturally occurring gingivitis and periodontitis, wound healing, and tissue regeneration (Wikesjö et al. 1994). The Beagle dog (*Canis lupus familiaris*) is commonly used because of its size and its cooperative nature, but several studies have also used mongrel dogs (Struillou et al. 2010). The characteristics of periodontal tissues and the size of teeth in dogs present, to a certain extent, some similarity to those of humans. However, dogs lack lateral jaw movements and premolar occlusal contacts (Kantarci et al. 2015). In dogs, the severity of periodontal disease increases with age and can result in tooth loss (Berglundh et al. 1991). In regenerative periodontal medicine, the dog model has been used for the histological demonstration of guided tissue regeneration (GTR) in various defect types, such as furcations, supracrestal, and infrabony defects (Caffesse et al. 1990). In addition, the dog model has been employed in studies which have led to our current understanding of the limitations of regenerative approaches, including membrane-associated properties (Araujo et al. 1998).

6.2.3 Miniature Pig Model

The miniature pig model has emerged as an alternative to the dog model. Varieties of miniature pig have been extensively used in biomedical research (Polejaeva et al. 2000). These animals have oral and maxillofacial structures similar to those of humans in terms of anatomy, physiology, and disease development (Wang et al. 2007). Natural gingivitis can be observed at 6 months of age. The pattern of disease progression follows the same stages as that in humans: gingival swelling, plaque accumulation, calculus formation, and bleeding on probing (Lang et al. 1998). Histologically, these clinical features are accompanied by inflammatory cell infiltration and vasodilatation. Starting at 16 months of age, miniature pigs may develop advanced periodontitis, with pocket depths up to 5 mm and alveolar bone resorption (Kantarci et al. 2015).

6.3 Defect Types

Four types of experimentally induced furcation defects have been used for testing the effects of different therapeutic modalities in pre-clinical studies. These include defects resulting from naturally occurring periodontitis and three types of experimentally produced defects: the acute defect, the chronic defect, and the combined acute/chronic defect.

6.3.1 Naturally Occurring Periodontitis Defects

Historically, periodontal defects caused by natural periodontal disease have been considered as a necessity in the study of periodontal regeneration (Haney et al. 1995). These defects occur late in the animal's life and the lesions are usually asymmetrical, as they result from a gradual and variable destruction of the periodontium, and include deposition of calculus and endotoxins on the root surface (Haney et al. 1995). In addition, they feature compromised mucogingival dimensions, which is a confounding factor when these models are used to study the biological potential of regeneration under optimized conditions of wound healing (Wikesjö et al. 1994). Taking into account the aforementioned limitations, the rationale for using these types of defects to study periodontal wound healing/regeneration appears to be limited (Caton et al. 1994).

6.3.2 Experimentally Induced Defects

6.3.2.1 The Acute Defect Model

In this model, mucoperiosteal flaps are elevated and the bone, the periodontal ligament, and cementum are surgically removed to create the defect type of the desired shape and dimension. Reference notches are usually created by a round bur on the roots, at the level of the reduced alveolar bone. These notches start on the buccal aspect of the root and extend into the furcation area, and they are used as a reference point for the histological analysis. The major drawback of the acute defect model is that approximately 50–70% of spontaneous regeneration can be expected, thus creating an important source of bias when studying the effect of different surgical techniques and biomaterials on tissue regeneration (Caton et al. 1994; Mardas et al. 2012).

6.3.2.2 The Chronic Defect Model

These defects are created by placing orthodontic elastics or ligatures around the circumference of teeth, or slightly apical to the gingival margin. The elastics/ligatures gradually migrate apically, as plaque-induced inflammation destroys the periodontal ligament and supporting bone in 3–6 months (Caton and Kowalski 1976). Then, the root surfaces are carefully scaled and planed and a notch is placed on the roots, at the base of the defect, as a reference for the histological analysis. The advantage of this model is that spontaneous healing is not observed, but the disadvantages include the considerable time needed for the creation of the defects and the asymmetrical nature of the defects. In addition, conventional root debridement produces root surface conditions similar to those of surgically induced (acute) defects. Taking into account these limitations, the relevance for using this type of defect to study periodontal wound healing/regeneration appears to be limited (Caton et al. 1994).

6.3.2.3 The Acute/Chronic Defect Model

The majority of the available pre-clinical studies use this model to study wound healing/periodontal regeneration in class II or III furcation defects. This defect is developed by surgically removing alveolar bone, periodontal ligament, and cementum in the experimental site. Prior to flap closure, the defect is placed into a chronically inflamed state to reduce spontaneous regeneration by placing a foreign body, such as metal strips, orthodontic wires and bands, impression material, or gutta-percha for 1–3 months (Caton et al. 1994). At surgical re-entry, the foreign bodies are removed, and the lesions are debrided from granulation tissue, plaque biofilm, and calculus. After the root surface is scaled, the tested biomaterial/active principle can eventually be delivered into the defect (Araújo and Lindhe 1997; Takayama et al. 2001; Donos et al. 2003b). The advantages of this model are that defects are produced rapidly, they do not heal spontaneously, and bilateral symmetrical periodontal tissue loss can be predictably induced.

6.3.3 The Critical Size Defect Concept in Furcation Studies

A critical size defect (CSD) is defined as 'the smallest size intra-osseous wound in a particular bone and species that will not heal spontaneously during the lifetime of the animal' (Schmitz and Hollinger 1986). Even if a certain biological variability exists between different animal models, it is of the outmost importance that the experimental bone defect created is of a critical size for the animal model used, thus avoiding the occurrence of spontaneous periodontal regeneration and allowing testing of the true regenerative potential of the biomaterials and surgical techniques investigated. However, because most pre-clinical studies have an evaluation time limit, Gosain et al. (2000) state that the CSD in animal research refers to the size of a defect that will not heal over the duration of the study.

6.3.3.1 Furcation Degree II CSD

In order to test the regenerative potential of different regenerative treatments in class II furcation defects, the majority of studies have used surgically created CSDs measuring 5 mm in height (from the roof of the bifurcation) and 2 mm in depth (Lekovic and Kenney 1993; Hürzeler 1997; Deliberador et al. 2006). After intrasulcular incisions were made from the mesial side of the involved teeth (mainly premolars) to the distal side of the molars, a mucoperiosteal flap was elevated to expose both buccal and lingual alveolar bone plates. The defects were then created by using carbide round burs under abundant saline irrigation. The interproximal bone remained intact. Then, the surfaces were carefully scaled and root planed. Following removal of granulation tissue and complete root instrumentation, reference notches were placed in the roots at the level of the alveolar bone crest, using a number 1/2 round bur. These notches were positioned on the buccal aspects of the roots and extended interproximally and into the furcation areas, as deep as the involvement of the class II furcation permits. After the root surface is scaled, the tested biomaterial/active principle can be delivered into the defect.

6.3.3.2 Furcation Degree III CSD

The first attempts to create defects that would not heal spontaneously were made by the team of Ellegaard et al. (1974), who induced through-and-through bifurcation defects in posterior teeth of Rhesus monkeys by passing a round bur through surgically denuded bifurcations. The size of the openings was approximately 2 mm in diameter. To avoid spontaneous healing, a steel wire of periodontal dressing was placed in the defects for four weeks. This study has shown that following surgical removal of the interradicular septum and the promotion of plaque retention in the monkey's posterior teeth, bifurcation defects may develop into lesions, which after six weeks of healing display features similar to those of interradicular pockets in humans. Six weeks postoperatively the height of the bone in the lesions produced was essentially maintained at the level determined at the time of surgery. The lesions were characterized by chronically inflamed connective tissue covered with epithelium of varying thickness, and they showed no tendency for spontaneous healing.

Based on this concept, Klinge et al. (1981), by using two different animal models (dog model and non-human primate model), examined the influence of different defect sizes and different flap management techniques on the healing potential after reconstructive surgery using citric acid conditioning. Chronic through-and-through defects of different sizes were created.

Specifically, bone was surgically removed from the furcation area and around the circumference of the tooth, including the proximal bone (horizontal defect). Three different levels of bone reduction were studied (2 mm, 3.5 mm, and 5 mm high). In addition, two different positions of the flap were studied (coronally positioned flap and replaced flap). It was demonstrated that new attachment occurred for teeth treated with coronally positioned flaps regardless of the defect size. This implied that variations in the dimension of the defects played a secondary role in the healing potential, and that the adequate post-operative flap coverage of the furcation was the critical step for the successful healing of through-and-through defects.

In a subsequent study by Klinge et al. (1985a), it was shown that healing was accomplished in even larger defects (~9 mm) when a coronal flap placement was used. It is possible that the magnitude of coronal flap positioning is of limited importance, provided a certain amount of coverage of the furcation is accomplished. It was also noticed that one important reason for the failure at larger defects was found to be recession of the flap, which resulted in early exposure of the furcation site (Klinge et al. 1985a). To counteract such soft tissue recession, the authors developed a technique which involved the utilization of 'crown attached' sutures and reported that, provided flap recession was prevented, new attachment occurred at both large and small defects (Klinge et al. 1985a). Similar results were obtained by Lindhe et al. (1995), who showed that comparatively large furcation defects ('key-hole' defects with cross-section dimensions of > 11 mm^2) could be successfully regenerated by GTR therapy provided that the soft-tissue flaps covering the membranes are prevented from receding apical of the furcation fornix during healing, and that the clot in the furcation defect remains non-infected.

The potential for new attachment formation after GTR was examined by Pontoriero et al. (1992) in three differently shaped furcation defects: (i) a small, 2×2 mm key-hole furcation defect, where the removal of the supporting bone and root cementum was confined to the furcation area, thus leaving intact the interdental alveolar bone; (ii) a large key-hole defect about 3 mm in the apico-coronal direction and 4 mm in the mesio-distal direction; and (iii) a large 'horizontal' defect about 5 mm in the apico-coronal direction and about 4 mm in the mesio-distal direction, where the removal of bone and root cementum was performed within the furcation area and extended at the buccal/lingual and interproximal surfaces. It was observed that small key-hole, degree III furcation defects healed following GTR treatment with complete new attachment. At control sites, only minor amounts of new attachment formation occurred. In larger defects, it was observed that GTR therapy failed to generate new attachment to a degree where the furcation defects became closed. It was also observed clinically that at such sites, extensive flap recession occurred following suture removal. The study revealed that the size of the furcation defect and the degree of bone loss adjacent to the defect were determining factors for the outcome of this kind of treatment. Thus, if the furcation defect was associated with circumferential bone loss, or if the defect was more than 3 mm in the apico-coronal direction, complete new attachment failed to occur. Thus, while small key-hole defects – that is, small vertical defects – healed, large key-hole defects and horizontal defects were consistently associated with flap recession and failure. Taking into consideration the CSD concept (smallest bone defect created), the key-hole defect was optimal for testing the regenerative potential of different materials, and the approach based on this study was adopted in clinical studies as well.

The most widely used model in regenerative studies remains the critical size supra-alveolar periodontal defect model, which was developed in beagle dogs by Wikesjö and his team (Wikesjö et al. 1999). Supra-alveolar critical size periodontal defects are produced by the resection of the buccal and lingual/ palatal bone of premolar teeth. Osseous resection can be restricted to the interdental area, which measures approximately 4–5 mm (height) and 3 mm (width; Araújo et al. 1998), or extended to create a horizontal circumferential defect up to 5–6 mm below the fornix of furcation (Giannobile et al. 1998; Wikesjö et al. 2003a, b). In this model, innate regeneration of alveolar bone and cementum does not exceed 25% of the defect height over a three-week healing interval following wound closure or primary intention healing. Extending the healing interval to eight weeks does not result in additional regeneration (Wikesjö et al. 1994, 2003a, b; Koo et al. 2004). This defect is a valuable model to test the regenerative potential of candidate treatments on class III furcation defects, as it allows evaluation of the regenerative potential of experimental treatments under optimal conditions and in a biologically controlled environment. By applying this model, different studies have evaluated root-conditioning protocols, bone grafts and bone substitutes, biological substances, and different barrier membranes (GTR) as stand-alone protocols or in combination (Sanz et al. 2015).

6.4 Regeneration Treatments of Class II Furcation Defects

6.4.1 Guided Tissue Regeneration

The potential to regenerate furcation defects in a predictable manner emerged with the development of the concept of GTR more than 30 years ago (Karring and Warrer 1992; Karring et al. 1993). The use of a barrier membrane prevents both gingival epithelial cells and connective tissue cells from repopulating the root surface during healing, and allows repopulation only by cells from the periodontal ligament or the alveolar bone marrow, thus inducing the formation of new cementum and connective tissue attachment (Nyman et al. 1980; Karring et al. 1980, 1993;

Sander and Karring 1995; Sanz et al. 2015). A variety of biocompatible barriers, non-absorbable (Caffesse at al. 1990, 1994; Danesh-Meyer et al. 1997; Bogle et al. 1997; Lekovic et al. 1998; Macedo et al. 2006) or bioabsorbable (Cirelli et al. 1997; Hürzeler et al. 1997; de Andrade et al. 2007; Wang et al. 2014) has been used for the regeneration of class II furcation defects. From a clinical and histological point of view, similar results can be achieved in GTR, whether bioabsorbable (such as collagen-based) or nonabsorbable (such as polytetrafluoroethylene, ePTFE) membranes are applied (Murphy and Gunsolley 2003). However, the bioabsorbable membranes do not require a second surgery for their retrieval, thus reducing the patient's discomfort and morbidity. The studies applying non-resorbable and resorbable membranes in critical size (5 mm in height × 2 mm in depth), surgically created furcation II defects showed a mean percentage of bone fill and new cementum formation ranging between 60 and 80% (Caffesse at al. 1990, 1994; Cirelli et al. 1997; Danesh-Meyer et al. 1997; Bogle et al. 1997; Hürzeler et al. 1997; Lekovic et al. 1998; Macedo et al. 2006; de Andrade et al. 2007; Wang et al. 2014). The results of these studies are presented in detail in Table 6.1.

6.4.2 Bone Grafts and GTR

The placement of bone grafts or alloplastic materials in furcation defects in association with flap surgery or GTR has been extensively evaluated in animal experiments. The biological rationale behind the use of grafts is the assumption that the material may contain bone-forming cells (osteogenesis) or serve as a scaffold for bone formation (osteoconduction), or that the matrix may contain bone-inductive substances (osteoinduction), which could stimulate both the regrowth of bone and the formation of new attachment (Karring and Cortellini 1999).

Limited studies in naturally occurring defects showed that bone grafts combined with different barrier membranes did not enhance the regeneration process of

Table 6.1 Guided tissue regeneration (GTR) in class II furcation defects.

Study	Model	Tooth	Type of membrane	Healing time (months)	Histomorphometric results
NATURALLY OCCURING PERIODONTITIS					
Bogle et al. 1997	Dog	Mandibular premolars	Control: Open-flap debridement Experimental group: Bioabsorbable polylactic acid–based membrane	6	Cementum formation (%) Control: 71 Test: 17* Bone filling (%) Control: 74 Test: 14*
ACUTE DEFECT MODEL					
Caffesse et al. 1994	Dog	Mandibular premolars	Control: PTFE non-resorbable membrane Test 1: Bioabsorbable type I barrier Test 2: Bioabsorbable type II barrier	6	**Notch to new cementum (mm)** Control: 4.42 ± 1.40 Test 1: 4.42 ± 1.08 Test 2: 5.80 ± 0.68 **Notch to bone crest (mm)** Control: 2.72 ± 1.43 Test 1: 2.95 ± 1.24 Test 2: 4.55 ± 1.05
Danesh-Meyer et al. 1997	Sheep	Mandibular premolars	Control: Open-flap debridement Test 1: PTFE non-resorbable membrane Test 2: PTFE non-resorbable soft-tissue patch	2	**Alveolar bone height (%)** Control: 61.5 ± 7.13 Test 1: $78.4 \pm 6.89*$ Test 2: 71.7 ± 6.73 **Cementum height (%)** Control: 93.0 ± 4.34 Test 1: $98.5 \pm 1.01*$ Test 2: $98.4 \pm 1.03*$
ACUTE/CHRONIC DEFECT MODEL					
Cirelli et al. 1997	Mongrel dogs	Mandibular premolars	Control: Open-flap debridement Test: GTR with anionic collagen membrane	3	**Cementum formation (%)** Control: 59.34 Test: 92.35* **Bone filling (%)** Control: 48.58 Test: 56.33
Macedo et al. 2006	Dog	Mandibular bicuspids	Control: PTFE non-resorbable (Gore-Tex$^+$) removed at 2 weeks Test: PTFE non-resorbable (Gore-Tex$^+$) removed at 4 weeks	3	**New tissue (mm^2)** Control: 12.45 ± 3.54 Test: 14.32 ± 4.01 **Bone height (mm)** Control: 3.56 ± 1.21 Test: 4.03 ± 0.94
de Andrade et al. 2007	Dog	Mandibular premolars	Control: Bioabsorbable membrane (polyglycolic acid) Test: Acellular dermal matrix	3	**New tissue (mm^2)** Control: 8.01 ± 2.69 Test: 7.21 ± 1.33 **Bone height (mm)** Control: 2.56 ± 0.84 Test: 2.86 ± 0.32

(Continued)

Table 6.1 (Continued)

Study	Model	Tooth	Type of membrane	Healing time (months)	Histomorphometric results
Wang et al. 2014	Dog	Mandibular premolars	Control: Open-flap debridement Test 1: Open-flap debridement + LIPUS Test 2: Resorbable bovine collagen membrane (BioGide[†]) Test 3: Resorbable bovine collagen membrane (BioGide[†]) + LIPUS	2	**Micro-CT scanning** **New alveolar bone surface (mm^2)** Control: 82.84 ± 16.67 Test 1: 98.44 ± 18.57 Test 2: 132.11 ± 22.76* Test 3: 150 ± 21.20*
Hürzeler et al. 1997	Monkey	Mandibular molars	Control: Open-flap debridement Test: Synthetic resorbable membrane Resolute[‡] (glycolide/lactic copolymer)	5	**Cementum deposition (mm)** Initial defect size: 5.05 ± 0.45 Control: 0.83 ± 0.19 Test: 2.88 ± 0.63* **Bone formation (mm)** Initial defect size: 2.81 ± 0.65 Control: 1.14 ± 0.35 Test: 2.78 ± 0.53*
CHRONIC DEFECT MODEL					
Caffesse et al. 1990	Dog	Mandibular premolars, molars	Control: Open-flap debridement Test: PTFE non-resorbable membrane (Gore-Tex[+])	3	**Furcation fill (mm^2)** Control: Ep + CT + B = 1.94 Experimental: Ep + CT + B = 3.38 (no statistical analysis)
Lekovic et al. 1998	Dog	Mandibular premolars, molars	Control: Open-flap debridement Test 1: PTFE non-resorbable membrane Test 2: Silicone rubber barrier material Test 3: Polycarbonate filter with pore size of 0.45 barrier material Test 4: Polycarpolactone barrier material	6	**Notch to new cementum (mm)** Control: 0.24 ± 0.007 Test 1: 1.96 ± 0.031* Test 2: 2.16 ± 0.011* Test 3: 2.18 ± 0.015* Test 4: 2.04 ± 0.037* **Notch to bone crest (mm)** Control: 0.32 ± 0.017 Test 1: 1.18 ± 0.019* Test 2: 1.44 ± 0.014* Test 3: 1.32 ± 0.015* Test 4: 1.2 ± 0.010*

*Statistically significant difference from control;
[+]Gore-Tex, W.L. Gore and Assoc., Flagstaff, AZ, USA;
[†]Biogide, Geistlich Biomaterials, Wolhusen, Switzerland;
[‡]Resolute, W.L. Gore and Assoc., Flagstaff, AZ, USA.
CT = computed tomography; LIPUS = low-intensity pulsed ultrasound; PTFE = polytetrafluoroethylene.

furcation class II defects (Caffesse et al. 1993; Lekovic and Kenney 1993). Likewise, in critical size acute defects in the dog model, Deliberador et al. (2006) compared the results of autogenous bone (AB) alone and in combination with a calcium sulphate paste as a barrier to an empty defect (control). At three months, most specimens failed to show complete bone fill of the furcation. New bone formation was moderate and restricted between the notch areas to the mid portion of the defect. The amount of periodontal regeneration in the three groups was approximately 50% of the root length, without differences between the groups. Areas of ankyloses were also present in some sections, but no active root resorption was observed. More recently, Struillou et al. (2011) investigated the regenerative capacity of injectable biphasic calcium phosphate (BCP) in combination with injectable polymer (Si-HPMC) in critical size (5 mm high, 3 mm deep), acute surgically created defects in premolar furcation of beagle dogs. Three months after treatment, a bone in-growth of $23\% \pm 10\%$ and $35.5\% \pm 13.9\%$ was observed in the empty and biomaterial-filled defects, respectively. Although a tendency for higher bone in-growth was observed in the defects filled with the biomaterial, this difference did not reach statistical significance.

Deproteinized bovine bone mineral (DBBM) is an extensively used bone substitute with documented reconstructive potential (Baldini et al. 2011). In a mini-pig animal model, the potential of porous titanium granules (PTGs) and DBBM in the reconstructive treatment of surgically created acute buccal degree II furcation defects was tested. Six weeks after treatment, the histological analysis showed significantly increased vertical bone formation in both the PTG (62.5%) and control (empty; 64.3%) groups compared to the DBBM-treated defects (41.9%, $p < 0.01$), which, on the contrary, had a reduced regenerative response. The micro-computed tomography (CT)

analysis showed significantly more buccal-palatal defect fill in furcation defects treated with PTG (96.8%) compared to the DBBM (62%) and control groups (72.2%, $p < 0.05$; Wohlfart et al. 2012). It should be noted that in this study, degree II furcation defects larger than what was typically used were surgically created (buccal bone was removed to half of the root width) and this might have affected their regenerative potential.

6.4.3 Enamel Matrix Proteins

Biomimetic substances have been tested in experimental studies to assess their regenerative capability in furcation lesions. This group of proteins, which play a key role in root formation during odontogenesis, have demonstrated in both in vitro and in vivo studies a capacity to attract and increase the migration and proliferation of undifferentiated mesenchymal cells, which then form acellular cementum, periodontal ligament, and alveolar bone (Zetterström et al. 1997; Amin et al. 2012, 2013, 2014, 2016). Remarkably, not only did regenerative techniques using enamel matrix derivatives show enhanced hard-tissue formation, they also reported increased gingival tissue thickness using the beagle dog model (Al Hezaimi et al. 2012). As class II furcation defects are non-containing defects, it has been suggested that the use of biological substances may be clinically applied in combination with different bone graft materials, although this combination therapy has not yet been experimentally evaluated to provide histological outcomes (Sculean et al. 2007; Trombelli and Farina 2008). In an experimental study in mongrel dogs, the use of enamel matrix derivative (EMD) alone was associated with better regenerative outcomes in comparison to its combined use with ePTFE membranes in critical size acute/chronic surgically created buccal class II furcation defects. Following eight weeks of healing, the EMD group resulted in 67% new bone formation and 94% new cementum. The combined approach resulted in compromised healing due to membrane exposure (28% new bone, 80% new cementum; Regazzini et al. 2004).

6.4.4 Growth Factors

Growth factors form a class of natural polypeptides that act as biological mediators regulating cell proliferation, chemotaxis, differentiation, and synthesis. These factors also play a major role during tissue regeneration, by binding to specific receptors on the cell surface. Growth and differentiation factor technologies have been evaluated for their potential to enhance periodontal wound healing/regeneration in healthy and systemically compromised conditions (Stavropoulos and Wikesjö 2012; Bizenjima et al. 2015). Such biologically active substances, used either alone or in combination with GTR, have also been tested for their efficacy in improving regeneration outcomes in critical size furcation lesions. In particular, fibroblast growth factor (FGF; Murakami et al. 1999, 2003; Takayama et al. 2001), bone morphogenetic proteins (BMPs; Ripamonti et al. 1996, 2001), transforming growth factor-β (TGF-β; Teares et al. 2008, 2012), insulin growth factor (IGF-1), and platelet-derived growth factor (PDGF; Soares et al. 2005) are the most studied. The results of the application of growth factors in class II furcation defects are presented in Table 6.2.

6.4.5 Cell Therapy

The most common cells applied for regeneration are mesenchymal stem cells (MSCs), as these pluripotent cells can differentiate into a significant number of cell types, including osteoblasts, fibroblasts, and cementoblasts (Risbud and Shapiro 2005). MSCs have been isolated from periodontal ligament (PDL; Seo et al. 2004; Trubiani et al. 2005) and it was demonstrated that, when they are cultured in contact with native PDL cells, MSCs acquire the characteristics of PDL cells, making them suitable for periodontal regeneration purposes (Kramer et al. 2004). Dogan and co-workers retrieved cells from regenerated

periodontal defects in dogs, which were then expanded in culture and transplanted into critical size surgically created class II furcation defects in the same animals. At 42 days post-surgery, a trend towards better bone formation (control 32.9% vs test 51.2%) and less cementum formation (control 71.7% vs test 75.5%) in the test group was reported, but no statistical analysis was performed in the study (Dogan et al. 2002).

The successful use of PDL cells to regenerate class II furcation defects was documented by Suaid and co-workers in a dog model. PDL cells obtained from extracted teeth were cultured in vitro and phenotypically characterized with regard to their biological properties. Acute CSDs were then surgically created and treated with either GTR (control group) or GTR associated to a cell-seeded collagen sponge (test group). Three months after treatment, the histomorphometric analysis showed that the cell-treated group presented a superior length of new cementum (8.08 ± 1.08 mm vs 6.00 ± 1.5), a greater extension of periodontal regeneration (7.28 ± 1.00 mm vs 3.94 ± 1.20, $p < 0.05$), a lower formation of connective tissue/epithelium (0.60 ± 0.99 mm vs 2.15 ± 1.92, $p < 0.05$), a larger area of new bone (9.02 ± 2.30 mm^2 vs 7.01 ± 0.61, $p < 0.05$), and a smaller area of connective tissue/epithelium (4.22 ± 0.95 mm^2 vs 5.90 ± 1.67, $p > 0.05$), compared with the control group (Suaid et al. 2011). More recently, Chantarawaratit et al. (2014) employed primary human PDL cells treated with acemannan, a polysaccharide extracted from aloe vera gel, for the regeneration of critical size acute class II furcation defects in mongrel dogs. It was observed that acemannan significantly increased the percentage of new bone formation at 30 and 60 days post-operatively, as well as the percentage of new cementum formation at 60 days post-operatively (Chantarawaratit et al. 2013).

Simsek et al. (2012) compared the effectiveness of MSCs with platelet-rich plasma (PRP) as a scaffold to PRP alone, autogenous cortical bone (ACB) graft alone, and the combination of ACB with PRP in the treatment of acute/chronic class II furcation defects versus open flap debridement

Table 6.2 Growth factors in class II furcation defects.

Study	Model	Tooth	Type of membrane	Healing time (months)	Histomorhometric results
ACUTE/CHRONIC DEFECT MODEL					
Murakami et al. 1999	Dog	Mandibular premolars, molars	Test 1: Gelatinous carrier (fibrin gel) alone Test 2: b-FGF + carrier	1.5	**New bone formation rate (%)** Test 1: 42.8 ± 10.7 Test 2: 79.6 ± 16.8* **New cementum formation rate (%)** Test 1: 34.3 ± 14.5 Test 2: 75.8 ± 22.7*
Murakami et al. 1999	Non-human primates	Mandibular molars	Test 1: Carrier alone Test 2: b-FGF + carrier	2	**New bone formation rate (%)** Test 1: 54.3 ± 8.0 Test 2: 71.3 ± 13.5* **New cementum formation rate (%)** Test 1: 38.9 ± 9.2 Test 2: 71.2. ± 15.2*
Murakami et al. 2003	Dog	Mandibular molars	Control: Gelatinous carrier (fibrin gel) alone Test 1: 0.1% b-FGF + gelatinous carrier	1.5	**New bone formation rate (%)** Test 1: 35.4 ± 8.9 Test 2: 83.6 ± 14.3* **New cementum formation rate (%)** Test 1: 37.2 ± 15.1 Test 2: 97.7 ± 7.5*
Takayama et al. 2001	Non-human primates	Maxillary, mandibular molars	Control: Open-flap debridement Test 1: Gelatinous carrier Test 2: 0.1% FGF-2 Test 3: 0.4% FGF-2	2	**New bone formation rate (%)** Control: 44.7 ± 6.2 Test 1: 54.3 ± 8.0 Test 2: 58.0 ± 21.9 Test 3: 71.3 ± 13.5* **New cementum formation rate (%)** Control: 46.7 ± 12.1 Test 1: 38.9 ± 9.2 Test 2: 79.1 ± 23.9* Test 3: 72.2 ± 14.4*
Keles et al. 2009	Dog	Mandibular premolars	Control: Open-flap debridement Test 1: Platelet pellet Test 2: Platelet pellet + resorbable membrane of polylactic acid (Atrisorb+)	3	**New cementum (%)** Control: 45.60 ± 11.92 Test 1: 83.99 ± 7.70* Test 2: 81.63 ± 8.17* **New bone (%)** Control: 42.44 ± 6.07 Test 1: 62.64 ± 7.89 Test 2: 61.06 ± 7.90

(Continued)

Table 6.2 (Continued)

Study	Model	Tooth	Type of membrane	Healing time (months)	Histomorhometric results
Suaid et al. 2010	Dog	Mandibular premolars	Control: Synthetic resorbable membrane Resolute† (glycolide/lactic copolymer) + bioactive glass (Perioglas‡) Test: Synthetic resorbable membrane Resolute (glycolide/lactic copolymer) + bioactive glass (Perioglas) + PRP	3	**New bone (mm)** Control:4.33 ± 0.62 Test: 5.01 ± 0.63 **New cementum (mm)** Control: 9.20 ± 3.21 Test: 12.45 ± 1.73*
Teares et al. 2008	Baboon	Mandibular molars	Control: Carrier alone: Basement membrane matrix (Matrigel¶) Test 1: TGF-β3 with carrier Test 2: TGF-β3 with carrier and minced muscle tissue	2	**New cementum (mm)** Control: 3.7 ± 0.7 Test 1: 3.5 ± 0.6 Test 2: 6.1 ± 0.4* **New bone (mm):** Control: 2.3 ± 0.4 Test 1: 2.8 ± 0.8 Test 2: 4.7 ± 0.3*
Teares et al. 2012	Baboon	Mandibular molars	Test 1: Matrigel containing 25 μg of recombinant hOP-1 Test 2: Matrigel containing 75 μg TGF-β3 Test 3: Matrigel with 25 μg hOP-1 and 25 μg TGF-β3 (20:1 ratio) Test 4: Matrigel with 25 μg hOP-1 and 1.25 μg TGF-β3 (20:1 ratio) plus morcellated autogenous muscle	2	**New cementum (mm):** Test 1: 6.18 ± 0.33* Test 2: 3.65 ± 0.88 Test 3: 5.45 ± 0.89* Test 4: 2.69 ± 1.06 **New bone (mm):** Test 1: 5.93 ± 0.92 Test 2: 5.67 ± 1.17 Test 3: 7.07 ± 0.57* Test 4: 4.73 ± 1.08

ACUTE DEFECT MODEL

Study	Model	Tooth	Type of membrane	Healing time (months)	Histomorhometric results
Ripamonti et al. 1996	Baboon	Mandibular molars	Control: Carrier Test 1: Carrier + 0.1 μg/ml hOP-1 Test 2: Carrier + 0.5 μg/ml hOP-1	2	**No bone formation was detected** **New cementum formation (distal root)** Control: 2.6 ± 0.2 Test 1: 6.2 ± 0.5* Test 2: 6.7 ± 0.3*
Ripamonti et al. 2001	Baboon	Mandibular molars	Test 1: BMP$_2$ (100 μg/ml) Test 2: hOP-1 (100 μg/ml) Test 3: hOP-1 + BMP$_2$ (100 μg/ml)	2	**New bone formation** Test 1: 4.2 ± 0.2 Test 2: 3.7 ± 0.4 Test 3: 3.1 ± 0.2 **New cementum formation (distal root)** Test 1: 3.7 ± 0.4 Test 2: 5.7 ± 0.3* Test 3: 3.6 ± 0.2

Table 6.2 (Continued)

Study	Model	Tooth	Type of membrane	Healing time (months)	Histomorhometric results
Soares et al. 2005	Dog	Mandibular molars	Control: No graft Test: Reparative tissue of extraction socket enhanced with PDGF-BB + IGF	45 days	**New cementum** Control: 2.49 ± 0.82 Test: 2.48 ± 0.47 **New bone** Control: 2.73 ± 0.42 Test: 2.49 ± 0.71

*Statistically significant difference from control;
+Atrisorb, Atrix Laboratories, Fort Collins, CO, USA;
†Perioglas, US Biomaterials, Alachua, FL, USA;
‡Resolute, W.L. Gore and Assoc., Flagstaff, AZ, USA;
⁋Matrigel™, BD Biosciences, San Jose, CA, USA; b-FGF = basic fibroblast growth factor; BMP_2 = bone morphogenetic protein-2; hOP-1 = human osteogenic protein-1; IGF = insulin growth factor; PDGF = platelet-derived growth factor; PRP = platelet-rich plasma; TGF = transforming growth factor.

(control) in the dog model. At eight weeks, cementum formation was significantly higher in the ACB, combination of ACB/PRP, and combination of MSCs/PRP groups compared to the control group ($p < 0.05$). It was concluded that periodontal regeneration with complete filling of class II furcation defects can be obtained with the use of GTR, PPR, MSCs, and their combinations. Finally, it was shown that a collagen matrix overlaid with embryonic stem cells (ES) is able to improve the regeneration of class II furcation defects (4 mm wide, 5 mm deep) in mini-pigs (Yang et al. 2013).

6.5 Regeneration Treatments of Class III Furcation Defects

6.5.1 Guided Tissue Regeneration

Starting from the late 1980s, the effects of placing non-bioresorbable or bioabsorbable membranes on degree III furcation CSD defects (3 mm wide and 4 mm high) as compared with those in control sites was evaluated in dogs (Niederman et al. 1989; Pontoriero et al. 1992; White et al. 1994; Lindhe et al. 1995; Araújo et al. 1997, 1998).

The results of the different studies are presented in Table 6.3. GTR resulted in significantly more gain of connective tissue attachment and regrowth of alveolar bone than control therapy, where no membrane was used. Complete closure of class III furcation defects with the formation of periodontal ligament and regrowth of the bone was achieved. It was shown that the size of the defect and the shape of the surrounding bone determined the outcome of regeneration, as already mentioned. The treatment failures were consistently associated with recession of the covering flaps and exposure of the defect. In addition, the results also demonstrated that bioabsorbable membranes provided a barrier that was equally effective to that of non-bioabsorbable membranes (Lindhe et al. 1995; Araújo et al. 1998).

6.5.2 Bone Grafts

The first attempts to treat class III furcation defects with the use of bone grafts (fresh autogenous hip marrow grafts, autogenous cancellous bone grafts) were made by Ellegaard et al. (1974, 1975) in the monkey model and Nilvéus et al. (1978) in the dog model. Although a higher frequency of furcation closure occurred with the use of the

Table 6.3 Guided tissue regeneration (GTR) in class III furcation defects.

Study	Model	Tooth	Type of membrane	Healing time (months)	Histomorhometric results
ACUTE DEFECT MODEL					
White et al. 1994	Dog	Mandibular premolars	Control: Open-flap debridement Test: PTFE non-resorbable membrane	3	**Distance from notch to coronal extent of bone (mm)** Control: -0.21 ± 7.27 Test: 1.50 ± 4.31
ACUTE/CHRONIC DEFECT MODEL					
Pontoriero et al. 1992	Dog	Mandibular premolars	Control: No membrane Test: PTFE non-resorbable membrane (Gore-Tex[+]) • Small key-hole defect (2 × 2 mm) • Large key-hole defect (3 × 4 mm) • Furcation defect part of circumferential loss of attachment	4	**Surface area (mm^2)** **Small key-hole defect** Control: 4.8 ± 1.3 Test: 4.1 ± 1.4 **Large key-hole defect:** Control: 13.6 ± 1 Test: 12.8 ± 2.8 **Furcation defect part of circumferential loss** Control: 22.3 ± 2.8 Test: 20.9 ± 2.4
Lindhe et al. 1995	Dog	Mandibular premolars	**Study 1:** Control: No membrane Test: PTFE non-resorbable membrane **Study 2:** Control: PTFE non-resorbable membrane Test: Synthetic resorbable membrane made of glycolide/lactic copolymer (Resolute†)	5	*Study 1* **Amount of new cementum** Control: 43% (±12) Test: 74% (±11)* **Height of new bone (mm)** Control: 0.7 ± 0.6 Test: 1.7 ± 0.5 *Study 2* **Amount of new cementum** Control: 82% (±13) Test: 86% (±11) **Height of new bone (mm)** Control: 2.8 ± 1.4 Test: 3.1 ± 1.1
Araújo et al. 1997	Dog	Mandibular premolars	Synthetic resorbable membrane made of glycolide/lactic copolymer (Resolute)	5	**Mineralized bone (%)** 36 (±12.6) **PDL (%)** 20 (±11.1)

Table 6.3 (Continued)

Study	Model	Tooth	Type of membrane	Healing time (months)	Histomorhometric results
Araújo et al. 1998	Dog	Mandibular premolars	Test 1: Synthetic resorbable membrane made of glycolide/lactic copolymer (Resolute) Test 2: Absorbable membrane made of polylactic acid (Guidor[†])	6	**Mineralized bone (%)** Test 1: 35 (±3) Test 2: 12 (±7)* **PDL (%)** Test 1: 19 (±4)* Test 2: 6 (±2)
Araújo et al. 1999	Dog	Mandibular premolars	Synthetic resorbable membrane made of glycolide/lactic copolymer (Resolute)	6	**Bone tissue (%)** 78 (±4.8)
CHRONIC DEFECT MODEL					
Gonçalves et al. 2006	Dog	Mandibular premolars	Control: Synthetic resorbable membrane made of glycolide/lactic copolymer (Resolute) + removal of cementum (scaling and root planing) Test: Synthetic resorbable membrane made of glycolide/lactic copolymer (Resolute) + preservation of cementum (polishing)	4	**New cementum (mm)** Control: 3.59 ± 1.67 Test: 6.20 ± 2.26 mm* **New bone (mm)** Control: 1.86 ± 1.76 Test: 4.62 ± 3.01 mm*

*Statistically significant difference from control;
+Gore-Tex, W.L. Gore and Assoc., Flagstaff, AZ, USA;
†Resolute, W.L. Gore and Assoc., Flagstaff, AZ, USA;
‡Guidor, Sunstar Americas Inc., Schaumburg, IL, USA; PDL = periodontal ligament; PTFE = polytetrafluoroethylene.

grafts, ankyloses and root resorption were documented as well. By using acute/chronic surgically created class III defects (larger than CSD) in dogs, Roriz et al. (2006) studied the regenerative potential of bovine-derived bone matrix with or without ePTFE membrane. Twelve weeks after treatment, it was concluded that both treatments had similar results and were not able to result in closure of class III furcation defects. It should be noted that in this study, the size of the defect (more than 4 mm in height) may have contributed to the lack of complete fill of the furcation in both groups. Another pre-clinical study using the dog model showed that implantation of beta tricalcium phosphate (β-TCP) with a tunnel pipe structure resulted

in new bone formation and new cementum in acute surgically created lesions (defect height was 4 mm) after eight weeks of treatment, but total closure of the furcation was not achieved (Saito et al. 2012).

6.5.3 Enamel Matrix Proteins

The first study evaluating the effect of EMD in combination with GTR versus GTR alone in class III furcation defects was performed by Araújo and Lindhe (1997) in surgically created acute/chronic lesions in the dog model. At four months, the central portion of both control and test furcation defects (4 mm high, 3 mm wide) was closed and the relative amounts of mineralized bone, bone marrow, and periodontal ligament were similar in both groups.

In a subsequent study, Donos et al. (2003b) evaluated the healing of mandibular degree III furcation treated with GTR, EMD, or a combination in monkeys. The dimensions of the furcation defects were approximately 4 mm wide and 3 mm high, corresponding to the CSD. The alveolar bone on the buccal and lingual aspect of the mesial and distal root of each molar was also removed, creating a 'horizontal' pattern of bone loss. However, the height of alveolar bone on the mesial and distal interproximal aspect of each experimental tooth was maintained. At five months of healing, similar results in terms of quality of the regenerated periodontal tissues were reported in the sites treated with GTR alone or in combination with EMD. Remarkably, the application of EMD alone resulted in unpredictable amounts of regenerated periodontal tissues and defect closure by newly formed bone (Figure 6.1). The same group also showed that only when GTR or GTR associated with EMD was applied was it possible to obtain complete defect regeneration (up to the fornix; Donos et al. 2003b; Gkranias et al. 2012). Moreover, they demonstrated different histological features in relation to the different treatment modalities. The sites treated according to the GTR principle showed a predominance of cellular cementum with extrinsic fibres or mixed fibres, while in the sites that were treated with EMD or a combination of GTR and EMD, the cementum was characterized apically as acellular and with extrinsic fibres and coronally as mixed with stratified fibres. In a recent investigation in dogs, the combined use of EMD with a synthetic bone graft (Emdogain Plus, Institut Straumann AG, Basel, Switzerland) was compared to coronally repositioned flap for the treatment of surgically created acute class III furcation in dogs. After two months of healing, in the experimental group, a significant amount of new attachment and bone formation was observed in the majority of the specimens (Mardas et al. 2012).

A new liquid carrier for EMD, Osteogain (Institut Straumann AG, Basel, Switzerland), specifically designed for mixing with different biomaterials, has also been for the first time tested in the regeneration of acute/chronic class III furcation defects in monkeys (Shirakata et al. 2017). The dimensions of the exposed furcation defects were 5 mm wide and 5 mm high (Figure 6.2). When comparing the histological outcome of defects treated with open-flap debridement (OFD; control), OFD and a collagen sponge saturated with EMD (OFD/EMD), and OFD and a collagen sponge saturated with Osteogain (OFD/Osteogain), higher amounts of connective tissue were observed in both test groups. Furthermore, the OFD/Osteogain group showed higher new attachment formation, cementum, and new bone area. None of the treatments achieved complete regeneration; that is, class III furcation persisted after treatment (Figure 6.3).

6.5.4 Growth Factors

These biologically active substances, used either alone or in combination with GTR, have been tested for their efficacy in improving regenerative outcomes in class III furcation lesions. Rossa et al. (2000) combined the use of b-FGF with GTR for the treatment of acute/chronic surgically created defects in dogs. The defects had a vertical height of 5 mm and a horizontal width of 7 mm. The proximal bone crest was not removed, resulting in an angular-type defect rather than a horizontal one. The study showed improvements in histological outcomes, such as newly formed cementum, and lower extent of epithelial migration when b-FGF was associated with GTR in comparison to GTR alone. However, differences between experimental and control groups did not reach statistical significance (this might be due to the large size of the created defects) and full closure of the furcation was not achieved in any of the specimens. Conversely, the combination of b-FGF with β-TCP was shown to enhance connective tissue attachment and to

(a)

(b)

(c)

(d)

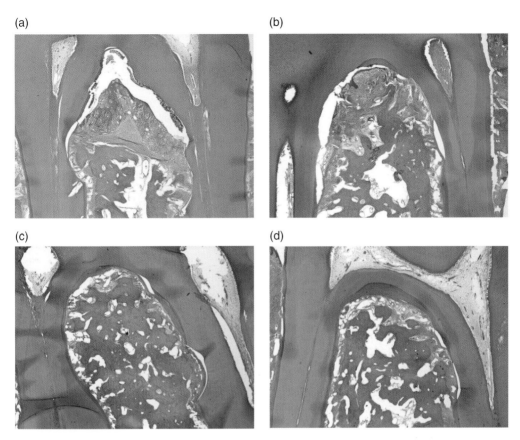

Figure 6.1 Overview photomicrographs of all class III furcation defects in different groups. (a) Furcation treated with ethylenediaminetetraacetic acid (EDTA). Regeneration was observed only at the level of the notch, with connective tissue and granulation tissue plus epithelium covering the rest of the space. (b) Furcation treated with enamel matrix derivative (EMD). The furcation was partially closed and a layer of new cementum with inserting fibres identified coronal to the notch. Regenerated bone filled most of the furcation area. (c) Guided tissue regeneration (GTR)-treated furcation where the membrane remained covered. The entire circumference of the defect is covered with a layer of new cementum. Regenerated alveolar bone fills the furcation defect completely. (d) Furcation treated with GTR + EMD. The furcation was closed and new cementum can be seen on most of the circumference of the defect. The defect was filled with new bone up to the fornix.

induce higher bone formation (up to the fornix) compared to b-FGF alone in class III furcation acute smaller defects (4 mm high) created in dogs (Saito et al. 2013).

By using the supra-alveolar, critical size model, the effect of recombinant human bone morphogenetic protein ($rhBMP_2$) was tested and substantial regeneration of alveolar bone and cementum was demonstrated (Wikesjö et al. 1994). However, treatment with $rhBMP_2$ did not appear to induce a functionally oriented periodontal ligament,

and resulted in ankyloses and root resorption (Wikesjö et al. 1999, 2003a; Takahashi et al. 2005). The use of PDGF in combination with GTR has been successfully tested by Park et al. (1995) in acute/chronic supra-alveolar, critical size surgically created defects in beagle dogs. They reported almost complete closure of the lesions without the occurrence of resorption or ankyloses. Using the supra-alveolar, critical size model, different concentrations of osteogenic protein-1 (OP-1) were evaluated in acute lesions in the dog.

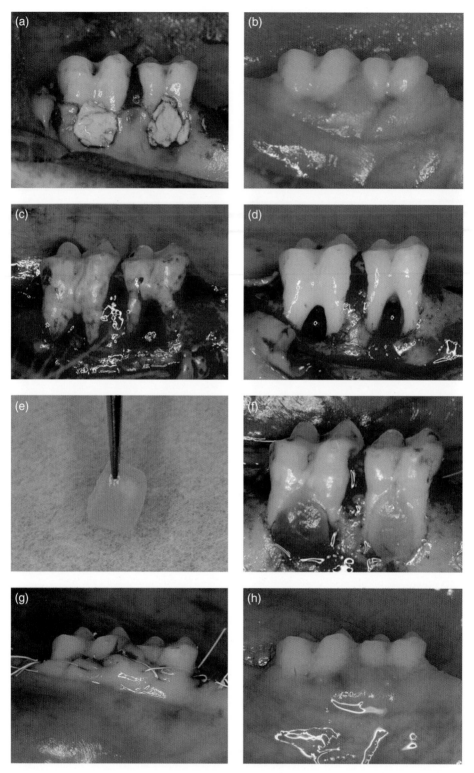

Figure 6.2 Clinical appearance of the mandibular buccal aspect of *Macaca fascicularis*. (a) Induction of chronic inflammation. After fabrication of class III furcation defects, impression materials were placed to encourage growth of oral microflora along the exposed root surfaces. (b) Prior to reconstructive surgery. (c) Immediately after flap reflection. Note the excessive granulation tissue in the chronic defects. (d) Defects were exposed and debrided again at the time of reconstructive surgery. (e) Osteogain/absorbable collagen sponge (ACS) construct before surgical implantation. (f) Left (second molar): ACS alone; right (first molar): placement of Osteogain/ACS. (g) Flaps coronally repositioned and sutured. (h) 16 weeks after reconstructive surgery.

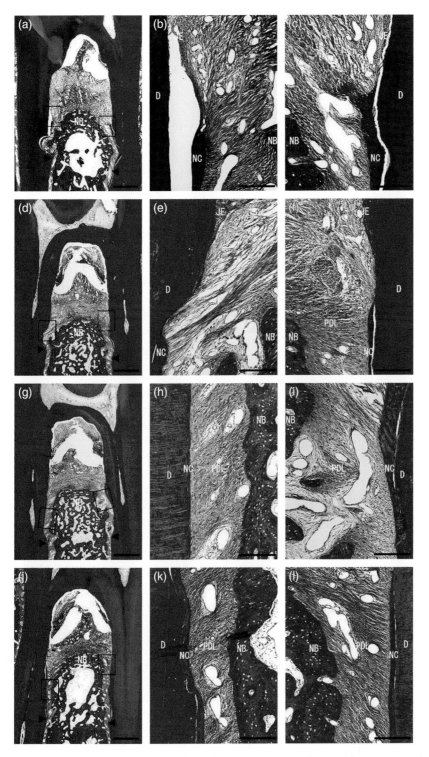

Figure 6.3 Overview photomicrographs of all class III furcation defects in different groups (Azan-Mallory staining). (a) OFD (open-flap debridement) group overview (scale bar: 1 mm). (b) Higher magnification of framed area (left) in (a) (scale bar: 200 μm). (c) Higher magnification of framed area (right) in (a) (scale bar: 200 μm). (d) Absorbable collagen sponge (ACS) group overview (scale bar: 1 mm). (e) Higher magnification of framed area (left) in (d) (scale bar: 200 μm). (f) Higher magnification of framed area (right) in (d) (scale bar: 200 μm). (g) Emdogain/ACS group overview (scale bar: 1 mm). (h) Higher magnification of apical framed area (left) in (g) (scale bar: 200 μm). (i) Higher magnification of framed area (right) in (g) (scale bar: 200 μm). (j) Osteogain/ACS group overview (scale bar: 1 mm). Arrowhead: notch (apical extent of root planing). (k) Higher magnification of framed area (left) in (j) (scale bar: 200 μm). (l) Higher magnification of framed area (right) in (j) (scale bar: 200 μm). JE = junctional epithelium, NB = new bone; NC = new cementum; PDL = periodontal ligament.

At a dose of 7.5 μg/ml of OP-1 in a collagen carrier 3.9 ± 1.7 mm and 6.1 ± 3.4 mm^2 of linear bone height and bone area were achieved. These outcomes were significantly improved in comparison to the outcomes achieved in the defects treated with surgery only or with carrier only (Giannobile et al. 1998).

6.5.5 Cell Therapy

Only limited studies have investigated the use of cell therapy in the treatment of class III furcation defects. Autogenous periosteal cells combined with the application of β-TCP have shown improved periodontal tissue regeneration in acute/chronic surgically created defects compared to β-TCP-treated and empty defects in a dog model. The furcation defects were approximately 3 mm wide and 4 mm high (Jiang et al. 2010). More recently, Nagahara et al. (2015), using the same defect size, also confirmed that applying a β-TCP scaffold to bone marrow mesenchymal stem cells helps enhance new bone formation in class III furcation defects exposed to inflammation in beagle dogs.

Using the supra-alveolar, critical size model, autologous periodontal ligament cells were isolated from extracted teeth, cultured and phenotypically characterized, and eventually applied on a collagen sponge carrier alone or in combination with GTR in surgically created acute/chronic defects in the beagle dog model (Murano et al. 2006; Suaid et al. 2012). After three months of healing, both groups resulted in additional new cementum and new periodontal ligament production, together with a larger area of new bone formation.

6.6 Discussion

It is well accepted that there is no single animal model that represents all aspects of periodontal human disease, tissue architecture, and the healing and ageing processes. However, human studies cannot always be coupled with tissue harvesting, which is however necessary for microscopic and histological analyses that define the biological impact of the regenerative methods and materials applied (Kantarci et al. 2015). Therefore, it has been suggested that animal studies are still an important step for establishing cause-and-effect relationships and for the initial evaluation of principles in the development of new regenerative devices and advanced therapeutics.

Regenerative therapy of advanced furcation involvement (classes II and III) has been extensively studied in pre-clinical models, but the question remains whether this pre-clinical evidence is enough to support the clinical use of the different techniques and materials investigated in regenerative periodontal therapy. The clinical challenge in furcation involvement is the destruction of the horizontal component, but also the combined need for vertical periodontal regeneration within the same area. There is extensive evidence that, independent of the defect type and animal model adopted, regenerative periodontal surgery using a combination of barrier membranes and grafting materials may result in periodontal regeneration to a varying extent (Sculean et al. 2008). GTR is more predictable in class II furcation than in class III furcation defects. Some studies reported failures in the closure of the furcation, often associated with recession of the covering tissue flaps, which subsequently resulted in exposure of the membrane. These results suggested that regenerative outcomes in the treatment of furcation defects are only possible if the healing environment under the membrane is well protected by the flaps during healing, and the barrier membranes are not exposed and hence contaminated by the oral micro-environment (Klinge et al. 1981, 1985a, b; Lindhe et al. 1995). Superior histological outcomes, predominantly bone repair, following the use of a combination of grafting materials and barrier membranes, compared with grafting materials alone or membranes alone, were only found in non-contained periodontal defects (class III furcation defects). However, in contained defects, such as class II furcation lesions, no additional advantage of a combined treatment was suggested overall. This implies that the principal mechanism by which a graft material supports regeneration may not be its osteoconductivity, but rather its space provision capacity, a question which warrants further investigation (Polimeni at al. 2004).

Biological and biomimetic substances, such as EMD, have also been tested in experimental studies to assess their regenerative capability in furcation lesions. As class III furcation defects are non-contained defects, the use of biologics is associated with important limitations. Owing to their liquid/gel-like consistency, any space-making effect is in fact prevented, and therefore the regenerative potential of such materials may be limited in furcation defects. Remarkably, in some studies, the use of EMD in combination with GTR in class III furcation defects resulted in some periodontal regeneration. However, there should always be caution in extrapolating results from experimental studies in animals to the clinical scenario, where it has been shown that the same treatment principles may not apply in class III clinical cases (Donos et al. 2003a, 2004).

Growth and differentiation factor technologies have also been evaluated for their potential to enhance periodontal wound healing/regeneration in furcation lesions (Stavropoulos and Wikesjö 2012). Such biologically active substances, used either alone or in combination with GTR, seem to be promising in enhancing the regenerative outcomes in class II and III furcation defects, but further pre-clinical and clinical research is needed to adequately evaluate the efficacy of these novel treatments in periodontal wound healing/regeneration. Cell-based therapies have also received considerable attention in regenerative medicine, but their experimental evaluation in the treatment of periodontal furcation lesions is still at a very early stage of development.

In recent years, due to the low rate of cell survival after cell implantation, the paracrine functions of mesenchymal stem cells have received increasing attention as a regenerative mechanism (Nagata et al. 2017). The possibility of enhancing the regeneration of furcation defects with the help of transplanted conditioned medium obtained from cultured periodontal stem cells is certainly an interesting and stimulating area for future research.

6.6.1 Limitations of Pre-clinical Studies

It is important to recognize the limitations of animal studies, as answers obtained from experiments performed under standardized conditions are specific to the questions posed, and do not necessarily translate into the clinical setting (Donos et al. 2003a). In addition, 'biological variability' is still a concern and is often resorted to as an explanation for divergent experimental results. This variability may be due to the erratic behaviour of genetic, biochemical, physiological, or immunological host factors, or to the microbial flora associated with the individual animal. The lack of genetically defined stocks within dogs and primates (the animals mainly used in this field of research), together with the ethical concerns, may represent an important limiting factor in our attempts to reduce the effect of biological variability.

As mentioned previously, regenerative therapies require a histological demonstration of the actual outcome of periodontal regeneration by measuring the tooth-supporting tissues (i.e. cementum, periodontal ligament, and alveolar bone) over a previously diseased root surface (Sanz et al. 2015). The heterogeneity of the available studies in terms of species, study design, observation period, and materials makes them difficult to compare. The evaluation of the results may also be impaired by the difficulty in standardizing the defect morphology and the extent of bone loss (horizontal and non-horizontal), as well as by the different nature of the defects (naturally occurring vs ligature induced, or acute vs chronic).

The different anatomy and dimensions of teeth and alveolar processes in the available experimental animal models may reduce the clinical value of the outcomes. For example, experimental procedures performed in narrow and shallow two-rooted canine mandibular and maxillary premolar furcation defects with short trunks might translate poorly to clinical furcation defects in humans, especially when considering the large three-rooted maxillary molars.

Another important factor affecting the outcome of pre-clinical studies is the concept of the CSD. It was shown that degree III furcation involvements with a cross-section dimension larger than 4 mm are more difficult to regenerate than smaller ones (Pontoriero et al. 1989, 1992). On the other hand, complete healing was reported in larger degree III furcation involvements when the membrane was kept completely covered by the flap during healing (Lindhe et al. 1995; Araújo et al. 1997, 1998; Araújo and Lindhe 1997). These results indicate that defect morphology might be less important than post-surgical flap dehiscence and consequent exposure of the membrane. The complete closure of degree III furcation is unpredictable and depends on the size of the entrance of the defect (Pontoriero et al. 1989, 1992), the height of the defect, and the complete flap coverage of the membrane during the healing period (Lindhe et al. 1995). Keyhole furcation defects without concomitant horizontal bone reduction seemed to provide better post-operative support to the flaps and prevent recession. In addition, taking into consideration that the healing process in dogs is more rapid compared to humans (Cardarapoli et al. 2003; Mardas et al. 2012), the development of new, more challenging CSDs (width, height) should be considered to evaluate the regenerative potential of different materials.

The lack of standardization in terms of sample orientation for histological evaluation and quantitative assessment is another potential source of bias. In the early studies, the mesial-distal section plane was the one most commonly employed (Crigger et al. 1978). The true value of the histological analysis of mesial-distal sections in class II and III furcation has been questioned by Selvig (1994). This plane might impair interpretation, since it is very difficult to determine at which point in the buccal-lingual direction the section was obtained. When the section is obtained at the most proximal point from the intact attachment apparatus (e.g. from the lingual wall of the buccal furcation defect), analysis might provide a false idea of a greater regenerative response than a section obtained at a more distant point from the remaining periodontium, simply because of a smaller distance from precursor cells in the first case. According to Bogle et al. (1997), for a more precise histomorphometric evaluation of the whole regenerative process of furcation lesions, buccal-lingual histological sections must be obtained, because they allow for an analysis of the healing response from the lingual limits of the defect to the buccal cemento-enamel junction.

Another difficulty when trying to compare pre-clinical studies is the different ways of calculating the results. In some studies the attachment gain is measured in millimetres, while in others it is calculated as a percentage of the original defect height. The use of percentages compensates for differences in size between different experimental teeth and defects, but tends to mask the fact that a large percentage change may reflect a very small change in real units of measurement (Selvig 1994).

Furthermore, it is still unclear what is the necessary minimum observation period to ensure that the observed result is, in fact, the endpoint of the healing process. The observation period in most pre-clinical studies varies from a couple of weeks up to three or six months. If the aim is to record the maximum extent of repair, including cementum and bone regeneration, a longer observation period should be recorded. Cementum does not form on root-planed surfaces in the dog before approximately three weeks after surgery. At six weeks, considerable amounts of new cementum may have formed. Connective tissue attachment may be well established at its final level six months after surgery, but the final picture of mature cementum and bone formation may not be expressed until a later stage. It has been reported that regenerated tissues continue their formation and/or remodelling even after three months of wound healing, and that this process can continue for up to six months (Araújo et al. 1997).

6.6.2 Ethical Codes for Animal Experimentation

There is increasing concern in society and the medical profession regarding animal welfare, with significant controversy surrounding the use of animals in research and testing (Biller-Andorno et al. 2015). It has been suggested that animal experiments can be sanctioned if there is no alternative means of achieving the same scientific or educational objective, and if the benefits to society outweigh the costs in terms of animal harm (Rusche 2003). Harming animals is highly undesirable and experiments can only be justified if the social good derived from this type of use actively outweighs the negative aspect of harming a sensitive creature (Kolar 2006). Whenever possible, alternative methods should be sought. The three Rs (3Rs) principle, which should be applied as a guide when conducting animal research, includes replacement, reduction, and refinement:

- *Replacement*: Using an experimental subject that is phylogenetically lower or using non-animal systems. A few promising alternative methods put forward recently are in vitro techniques; tissue culture methods; use of lower organisms including microbes, tissues from slaughter, and autopsy embryos; and non-animal systems such as computers or mathematical modelling.
- *Reduction*: Before proposing to conduct animal experimentation, efforts should be made to ascertain that the proposed

animal experiment has not been done previously. Also, the minimum possible number of animals required should be used to yield meaningful data and not maximum precision.
- *Refinement*: A multitude of refinements of technique that would reduce animal harm are ready for immediate application in biomedical research.

Since 1986, the European Union (EU) has had specific legislation covering the use of animals for scientific purposes.

The Council for International Organizations of Medical Sciences (COIMS) is an international non-governmental representative of many branches of medicine and cognate disciplines, which has laid down the guiding principles to provide a conceptual ethical framework acceptable to both the international biomedical community and animal welfare groups. COIMS set the following international guiding principles (Howard-Jones 1985):

- The use of animals for scientific purposes is innately undesirable.
- Another method should be used whenever possible.
- The use of animals in the present state of knowledge is unavoidable.
- Scientists should have a moral obligation in designing the plan for the minimal number of animals to be employed.

The guiding principles are the product of consultation with a large and representative sample of the biomedical community, including experts from the World Health Organization (WHO) and representatives of animal welfare groups.

6.7 Conclusions

Furcation involvement poses one of the most difficult challenges in periodontal therapy. Based on the available data, if one considers closure of the furcation defect as the main endpoint of therapy, then the results of regeneration have to be regarded as satisfying and predictable only for class II furcation involvements. Conversely, class III furcation defects are still considered a great challenge in terms of periodontal regeneration and, although the efficacy of different treatments has been demonstrated in some pre-clinical studies, the effectiveness and relevance for clinical practice may be questioned. In the future, new regenerative treatment modalities and the development of more challenging CSDs in pre-clinical studies are clearly needed to improve the predictability of complete resolution of class III furcation defects.

Summary of Evidence

- Animal studies, despite their limitations, are an important step for establishing cause-and-effect relationships and for the initial evaluation of principles in the development of new regenerative devices and advanced therapeutics.
- Independent of the defect type and animal model adopted, regenerative periodontal surgery using a combination of barrier membranes and grafting materials may result in periodontal regeneration to a variable extent in furcation involvements.
- The results of regeneration have to be regarded as satisfying and predictable only for class II furcation involvements, as class III furcation defects are still considered a great challenge in terms of periodontal regeneration, although the efficacy

of different treatments has been demonstrated in some pre-clinical studies.
- The concept of the critical size defect (CSD) is an important factor affecting the outcome in pre-clinical studies, and new, more challenging CSDs (in width and height) should be developed to evaluate the regenerative potential of different materials in furcation involvement. This is in particular consideration of the higher regeneration ability of animals in comparisons to humans.
- Growth and differentiation factor technologies and cell-based therapies have also received considerable attention in regenerative medicine, but their experimental evaluation in the treatment of periodontal furcation lesions is still at a very early stage of development.

References

Al-Hezaimi, K., Al-Fahad, H., O'Neill, R. et al. (2012). The effect of enamel matrix protein on gingival tissue thickness in vivo. *Odontology* 100, 61–66.

Amin, H.D., Olsen, I., Knowles, J.C. and Donos, N. (2012). Differential effect of amelogenin peptides on osteogenic differentiation in vitro: Identification of possible new drugs for bone repair and regeneration. *Tissue Engineering Part A* 18, 1193–1202.

Amin, H.D., Olsen, I., Knowles, J.C. et al. (2013). Effects of enamel matrix proteins on multi-lineage differentiation of periodontal ligament cells in vitro. *Acta Biomaterialia* 9, 4796–4805.

Amin, H.D., Olsen, I., Knowles, J. et al. (2014). A tyrosine-rich amelogenin peptide promotes neovasculogenesis in vitro and ex vivo. *Acta Biomaterialia* 10, 1930–1939.

Amin, H.D., Olsen, I., Knowles, J. et al. (2016). Interaction of enamel matrix proteins with human periodontal ligament cells. *Clinical Oral Investigation* 20, 339–347.

Araújo, M.G., Berglundh, T., Albrekstsson, T., and Lindhe, J. (1999). Bone formation in furcation defects: An experimental study in the dog. *Journal of Clinical Periodontology* 26, 643–652.

Araújo, M.G., Berglundh, T., and Lindhe, J. (1997). On the dynamics of periodontal tissue formation in degree III furcation defects: An experimental study in dogs. *Journal of Clinical Periodontology* 24, 738–746.

Araújo, M.G., Berglundh, T., and Lindhe, J. (1998). GTR treatment of degree III furcation defects with 2 different resorbable barriers: An experimental study in dogs. *Journal of Clinical Periodontology* 25, 253–259.

Araújo, M.G., and Lindhe, J. (1997). GTR treatment of degree III furcation defects following application of enamel matrix proteins: An experimental study in dogs. *Journal of Clinical Periodontology* 25, 524–530.

Avila-Ortiz, G., De Buitrago, J.G., and Reddy, M.S. (2015). Periodontal regeneration – furcation defects: A systematic review from the AAP Regeneration Workshop. *Journal of Periodontology* 86 (Suppl. 2), 69–77.

Baldini, N., De Sanctis, M., and Ferrari, M. (2011). Deproteinized bovine bone in periodontal and implant surgery. *Dental Materials* 27, 61–70.

Berglundh, T., Lindhe, J., and Sterrett, J.D. (1991). Clinical and structural characteristics of periodontal tissues in young and old dogs. *Journal of Clinical Periodontology* 18, 616–623.

Biller-Andorno, N., Grimm, H., and Walker, R.L. (2015). Professionalism and ethics in animal research. *Natural Biotechnology* 33, 1027–1028.

Bizenjima, T., Seshima, F., Ishizuka, Y. et al. (2015). Fibroblast growth factor-2 promotes healing of surgically created periodontal defects in rats with early, streptozotocin-induced diabetes via increasing cell proliferation and regulating angiogenesis. *Journal of Clinical Periodontology* 42, 62–71.

Bogle, G., Garrett, S., Stoller, N.H. et al. (1997). Periodontal regeneration in naturally occurring Class II furcation defects in beagle dogs after guided tissue regeneration with bioabsorbable barriers. *Journal of Periodontology* 68, 536–544.

Caffesse, R.G., Dominguez, L.E., Nasjleti, C.E., et al. (1990). Furcation defects in dogs treated by guided tissue regeneration (GTR). *Journal of Periodontology* 61, 45–50.

Caffesse, R.G., Nasjleti, C.E., Morrison, E.C., and Sanchez, R. (1994). Guided tissue regeneration: Comparison of bioabsorbable and non-bioabsorbable membranes. Histologic and histometric study in dogs. *Journal of Periodontology* 65, 583–591.

Caffesse, R.G., Nasjleti, C.E., Plotzke, A.E., et al. (1993). Guided tissue regeneration and bone grafts in the treatment of furcation defects. *Journal of Periodontology* 64 (Suppl. 11), 1145–1153.

Cardaropoli, G., Araújo, M., and Lindhe, J. (2003). Dynamics of bone tissue formation in tooth extraction sites: An experimental study in dogs. *Journal of Clinical Periodontology* 30, 809–818.

Caton, J.G., and Kowalski, C.J. (1976). Primate model for testing periodontal treatment procedures: II. Production of contralaterally similar lesions. *Journal of Periodontology* 47, 506–510.

Caton, J., Mota, L., Gandini, L., and Laskaris, B. (1994). Non-human primate models for testing the efficacy and safety of periodontal regeneration procedures. *Journal of Periodontology* 65, 1143–1150.

Chantarawaratit, P., Sangvanich, P., Banlunara, W. et al. (2014). Acemannan sponges stimulate alveolar bone, cementum and periodontal ligament regeneration in a canine class II furcation defect model. *Journal of Periodontal Research* 49, 164–178.

Cirelli, J.A., Marcantonio, E., Jr, Adriana, R. et al. (1997). Evaluation of anionic collagen membranes in the treatment of class II furcation lesions: A histometric analysis in dogs. *Biomaterials* 18, 1227–1234.

Crigger, M., Bogle, G., Nilvéus, R. et al. (1978). The effect of topical citric acid application on the healing of experimental furcation defects in dogs. *Journal of Periodontal Research* 13, 538–549.

Danesh-Meyer, M.J., Pack, A.R., and McMillan, M.D. (1997). A comparison of 2 polytetrafluoroethylene membranes in guided tissue regeneration in sheep. *Journal of Periodontal Research* 32, 20–30.

de Andrade, P.F., de Souza, S.L., de Oliveira, M.G. et al. (2007). Acellular dermal matrix as a membrane for guided tissue regeneration in the treatment of Class II furcation lesions: A histometric and clinical study in dogs. *Journal of Periodontology* 78, 1288–1299.

Deliberador, T.M., Nagata, M.J., Furlaneto, F.A. et al. (2006). Autogenous bone graft with or without a calcium sulfate barrier in the treatment of Class II furcation defects: A histologic and histometric study in dogs. *Journal of Periodontology* 77, 780–789.

De Santana, R.B., Gusman, H.C., and Van Dyke, T.E. (1999). The response of human buccal maxillary furcation defects to combined regenerative techniques: Two controlled clinical studies. *Journal of the International Academy of Periodontology* 1, 69–77.

Dogan, A., Ozdemir, A., Kubar, A., and Oygür, T. (2002). Assessment of periodontal healing by seeding of fibroblast-like cells derived from regenerated periodontal ligament in artificial furcation defects in a dog: aA pilot study. *Tissue Engineering* 8, 273–282.

Donos, N., Glavind, L., Karring, T., and Sculean, A. (2003a). Clinical evaluation of an enamel matrix derivative in the treatment of mandibular degree II furcation involvement: A 36-month case series. *International Journal of Periodontics and Restorative Dentistry* 23, 507–512.

Donos, N., Glavind, L, Karring T., and Sculean A. (2004). Clinical evaluation of an enamel matrix derivative and a bioresorbable membrane in the treatment of degree III mandibular furcation involvement: A series of nine patients. *International Journal of Periodontics and Restorative Dentistry* 200, 362–369.

Donos, N., Sculean, A., Glavind, L. et al. (2003b). Wound healing of degree III furcation involvements following guided tissue regeneration and/or Emdogain: A histologic study. *Journal of Clinical Periodontology* 30, 1061–1068.

Ellegaard, B., Karring, T., Davies, R., and Löe, H. (1974). New attachment after treatment of intrabony defects in monkeys. *Journal of Periodontology* 45, 368–377.

Ellegaard, B., Karring, T., and Löe, H. (1975). The fate of vital and devitalized bone grafts in the healing of interradicular lesions. *Journal of Periodontal Research* 10, 88–97.

Giannobile, W.V., Finkelman, R.D., and Lynch, S.E. (1994). Comparison of canine and non-human primate animal models for periodontal regenerative therapy: Results following a single administration of PDGF/IGF-I. *Journal of Periodontology* 65, 1158–1168.

Giannobile, W.V., Ryan, S., Shih, M.S. et al. (1998). Recombinant human osteogenic protein-1 (OP-1) stimulates periodontal wound healing in class III furcation defects. *Journal of Periodontology* 69, 129–137.

Gkranias, N.D., Graziani, F., Sculean, A., and Donos, N. (2012). Wound healing following regenerative procedures in furcation degree III defects: Histomorphometric outcomes. *Clinical Oral Investigation* 16, 239–249.

Gonçalves, P.F., Gurgel, B.C., Pimentel, S.P. et al. (1996). Root cementum modulates periodontal regeneration in Class III furcation defects treated by the guided tissue regeneration technique: A histometric study in dogs. *Journal of Periodontology* 77, 976–982.

Gosain, A.K., Song, L., Yu, P. et al. (2000). Osteogenesis in cranial defects: Reassessment of the concept of critical size and the expression of TGF-beta isoforms. *Plastic Reconstructive Surgery* 106, 360–371.

Graves, D.T., Fine D., Teng, Y.T. et al. (2008). The use of rodent models to investigate host–bacteria interactions related to periodontal diseases. *Journal of Clinical Periodontology* 35, 89–105.

Haney, J.M., Zimmerman, G.J., and Wikesjö, U.M. (1995). Periodontal repair in dogs: Evaluation of the natural disease model. *Journal of Clinical Periodontology* 22, 208–213.

Howard-Jones, N.A. (1985). CIOMS ethical code for animal experimentation. *WHO Chronicles* 39, 51–56.

Hürzeler, M.B., Quiñones, C.R., Caffesse, R.G. et al. (1997). Guided periodontal tissue regeneration in Class II furcation defects following treatment with a synthetic bioabsorbable barrier. *Journal of Periodontology* 68, 498–505.

Ivanovic, A., Nikou, G., Miron, R.J. et al. (2014). Which biomaterials may promote periodontal regeneration in intrabony periodontal defects? A systematic review of preclinical studies. *Quintessence International* 45, 385–395.

Jiang, J., Wu, X., Lin, M. et al. (2010). Application of autologous periosteal cells for the regeneration of class III furcation defects in beagle dogs. *Cytotechnology* 62, 235–243.

Kantarci, A., Hasturk, H., and Van Dyke, T.E. (2015). Animal models for periodontal regeneration and peri-implant responses. *Periodontology* 2000 68, 66–82.

Karring, T., and Cortellini, P. (1999). Regenerative therapy: Furcation defects. *Periodontology 2000* 19, 115–137.

Karring, T., Nyman, S., Gottlow, J., and Laurell, L. (1993). Development of the biological concept of guided tissue regeneration: Animal and human studies. *Periodontology 2000* 1, 26–35.

Karring, T., Nyman, S., and Lindhe, J. (1980). Healing following implantation of periodontitis affected roots into bone tissue. *Journal of Clinical Periodontology* 7, 96–105.

Karring, T., and Warrer, K. (1992). Development of the principle of guided tissue regeneration. *Alpha Omegan* 85, 19–24.

Keles, G.C., Cetinkaya, B.O., Baris, S. et al. (2009). Comparison of platelet pellet with or without guided tissue regeneration in the treatment of class II furcation defects in dogs. *Clinical Oral Investigation* 13, 393–400.

Klinge, B., Nilvéus, R., and Egelberg, J. (1985a). Effect of crown-attached sutures on healing of experimental furcation defects in dogs. *Journal of Clinical Periodontology* 12, 369–373.

Klinge, B., Nilvéus, R., and Egelberg, J. (1985b). Bone regeneration pattern and ankylosis in experimental furcation defects in dogs. *Journal of Clinical Periodontology* 12, 456–464.

Klinge, B., Nilvéus, R., Kiger, R.D., and Egelberg, J. (1981). Effect of flap placement and defect size on healing of experimental furcation defects. *Journal of Periodontal Research* 16, 236–248.

Kolar, R. (2006). Animal experimentation. *Science and Engineer Ethics* 12, 111–122.

Koo, K.T., Polimeni, G., Albandar, J.M., and Wikesjö, U.M. (2004). Periodontal repair in dogs: Analysis of histometric assessments in the supraalveolar periodontal defect model. *Journal of Periodontology* 75, 1688–1693.

Kramer, P.R., Nares, S., Kramer, S.F. et al. (2004). Mesenchymal stem cells acquire characteristics of cells in the periodontal ligament in vitro. *Journal of Dental Research* 83, 27–34.

Lang, H., Schuler, N., and Nolden, R. (1998). Attachment formation following replantation of cultured cells into periodontal defects: A study in minipigs. *Journal of Dental Research* 77, 393–405.

Lekovic, V., and Kenney, E.B. (1993). Guided tissue regeneration using calcium phosphate implants together with 4 different membranes: A study on furcations in dogs. *Journal of Periodontology* 64, 1154–1156.

Lekovic, V., Klokkevold, P.R., Kenney, E.B. et al. (1998). Histologic evaluation of guided tissue regeneration using 4 barrier membranes: A comparative furcation study in dogs. *Journal of Periodontology* 69, 54–61.

Lindhe, J., Pontoriero, R., Berglundh, T., and Araujo, M. (1995). The effect of flap management and bioresorbable occlusive devices in GTR treatment of degree III furcation defects: An experimental study in dogs. *Journal of Clinical Periodontology* 22, 276–283.

Macedo, G.O., Souza, S.L., Novaes, A.B., Jr et al. (2006). Effect of early membrane removal on regeneration of Class II furcation defects in dogs. *Journal of Periodontology* 77, 46–53.

Mardas, N., Kraehenmann, M., and Dard, M. (2012). Regenerative wound healing in acute degree III mandibular defects in dogs. *Quintessence International* 43, e48–e59.

Murakami, S., Takayama, S., Ikezawa, K. et al. (1999). Regeneration of periodontal tissues by basic fibroblast growth factor. *Journal of Periodontal Research* 34, 425–430.

Murakami, S., Takayama, S., Kitamura, M. et al. (2003). Recombinant human basic fibroblast growth factor (bFGF) stimulates periodontal regeneration in class II furcation defects created in beagle dogs. *Journal of Periodontal Research* 38, 97–103.

Murano, Y., Ota, M., Katayama, A. et al. (2006). Periodontal regeneration following transplantation of proliferating tissue derived from periodontal ligament into class III furcation defects in dogs. *Biomedical Research* 27, 139–147.

Murphy, K.G., and Gunsolley, J.C. (2003). Guided tissue regeneration for the treatment of periodontal intrabony and furcation defects: A systematic review. *Annals of Periodontology* 8, 266–302.

Nagahara, T., Yoshimatsu, S., Shiba, H. et al. (2015). Introduction of a mixture of β-tricalcium phosphate into a complex of bone marrow mesenchymal stem cells and type I collagen can augment the volume of alveolar bone without impairing cementum regeneration. *Journal of Periodontology* 86, 456–464.

Nagata, M., Iwasaki, K., Akazawa, K. et al. (2017). Conditioned medium from periodontal ligament stem cells enhances periodontal regeneration. *Tissue Engineering, Part A* 23, 367–377.

Niederman, R., Savitt, E.D., Heeley, J.D., and Duckworth, J.E. (1989). Regeneration of furca bone using Gore-Tex periodontal material. *International Journal of Periodontics and Restorative Dentistry* 9, 468–480.

Nilvéus, R., Johansson, O., and Egelberg, J. (1978). The effect of autogenous cancellous bone grafts on healing of experimental furcation defects in dogs. *Journal of Periodontal Research* 13, 532–537.

Nyman, S., Karring, T., Lindhe, J., and Plantén, S. (1980). Healing following implantation of periodontitis-affected roots into gingival connective tissue. *Journal of Clinical Periodontology* 7, 394–401.

Oz, H.S., and Puleo, D.A. (2011). Animal models for periodontal disease. *Journal of Biomedical Biotechnology* 2011, 754857.

Park, J.B., Matsuura, M., Han, K.Y. et al. (1995). Periodontal regeneration in class III furcation defects of beagle dogs using guided tissue regenerative therapy with platelet-derived growth factor. *Journal of Periodontology* 66, 462–477.

Polejaeva, I.A., Chen, S.H., Vaught, T.D. et al. (2000). Cloned pigs produced by nuclear transfer from adult somatic cells. *Nature* 407, 86–90.

Polimeni, G., Koo, K.T., Qahash, M. et al. (2004). Prognostic factors for alveolar regeneration: Effect of a space-providing biomaterial on guided tissue regeneration. *Journal of Clinical Periodontology* 31, 725–729.

Pontoriero, R., Lindhe, J., Nyman, S., et al. (1989). Guided tissue regeneration in the treatment of furcation defects in mandibular molars: A clinical study of degree III involvements. *Journal of Clinical Periodontology* 16, 170–174.

Pontoriero, R., Nyman, S., Ericsson, I., and Lindhe, J. (1992). Guided tissue regeneration in surgically-produced furcation defects: An experimental study in the beagle dog. *Journal of Clinical Periodontology* 19, 159–163.

Regazzini, P.F., Novaes, A.B. Jr, de Oliveira, P.T. et al. (2004). Comparative study of enamel matrix derivative with or without GTR in the treatment of class II furcation lesions in dogs. *International Journal of Periodontics and Restorative Dentistry* 24, 476–487.

Ripamonti, U., Crooks, J., Petit, J.C., and Rueger, D.C. (2001). Tissue regeneration by combined applications of recombinant human osteogenic protein-1 and bone morphogenetic protein-2: A pilot study in Chacma baboons (Papio ursinus). *European Journal of Oral Sciences* 109, 241–248.

Ripamonti, U., Heliotis, M., Rueger, D.C., and Sampath, T.K. (1996). Induction of cementogenesis by recombinant human osteogenic protein-1 (hop-1/bmp-7) in the baboon (Papio ursinus). *Archive of Oral Biology* 41, 121–126.

Risbud, M.V., and Shapiro, I.M. (2005). The effect of brain-derived neurotrophic factor on periodontal furcation defects: Stem cells in craniofacial and dental tissue engineering. *Orthodontic and Craniofacial Research* 8, 54.

Roriz, V.M., Souza, S.L., Taba, M., Jr, et al. (2006). Treatment of Class III furcation defects with expanded polytetrafluoroethylene membrane associated or not with anorganic bone matrix/synthetic cell-binding peptide: A histologic and histomorphometric study in dogs. *Journal of Periodontology* 77, 490–497.

Rossa, C., Marcantonio, E., Jr, Cirelli, J.A. et al. (2000). Regeneration of Class III furcation defects with basic fibroblast growth factor (b-FGF) associated with GTR: A descriptive and histometric study in dogs. *Journal of Periodontology* 71, 775–784.

Rusche, B. (2003). The 3Rs and animal welfare: Conflict or the way forward? *ALTEX* 20, 63–76.

Saito, A., Saito, E., Kuboki, Y. et al. (2013). Periodontal regeneration following application of basic fibroblast growth factor-2 in combination with beta tricalcium phosphate in class III furcation defects in dogs. *Dental Materials Journal* 232, 256–262.

Saito, E., Saito, A., Kuboki, Y. et al. (2012). Periodontal repair following implantation of beta-tricalcium phosphate with different pore structures in Class III furcation defects in dogs. *Dental Materials Journal* 31, 681–688.

Sander, L., and Karring, T. (1995). New attachment and bone formation in periodontal defects following treatment of submerged roots with guided tissue regeneration. *Journal of Clinical Periodontology* 22, 295–299.

Sanz, M., Jepsen, K., Eickholz, P., and Jepsen, S. (2015). Clinical concepts for regenerative therapy in furcations. *Periodontology 2000* 68, 308–332.

Schmitz, J.P., and Hollinger, J.O. (1986). The critical size defect as an experimental model for craniomandibulofacial nonunions. *Clinical Orthopaedics and Related Research* 205, 299–308.

Schou, S., Holmstrup, P., and Kornman, K.S. (1993). Non-human primates used in studies of periodontal disease pathogenesis: A review of the literature. *Journal of Periodontology* 64, 497–508.

Sculean, A., Nikolidakis, D., and Schwarz, F. (2008). Regeneration of periodontal tissues: Combinations of barrier membranes and grafting materials – biological foundation and preclinical evidence: A systematic review. *Journal of Clinical Periodontology* 35, 106–116.

Sculean, A., Windisch, P., Döri, F. et al. (2007). Emdogain in regenerative periodontal therapy: A review of the literature. *Fogorvosi Szemle* 100, 220–232.

Selvig, K.A. (1994). Discussion: Animal models in reconstructive therapy. *Journal of Periodontology* 65, 1169–1172.

Seo, B.M., Miura, M., Gronthos, S. et al. (2004). Investigation of multipotent postnatal stem cells from human periodontal ligament. *Lancet* 10–16, 149–155.

Shirakata, Y., Miron, R.J., Nakamura, T. et al. (2017). Effects of EMD liquid (Osteogain) on periodontal healing in class III furcation defects in monkeys. *Journal of Clinical Periodontology* 44, 298–307.

Simsek, S.B., Keles, G.C., Baris, S., and Cetinkaya, B.O. (2012). Comparison of mesenchymal stem cells and autogenous cortical bone graft in the treatment of class II furcation defects in dogs. *Clinical Oral Investigation* 16, 251–258.

Soares, F.P., Hayashi, F., Yorioka, C.W. et al. (2005). Repair of Class II furcation defects after a reparative tissue graft obtained from extraction sockets treated with growth factors: A histologic and histometric study in dogs. *Journal of Periodontology* 76, 1681–1689.

Stavropoulos, A., and Wikesjö, U.M. (2012). Growth and differentiation factors for periodontal regeneration: A review on factors with clinical testing. *Journal of Periodontal Research* 47, 545–553.

Struillou, X., Boutigny, H., Badran, Z. et al. (2011). Treatment of periodontal defects in dogs using an injectable composite hydrogel/biphasic calcium phosphate. *Journal of Material Sciences Materials in Medicine* 22, 1707–1717.

Struillou, X., Boutigny, H., Soueidan, A., and Layrolle, P. (2010). Experimental animal models in periodontology: A review. *Open Dental Journal* 4, 37–47.

Suaid, F.A., Macedo, G.O., Novaes, A.B. et al. (2010). The bone formation capabilities of the anorganic bone matrix-synthetic cell-binding peptide 15 grafts in an animal periodontal model: A histologic and histomorphometric study in dogs. *Journal of Periodontology* 81, 594–603.

Suaid, F.F., Ribeiro, F.V., Gomes, T.R. et al. (2012). Autologous periodontal ligament cells in the treatment of Class III furcation defects: A study in dogs. *Journal of Clinical Periodontology* 39, 377–384.

Suaid, F.F., Ribeiro, F.V., Rodrigues, T.L. et al. (2011). Autologous periodontal ligament cells in the treatment of class II furcation defects: A study in dogs. *Journal of Clinical Periodontology* 38, 491–498.

Takahashi, D., Odajima, T., Morita, M. et al. (2005). Formation and resolution of ankylosis under application of recombinant human bone morphogenetic protein-2 (rhBMP-2) to class III furcation defects in cats. *Journal of Periodontal Research* 40, 299–305.

Takayama, S., Murakami, S., Shimabukuro, Y. et al. (2001). Periodontal regeneration by FGF-2 (bFGF) in primate models. *Journal of Dental Research* 80, 2075–2079.

Teares, J.A., Petit, J.C., and Ripamonti, U. (2012). Synergistic induction of periodontal tissue regeneration by binary application of human osteogenic protein-1 and human transforming growth factor-β3 in Class II furcation defects of Papio ursinus. *Journal of Periodontal Research* 47, 336–344.

Teares, J.A., Ramoshebi, L.N., and Ripamonti, U. (2008). Periodontal tissue regeneration by recombinant human transforming growth factor-beta 3 in Papio ursinus. *Journal of Periodontal Research* 43, 1–8.

Trombelli, L., and Farina, R (2008). Clinical outcomes with bioactive agents alone or in combination with grafting or guided tissue regeneration. *Journal of Clinical Periodontology* 35, 117–135.

Trubiani, O., Di Primio, R., Traini, T. et al. (2005). Morphological and cytofluorimetric analysis of adult mesenchymal stem cells expanded ex vivo from periodontal ligament. *International Journal of Immunopathology and Pharmacology* 18, 213–221.

Wang, S., Liu, Y., Fang, D., and Shi, S. (2007). The miniature pig: A useful large animal model for dental and orofacial research. *Oral Disease* 13, 530–537.

Wang, Y., Chai, Z., Zhang, Y. et al. (2014). Influence of low-intensity pulsed ultrasound on osteogenic tissue regeneration in a periodontal injury model: X-ray image alterations assessed by micro-computed tomography. *Ultrasonics* 54, 1581–1584.

White, C., Jr., Hancock, E.B., Garetto, L.P., and Kafrawy, A.A. (1994). A histomorphometric study on the healing of class III furcations utilizing bone labelling in beagle dogs. *Journal of Periodontology* 65, 84–92.

Wikesjö, U.M., Guglielmoni, P., Promsudthi, A. et al. (1999). Periodontal repair in dogs: Effect of rhBMP-2 concentration on regeneration of alveolar bone and periodontal attachment. *Journal of Clinical Periodontology* 26, 392–400.

Wikesjö, U.M., Kean, C.J., and Zimmerman, G.J. (1994). Periodontal repair in dogs: Supraalveolar defect models for evaluation of safety and efficacy of periodontal reconstructive therapy. *Journal of Periodontology* 65, 1151–1157.

Wikesjö, U.M., Lim, W.H., Thomson, R.C. et al. (2003a). Periodontal repair in dogs: Evaluation of a bioabsorbable space-providing macroporous membrane with recombinant human bone morphogenetic protein-2. *Journal of Periodontology* 74, 635–647.

Wikesjö, U.M., Xiropaidis, A.V., Thomson, R.C. et al. (2003b). Periodontal repair in dogs: Space-providing ePTFE devices increase rhBMP-2/ACS-induced bone formation. *Journal of Clinical Periodontology* 30, 715–725.

Wohlfahrt, J.C., Aass, A.M., Rønold, H.J. et al. (2012). Microcomputed tomographic and histologic analysis of animal experimental degree II furcation defects treated with porous titanium granules or deproteinized bovine bone. *Journal of Periodontology* 83, 211–221.

Yang, J.R., Hsu, C.W., Liao, S.C. et al. (2013). Transplantation of embryonic stem cells improves the regeneration of periodontal furcation defects in a porcine model. *Journal of Clinical Periodontology* 40, 364–371.

Zetterström, O., Andersson, C., Eriksson, L. et al. (1997). Clinical safety of enamel matrix derivative (EMDOGAIN) in the treatment of periodontal defects. *Journal of Clinical Periodontology* 24, 697–704.

Chapter 7

Regenerative Therapy of Furcations in Human Clinical Studies: What has been Achieved So Far?

Søren Jepsen and Karin Jepsen

Department of Periodontology, Operative and Preventive Dentistry, University of Bonn, Germany

7.1 Introduction

Different strategies are available to address the problem of furcation involvement (FI). One option is the elimination of the furcation defect. This can be achieved by removal of the involved root(s) using resective approaches (see Chapter 8). Alternatively, periodontal tissues that have been destroyed by periodontitis can be regenerated, thereby decreasing the lesion. Regenerative periodontal therapy of furcation defects has proven successful in many experimental pre-clinical studies (see Chapter 6).

This chapter reviews the evidence for the effectiveness of regenerative therapy for the treatment of furcation defects in different clinical scenarios, in order to address the question: 'What has been achieved so far?'

7.2 Outcome Measures for Regenerative Therapy in Furcation Defects

A variety of outcome measures can be considered to assess the effectiveness of regenerative furcation therapies.

7.2.1 Human Histology

Evidence for periodontal regeneration requires the histological demonstration of restored tooth-supporting tissues, including cementum, periodontal ligament, and alveolar bone, over a previously diseased root surface. Even though such outcomes have been demonstrated in well-controlled experimental animal studies for a variety of treatment modalities (see Chapter 6), information derived from human histology is scarce. Four histological studies investigated human degree II furcation defects (Harris 2002; Stoller et al. 2001; Camelo et al. 2003; Nevins et al. 2003), one studied degree III defects (Mellonig et al. 2009), while one presented data from degree II and III furcation defects (Gottlow et al. 1986).

7.2.1.1 Degree II Furcation Defects

Regarding degree II defects, all five studies reported partial regeneration of the periodontal tissues. Two studies applied demineralized freeze-dried bone allograft (DFDBA) combined with recombinant human platelet-derived growth factor-BB (rhPDGF-BB) and reported formation of bone, cementum, and periodontal ligament coronally to the notch (Camelo et al. 2003; Nevins et al. 2003). Two other studies used barrier membranes (guided tissue regeneration, GTR) and described formation of cementum, periodontal ligament, and bone (Gottlow et al. 1986; Stoller et al. 2001). Harris (2002) used a combination (DFDBA + polyhydroxyalkanoate [PHA] + tetracycline + resorbable

Diagnosis and Treatment of Furcation-Involved Teeth, First Edition. Edited by Luigi Nibali.
© 2018 John Wiley & Sons Ltd. Published 2018 by John Wiley & Sons Ltd.
Companion website: www.wiley.com/go/nibali/diagnosis

membrane) and observed partial defect closure with new bone, cementum, and connective tissue attachment coronal or limited to the notch area.

7.2.1.2 Degree III Furcation Defects

The two studies evaluating degree III furcation defects reported only partial regeneration. Gottlow et al. (1986), using barrier membranes (GTR), demonstrated 2.8 mm new cementum with inserting collagen fibres in a 7 mm furcation defect. Mellonig et al. (2009), using a combined technique (rhPDGF + beta-tricalcium phosphate [β-TCP] + collagen membrane) reported partial closure in three out of the four defects. The histomorphometric data revealed new cementum ranging from 0.0 to 5.5 mm, while the length of new bone and new collagen fibres ranged from 0.0 to 2.0 mm.

7.2.2 Clinical Outcomes

From a clinical point of view, complete elimination of the inter-radicular defect appears to be the most important outcome. Decreasing furcation degree is associated with a decreased long-term tooth loss risk (see Chapter 5). Thus, the main outcome variables for studies evaluating the efficacy of regenerative techniques in furcations are change of furcation status (conversion into class I or complete closure) and horizontal hard-tissue fill. As histological evidence for successful furcation regeneration is not a practical outcome variable for controlled clinical trials, changes in direct bone measurements (horizontal probing bone level, at surgery and during re-entry) serve as primary outcome variables for evaluating clinical success, while clinical attachment level gain (horizontal/vertical probing attachment level), probing depth reduction (horizontal/vertical), and radiographic assessments may serve as secondary outcomes (Machtei 1997). Bone fill during a re-entry procedure is the only component of a regenerated periodontium that can be accurately assessed clinically. In fact, it was stated at a European consensus conference that it would be desirable for all future

GTR studies to report the reduction in horizontal probing during re-entry, and also the frequency (predictability) of complete furcation closure (Jepsen et al. 2002).

As an alternative to open probing bone level assessments during a re-entry procedure, probing bone measurements were proposed and evaluated (Suh et al. 2002). In some clinical trials, horizontal probing bone level was assessed after only six months, and it may be speculated that this is too early for a final evaluation of bone fill in furcation defects. Patient-reported outcomes following regenerative furcation surgery may include postoperative pain, the rate of complications, perceived benefit, and change in quality of life (see Chapter 13).

7.3 Clinical Scenarios

Most of the currently available clinical studies to date have been devoted to mandibular molars with buccal/lingual degree II furcation defects and maxillary molars with buccal/interproximal degree II furcation defects. More limited information is available on mandibular degree III furcation defects and maxillary degree III furcation defects, whereas there is a paucity of data on regenerative treatment in degree I furcations and in maxillary premolars (Avila-Ortiz et al. 2015; Reddy et al. 2015).

The efficacy of various regenerative approaches in furcation defects has been evaluated by several systematic reviews with or without meta-analyses (Jepsen et al. 2002; Murphy and Gunsolley 2003; Reynolds et al. 2003; Kinaia et al. 2011; Chen et al. 2013; Avila-Ortiz et al. 2015) and has also been addressed in a recent comprehensive narrative review (Sanz et al. 2015), which served as a basis for this chapter.

7.3.1 Degree II Furcation Defects

7.3.1.1 Barrier Membranes (GTR)
After clinical case series (Becker et al. 1988) had demonstrated promising results for GTR

therapy in furcation defects using expanded PTFE barriers (Gore-Tex Periodontal Membrane, W.L. Gore and Assoc., Flagstaff, AZ, USA), several randomized controlled clinical trials compared GTR therapy with open-flap debridement (OFD, representing standard control treatment) in human degree II furcation defects. Several studies observed more favourable horizontal probing attachment level gain and horizontal probing bone level gain after GTR than after OFD in degree II furcation defects of mandibular molars (Pontoriero et al. 1988; Lekovic et al. 1989, 1991; Mellonig et al. 1994; Wang et al. 1994; Mombelli et al. 1996; Prathibha et al. 2002; Cury et al. 2003; Bremm et al. 2004; see also Table 7.1), of maxillary molars (Metzler et al. 1991; Mellonig et al. 1994; Pontoriero and Lindhe 1995a; Avera et al. 1998; see also Table 7.2), and of maxillary and mandibular molars (Flanary et al. 1991; Paul et al. 1992; Twohey et al. 1992; Caton et al. 1994; Yukna and Yukna 1996; see also Table 7.3). Whereas some authors observed more favourable results six months after GTR therapy in maxillary degree II furcations only in buccal sites (Pontoriero and Lindhe 1995a), others reported statistically better horizontal probing bone level gain also in mesiopalatal degree II furcations nine months following GTR (Avera et al. 1998).

A systematic review with meta-analyses assessed the efficacy of membrane therapy in the treatment of periodontal furcation defects measured against standard surgical periodontal treatment (i.e. OFD; Jepsen et al. 2002), and confirmed the superiority of GTR over OFD in class II furcation defects; however, the results also showed significant heterogeneity, indicating high variability. These results were subsequently also confirmed by other systematic reviews (Murphy and Gunsolley 2003; Kinaia et al. 2011). This variability may be explained by prognostic factors (e.g. smoking, peri-surgical antibiotics, or defect morphology; Bowers et al. 2003; Horwitz et al. 2004). Deep pockets at baseline facilitate more favourable results after regenerative therapy (Machtei et al. 1994;

Horwitz et al. 2004). However, other authors have found deep baseline pockets to be associated with significant reductions in the number of complete furcation closures (Bowers et al. 2003). This discrepancy may be a result of differences in bone morphology. Wide furcations respond less favourably and in deep degree II furcations (≥5mm) complete closure is less likely (Bowers et al. 2003). If the fornix of the furcation is located apically to the interproximal alveolar crest (key-hole defect), more horizontal attachment gain may be expected than in teeth with a furcation fornix located coronally of the interproximal bone level. If there is bone coronal of the furcation fornix adjacent to the tooth, coverage and stabilization of the membrane may be achieved by a coronal positioning of the flap. Under such conditions, the surface of the periodontal ligament to provide cells to colonize the blood clot within the defect is larger than in a tooth where the fornix is located coronal of the alveolar crest (Bowers et al. 2003; Horwitz et al. 2004).

When comparing the use of non-resorbable and biodegradable barrier membranes in the treatment of mandibular degree II furcation defects, similar horizontal defect fill has been reported (Blumenthal 1993; Bouchard et al. 1993; Christgau et al. 1995; Hugoson et al. 1995; Yukna and Yukna 1996; Caffesse et al. 1997; Eickholz et al. 1997, 1998; Garrett et al. 1997; Scott et al. 1997; Dos Anjos et al. 1998; Pruthi et al. 2002; see also Table 7.4). Only a few studies have compared the clinical efficacy of different bioabsorbable barrier membranes for treatment of Class II furcations; none found one bioabsorbable material to be superior to another (Vernino et al. 1999; Eickholz et al. 2000).

7.3.1.2 Combination Therapy (GTR and Bone Grafts)
The combination of a barrier membrane with a filler material may enhance the horizontal fill of molars with degree II FI as shown in a systematic review with meta-analysis (Chen et al. 2013). Out of four studies

Table 7.1 Comparison of clinical results after open-flap debridement and guided tissue regeneration in degree II furcation defects of mandibular molars.

Authors	Study type	Parameter	Open-flap debridement baseline (mm)	Gain (mm)	n	Guided tissue regeneration baseline (mm)	Gain (mm)	n	Barrier material/filler	Observation period
Lekovic et al. 1989	RCT	Horizontal probing bone level *Buccal*	No data	−0.14	12	No data	0.18	12[a]	Expanded polytetrafluoroethylene	6 months
Lekovic et al. 1991	RCT	Horizontal probing bone level *Buccal*	4.2	−0.2	15	4.2	1.6*	15[a]	Connective tissue graft including periosteum	6 months
Mellonig et al. 1994	RCT	Horizontal probing bone level	7.6	1.0	11	8.4	4.5*	11[a]	Expanded polytetrafluoroethylene	6 months
Wang et al. 1994	RCT	Horizontal probing bone level	5.58	1.08	12	6.00	2.04*	12[a]	BioMend[a,b]	12 months
Prathibha et al. 2002	RCT	Horizontal probing bone level	4.7	0.64	10	4.79	2.38*	10[a]	TefGen[c]	6 months
Comparison of open-flap debridement with guided tissue regeneration in combination with fillers										
Houser et al. 2001	RCT	Horizontal probing bone level	6.2	0.9	13	5.7	3.0*	18	BioGide[a,d] and BioOss®	
Tsao et al. 2006	RCT	Horizontal probing bone level	4.7	0.2	9	4.3 4.4	1.1* 1.1*	9 9	Puros[a,e] BioMend and Puros	6 months

*Statistically significant difference between open-flap debridement and guided tissue regeneration;
[a] split-mouth design;
[b] bovine type 1 collagen;
[c] polytetrafluoroethylene;
[d] deproteinized bovine bone mineral/porcine collagen;
[e] mineralized solvent-dehydrated bone allograft;
RCT = randomized controlled trial.

Table 7.2 Comparison of clinical results after open-flap debridement and guided tissue regeneration in degree II furcation defects of maxillary molars.

Authors	Study type	Parameter	Open-flap debridement baseline (mm)	Gain (mm)	n	Guided tissue regeneration baseline (mm)	Gain (mm)	n	Barrier material	Observation period
Metzler et al. 1991	RCT	Horizontal probing bone level *Buccal and interproximal*	3.7	0.3	17	3.7	0.9*	17[a]	Expanded polytetrafluoroethylene	6 months
Mellonig et al. 1994	RCT	Horizontal probing bone level	4.5	0.3	8	4.9	1.0*	8[a]	Expanded polytetrafluoroethylene	6 months
Pontoriero and Lindhe 1995a	RCT	Horizontal probing bone level						10[a]	Expanded polytetrafluoroethylene	6 months
		Buccal	3.2	0.3	10	3.2	1.1*	10[a]		
		Mesiolingual	3.4	0.2	8	3.5	0.4	8[a]		
		Distolingual	3.2	0.2	8	3.4	0.2	8[a]		
Avera et al. 1998	RCT	Horizontal probing bone level *Mesiolingual*	No data	-0.69		No data	1.19*		Expanded polytetrafluoroethylene	9 months

*Statistically significant difference between open-flap debridement and guided tissue regeneration;
[a] split-mouth design;
RCT = randomized controlled trial.

Table 7.3 Comparison of clinical results after open-flap debridement and guided tissue regeneration in degree II furcation defects of maxillary and mandibular molars.

Authors	Study type	Parameter	Open-flap debridement baseline (mm)	Gain (mm)	n	Guided tissue regeneration baseline (mm)	Gain (mm)	n	Barrier material	Observation period
Flanary et al. 1991	RCT	Horizontal probing bone level	2.9	0.8	19	3.3	1.5*	19[a]	Biobrane[a,b]	6 months
Paul et al. 1992 (132)	RCT	Horizontal probing bone level	3.86	0	7	4.71	0.86*	7[a]	Collistar[a,b]	6 months
Twohey et al. 1992	RCT	Horizontal probing bone level *Buccal*	2.6	0.3	8	3.3	1.4*	8[a]	Biobrane	6 months
Yukna and Yukna 1996	RCT	Horizontal probing bone level	5.3	1.1	27	5.0	2.0*	27[a]	BioMend[a,c]	6–12 months (mean = 11.1 months)

*Statistically significant difference between open-flap debridement and guided tissue regeneration;
[a]split-mouth design;
[b]poly-dimethyl-siloxane mechanically bonded to a fine-knit, flexible nylon fabric;
[c]bovine type 1 collagen;
RCT = randomized controlled trial.

Table 7.4 Comparison of clinical results after guided tissue regeneration using expanded polytetrafluoroethylene and biodegradable barriers in degree II furcation defects of maxillary and/or mandibular molars.

Authors	Defect type	Parameter	Expanded polytetrafluoroethylene baseline (mm)	Gain (mm)	n	Biodegradable baseline (mm)	Gain (mm)	n	Barrier material	Observation period
Bouchard et al. 1993	Mandibular molars *Buccal*	Horizontal probing bone level	No data	2.2	12	No data	*	12[a]	Connective tissue graft	12 months
Yukna and Yukna 1996	Maxillary and mandibular molars	Horizontal probing bone level	4.3	1.7	32	4.7	1.5	32[a]	BioMend[*,b]	6–12 months (mean = 11.1 months)
Scott et al. 1997	Mandibular molars	Horizontal probing bone level	5.0	2.2	12	5.4	2.0	12[a]	LamBone[c]	6 months
Dos Anjos et al. 1998	Mandibular molars	Horizontal probing bone level	3.8	2.87	15	4.0	2.93	15[a]	Gengiflex[d]	6 months
Pruthi et al. 2002	Mandibular molars	Horizontal probing bone level	2.00	0.41	17	2.00	0.41	17[a]	BioMend	12 months

*Statistically significant difference between expanded polytetrafluoroethylene and biodegradable barriers;
[a] split-mouth design;
[b] bovine type 1 collagen;
[c] laminar bone membrane and particulate decalcified freeze-dried bone;
[d] cellulose.

on mandibular molars, two showed statistically significantly more horizontal bone fill following the combination therapy (Wallace et al. 1994; Luepke et al. 1997; Simonpietri et al. 2000; Maragos et al. 2002; see also Table 7.5).

7.3.1.3 Long-term Results

Long-term data following GTR therapy in furcation defects are sparse (Figueira et al. 2014). Using GTR, horizontal probing attachment level gains from 0.75 to 4.1 mm and horizontal probing bone level gains from 0.2 to 4.5 mm may be achieved, and degree II furcation defects may be closed or converted to degree I. Molars with degree I FI have a better long-term prognosis than molars with degree II defects (McGuire and Nunn 1996), whereas a gradual increase in the risk of tooth loss was observed for molars with degree II and III FI (Nibali et al. 2016). To date there are only limited data on the long-term results (≥4 years) after GTR therapy in degree II furcations. Significant gains in horizontal attachment (2.59 mm) were obtained one year post surgery for GTR-treated sites. These changes were maintained over four years with a slight decline at the end of year 3 (Machtei et al. 1996). Mean horizontal probing attachment level gains after the use of non-resorbable and biodegradable barriers could be maintained for five years (Eickholz et al. 2001). A 10-year follow-up of 18 teeth in 9 patients revealed further stability of horizontal probing attachment level gains between 12 and 120 months. However, two molars were lost in one patient, and another molar lost more than 2 mm of horizontal probing attachment level (Eickholz et al. 2006).

7.3.1.4 Enamel Matrix Derivative (EMD)

Only a limited number of clinical studies have evaluated enamel matrix derivative (Emdogain, Straumann, Basel, Switzerland) for the treatment of FI, either alone or in combination with another regenerative therapy (for review Donos et al. 2010; Koop et al. 2012; Miron et al. 2014, 2016), and no meta-analyses have been performed.

Mandibular Molars

In a case series study with 36 months of follow-up on 10 patients with 8 buccal and 8 lingual degree II FI, the use of EMD was evaluated (Donos et al. 2003a). The follow-up periods were 6, 12, and 36 months. At the buccal furcation defects, the horizontal probing attachment level measurements were reduced from 4.0 mm at baseline to 2.6 mm at 6 months, demonstrating a mean horizontal probing attachment level change of 1.4 mm. However, at 12 and 36 months the change was reduced to 0.8 mm and 0.6 mm, respectively, and, as such, the horizontal probing attachment level changes were not adequate to transform the degree II FI to degree I. At the lingual sites, the horizontal probing attachment level changes were minimal. In all cases, following the 12-month healing period the furcation defects remained as degree II. This study was performed in a small number of mandibular molars, and it did not have a control group in which either OFD or another established regenerative procedure, such as GTR, was performed.

When investigating the adjunctive use of EMD with OFD in 10 patients with 20 degree II furcation defects on contralateral molars by re-entry after 6 months, a significantly enhanced horizontal bone gain (2 mm in the EMD vs 0.8 mm in the OFD group) of the bony defects was found in EMD-treated furcations (Chitsazi et al. 2007). Complete furcation closure was reported in 1 of the 10 defects treated with EMD. However, a re-entry at 6 months post-operatively may be too early to evaluate bone fill of a furcation lesion.

A multi-centre randomized controlled clinical trial compared EMD with GTR in the treatment of degree II buccal furcation defects in mandibular molars (Jepsen et al. 2004). In this study, the investigators treated 45 patients with a total of 90 similar degree II furcation defects on contralateral molars, either with EMD or with a bioresorbable membrane. The clinical measurements performed at baseline, 8 months, and 14 months following surgery included

Table 7.5 Comparison of clinical results after guided tissue regeneration using a barrier membrane alone and in combination with osseous grafts in degree II furcation defects of mandibular molars (all randomized controlled trials).

Authors	Defect type	Parameter	Guided tissue regeneration barrier material alone (baseline) (mm)	Gain (mm)	n	Guided tissue regeneration barrier material + osseous graft baseline (mm)	Gain (mm)	n	Osseous graft material	Observation period
Wallace et al. 1994	Mandibular molars	Horizontal probing bone level *Buccal*	Expanded polytetrafluoroethylene 6.0	2.3	7	6.5	2.4	10	Decalcified freeze-dried bone allograft[b]	12 months
Luepke et al. 1997	Mandibular molars	Horizontal probing bone level	Guidor[c] 6.03	1.80	14	5.90	2.1	14[a]	Decalcified freeze-dried bone allograft[b]	6 months
Simonpietri-C et al. 2000	Mandibular molars	Horizontal probing bone level	Gengiflex*[d] 5.0	2.47	15	5.53	3.27*	15[a]	Bon-Apatite*[e]	6 months
Maragos et al. 2002	Mandibular molars	Horizontal probing bone level	CaSO4 3.8	0.9	11	3.5 / 3.7	1.2 / 2.2	11 / 14	CaSO4/doxycycline CaSO4/decalcified freeze-dried bone allograft[b]	12 months

*Statistically significant difference between guided tissue regeneration and guided tissue regeneration + osseous grafts;
[a] split-mouth design;
[b] decalcified freeze-dried bone allograft;
[c] synthetic biodegradable polymer;
[d] cellulose;
[e] anorganic bovine bone.

gingival margin levels, pocket probing depth, bleeding on probing, vertical attachment levels, vertical bone sounding from a stent at five buccal sites per tooth, and horizontal bone sounding at the furcation area. Similar defect measurements were performed during a re-entry procedure on all defects at 14 months post surgery. Change of horizontal furcation depth (comparing intrasurgical baseline and re-entry measurements) served as the primary outcome variable. The results indicated that both regenerative procedures produced clinical improvement. More specifically, EMD demonstrated a mean reduction of horizontal probing bone level of 2.6 mm, whereas the GTR-treated sites showed a horizontal probing bone level reduction of 1.9 mm (Table 7.6). Complete furcation closure was achieved in 8 of the 45 furcation defects treated with EMD and in 3 of the 45 defects treated with GTR. Partial closure (resulting in a change from degree II to degree I) was the same (27 of 45) in both groups. No change in furcation status was observed in 9 of 45 and in 11 of 45 defects, respectively, and deterioration was observed in one of 45 EMD-treated sites and in four of 45 GTR-treated sites. Furthermore, less post-operative pain and swelling was reported following the use of EMD, which could be explained by the antibacterial (Sculean et al. 2001) or anti-inflammatory potential that EMD might possess (Myhre et al. 2006; Nokhbehsaim et al. 2012). The study concluded that the use of EMD not only has a similar effect to GTR in transforming degree II buccal furcation defects to degree I in a predictable manner, but it may also achieve complete closure of the furcation defects to a greater extent than GTR. Furthermore, for furcation defects at mid-buccal sites, the EMD-treated sites presented less gingival recession than the GTR-treated sites (Meyle et al. 2004). This could be attributed to the fact that no measurable bone resorption occurred in the EMD-treated sites, whereas slight bone resorption occurred in the GTR-treated sites.

From the same sample of patients, it was also observed that the best clinical outcome in buccal degree II furcation defects following treatment with EMD was in male patients over 54 years of age who were non-smokers (Hoffmann et al. 2006), which is in agreement with observations in previous studies with GTR (Machtei et al. 1994). However, these results need to be interpreted with caution, because the number of patients in each subgroup (age, gender, smoking habit, etc.) was relatively low. Furthermore, in this study patient selection was of paramount clinical importance, because all selected teeth presented with proximal levels at or above the fornix of the furcation and there was always a zone of keratinized tissue of at least 2 mm present, for covering the furcation following the application of EMD. Similar results, with regard to the treatment with EMD in mandibular degree II FI, were reported in another randomized controlled trial with re-entry after 12 months (Barros et al. 2005). In 10 patients with 20 paired furcation defects, GTR therapy using an expanded PTFE membrane led to a mean horizontal defect fill of 3.3 mm, whereas EMD application resulted in a mean horizontal defect fill of 2.2 mm, with no significant difference between the modalities (Table 7.6).

Maxillary Molars

A randomized controlled trial with a split-mouth design in 15 patients with one pair of contralateral degree II proximal FI compared the use of EMD with OFD in conjunction with conditioning of the root surfaces with ethylenediaminetetraacetic acid (EDTA) gel (Casarin et al. 2008). At 6 months, a mean horizontal bone gain was 1.0 mm for the control group and 1.1 mm for the test group. However, there was a statistically significant difference in the number of remaining degree II FI, in favour of EMD. Of 15 proximal degree II furcations, 2 were completely closed and 9 were converted into degree I, 6 months following EMD application. In contrast, following OFD, only 5 furcations were converted into degree I, with the other

Table 7.6 Comparison of clinical results after guided tissue regeneration or enamel matrix derivative (Emdogain) application in degree II furcation defects of mandibular molars.

Authors	Study type	Parameter	Guided tissue regeneration baseline (mm)	Gain (mm)	n	EMD baseline (mm)	Gain (mm)	n	Barrier material/ filler	Observation period
Jepsen et al. 2004	RCT	Horizontal probing bone level *Buccal*	No data	1.9	45	No data	2.6*	45[a]	Resolut*[b]	14 months
Barros et al. 2005	RCT	Horizontal probing bone level	No data	3.3	15	No data	2.2	15[a]	Expanded polytetrafluoro-ethylene	6 months

*Statistically significant difference between guided tissue regeneration and enamel matrix derivative;
[a]split-mouth design;
[b]synthetic biodegradable polymer;
RCT = randomized controlled trial.

10 defects remaining degree II. Of the 15 patients, 12 were followed up for 24 months (Casarin et al. 2010) and at this time point the test group presented with 5 remaining degree II furcations versus 10 degree II furcations in the control group (p < 0.05). Overall, the treatment response of proximal furcations in maxillary molars to EMD application was not as favourable as that of mandibular furcations. The authors attributed this to more difficult access and higher plaque retention during follow up.

7.3.1.5 Combination Therapy (EMD and Bone Grafts)

Only a few clinical studies have evaluated the combination of EMD with bone grafts or bone substitutes in furcation defects (Miron et al. 2014).

Mandibular Molars

In a case series of 11 patients, each contributing one buccal mandibular degree II furcation defect, a combination therapy of EMD and autologous bone grafts was evaluated (Aimetti et al. 2007). After two years, complete clinical closure was achieved in four sites and all residual defects were reduced to degree I.

A comparative study tested the effectiveness of EMD in combination with DFDBA and a resorbable membrane (GTR; Jaiswal and Deo 2013). Using a parallel design, 30 buccal or lingual mandibular degree II furcations in 30 patients received either EMD + DFDBA + GTR, DFDBA + GTR, or OFD. After 12 months, mean reductions in horizontal probing depths were 2.1 mm for the EMD + DFDBA + GTR group and 1.5 mm for the DFDBA + GTR group (p > 0.05). The number of degree II furcations that were closed or converted to class I was greater for EMD + DFDBA + GTR.

A recently published parallel group randomized controlled trial with 40 patients compared EMD, beta-tricalcium phosphate coated hydroxyapatite (ß-TCP/HA), and EMD + ß-TCP/HA in buccal mandibular degree II furcation defects (Queiroz et al. 2016). After 12 months, the mean horizontal clinical attachment level gain was 2.7 mm for EMD, 2.6 mm for β-TCP/HA, and 2.9 mm for EMD + β-TCP/HA, with no significant differences among the groups. After 12 months, 13 of 13 furcations in the EMD group, 10 of 14 furcations in the β-TCP/HA group, and 12 of 14 furcations in the β-TCP/HA + EMD group improved their diagnoses to degree I. However, complete furcation closure was not detectable during the study period.

Maxillary Molars

A randomized controlled trial evaluated the combination of EMD + ß-TCP/HA compared with ß-TCP/HA alone in 30 patients with 30 proximal class II furcation defects in maxillary molars (Peres et al. 2013). Mean horizontal bone level gains after 6 months were 1.7 mm for both treatment modalities. The EMD + ß-TCP/HA group showed 7 closed furcations and 7 converted to degree I, versus 4 closed furcations and 10 converted to degree I in the ß-TCP/HA group ($p > 0.05$).

At present, no long-term data (>3 years) are available for the effects of EMD application in the regenerative therapy of furcation defects.

7.3.1.6 Platelet Concentrates

Growth and differentiation factor technologies have been evaluated for their potential to enhance periodontal wound healing/regeneration (Stavropoulos and Wikesjö 2012). Autologous platelet concentrates, such as platelet-rich plasma (PRP) and platelet-rich fibrin (PRF), are a source for growth factors that can be applied to the periodontal wound (Dohan Ehrenfest et al. 2009; Del Fabbro et al. 2011). Very recently, systematic reviews with meta-analyses have evaluated the regenerative potential of these approaches for furcation defects (Troiano et al. 2016; Castro et al. 2017). While three original studies were included in one systematic review (Troiano et al. 2016), the other included only two of them (Castro et al. 2017). These studies are presented in more detail in what follows.

Mandibular Molars

In a randomized clinical trial of six months' duration using a split-mouth design (Pradeep et al. 2009), the effectiveness of autologous PRP was compared with OFD in the treatment of 20 patients with a total of 40 mandibular degree II furcation defects. Although there was significantly more horizontal clinical attachment level gain (2.5 mm vs 0.8 mm) and radiographic bone fill following the

application of PRP, all furcation defects retained their degree II status.

Another randomized controlled trial of nine months' duration evaluated in a split-mouth design the use of autologous PRF in the treatment of mandibular degree II furcation defects in comparison with OFD, in 18 patients with 36 furcations (Sharma and Pradeep 2011). Complete clinical closure was achieved in 12 of 18 test defects, whereas another 5 were reduced to degree I. Change in horizontal clinical attachment level amounted to 2.7 mm following PRF versus 1.9 mm following OFD ($p < 0.05$).

A randomized controlled trial compared PRP, PRF, and OFD in the treatment of 72 mandibular degree II furcations in 42 patients after nine months (Bajaj et al. 2013). In this study, both forms of autologous platelet concentrates led to significantly better outcomes in all clinical and radiographic parameters compared with the OFD control, with no differences between PRP and PRF. Horizontal clinical attachment gain amounted to 2.75 mm (PRF) and 2.5 mm (PRP).

It should be noted that all these studies are from the same centre. More recently the authors have published modified PRF protocols using the addition of synthetic statins and hydroxyapatite (HA) bone grafts (Pradeep et al. 2016), or the addition of alendronate gel (Kanoriya et al. 2017), thereby further enhancing the outcomes of PRF therapy. Finally, another group of authors (Siddiqui et al. 2016) evaluated in a six-month study the efficacy of PRF compared to ß-TCP and to OFD alone in the treatment of degree II mandibular furcation defects. Horizontal probing bone level changes amounted to 2.1 mm, 2.2 mm, and 1.0 mm, respectively.

7.3.2 Degree III Furcation Defects

7.3.2.1 Barrier Membranes (GTR)

Only two randomized controlled clinical trials have compared OFD and GTR in molars with degree III FI (Pontoriero et al. 1989; Pontoriero and Lindhe 1995b).

Mandibular Molars

The earlier study reported therapy in mandibular molars (Pontoriero et al. 1989). After assessing FI clinically, only 1 of 42 furcations was scored as 'through-and-through' (degree III). After flap elevation, but before debridement, all 42 furcations were scored as degree III. Six months after treatment, furcation involvement was assessed clinically (i.e. without elevation of a flap). In the GTR group, 3 molars remained as degree III, whereas in the OFD group, 11 remained as degree III, indicating better results with GTR.

Maxillary Molars

OFD and GTR were also compared in the treatment of maxillary interproximal degree III furcation defects (Pontoriero and Lindhe 1995b). Baseline and six-month examinations were performed by re-entry after flap elevation. Neither OFD nor GTR led to even partial closure of the 22 degree III furcations.

These results are supported by other clinical trials, which also demonstrated very low frequency and predictability of closure in degree III furcation defects after GTR therapy: no complete and 3 partial closures of 10 degree III furcations, 12 and 24 months following GTR (Eickholz et al. 1998); and 6 partial closures of 10 degree III furcations, 24 months after GTR (Eickholz and Hausmann). Complete closure of degree III furcations (as evaluated during re-entry) was never reported (Jepsen et al. 2002).

7.3.2.2 Enamel Matrix Derivative

One case series study evaluated the treatment of degree III mandibular furcation defects by the use of EMD alone or in combination with a bioresorbable membrane (Donos et al. 2004). Nine patients with a total of 14 degree III mandibular furcation defects were assigned to one of three groups: EMD in four defects; GTR in three defects; and EMD + GTR in seven defects. None of the treatments resulted predictably in complete healing of the defects, and there was no obvious difference between the various treatment modalities. At 6 and 12 months, partial closure of the degree III involvements had occurred in 6 of the 14 treated furcations. The remaining teeth still presented through-and-through furcation defects. Within the limits of this case series, and taking into account the small number of patients and furcations included in each treatment group, it was concluded that the use of EMD alone or in combination with GTR did not result in predictable regeneration of degree III mandibular defects.

7.4 Furcation Regeneration: Step-by-step Procedure

The suggested treatment sequence is as follows:

1) *Patient selection.* Systemic factors that limit the success of periodontal surgery, such as uncontrolled diabetes and immunocompromised status, must be considered. Poor patient compliance, inadequate oral hygiene, and smoking are the most frequent patient factors limiting the selection of this procedure. Treatment options and alternatives must be presented to the patient and the potential problems and the additional costs should be discussed. Regenerative furcation surgery should be part of a comprehensive treatment plan aiming at complete periodontal and functional rehabilitation.

2) *Tooth selection.* Adequate access to the surgical site and also for future maintenance is extremely important. Molars with degree II furcations (mandibular and buccal maxillary FI) are the best candidates to be considered for a regenerative procedure. Based on the available evidence, interproximal maxillary degree II furcation defects are significantly less suited, most likely due to limited access. Degree III mandibular and maxillary furcations have shown various treatment responses and in general there are no

significant differences in treatment outcomes comparing regenerative therapy with conventional surgery. Defect and site characteristics have been identified that have impacts on the outcomes of regenerative furcation surgery (Reddy et al. 2015). For example, a thicker biotype and the absence of soft-tissue recession can positively influence healing following GTR procedures. More favourable outcomes can be expected in sites in which the remaining interproximal bone height is coronal to the entrance of the furcation defect, compared to those in which the bone is at or apical to the furcation entrance (Figure 7.1). Interdental root proximity may impair proper defect debridement. Presence of a root canal filling is not a contraindication to furcation regeneration per se, provided there are no signs of apical pathology.

3) *Regenerative periodontal surgery.* The goal is to obtain sufficient access to the defect for meticulous debridement and application of the regenerative device. In the case of isolated defects, vertical releasing incisions may be used (Figure 7.2). Alternatively, the flap can be extended laterally (Figure 7.1). Keratinized tissues should be preserved by intrasulcular incision and the elevation of a full-thickness mucoperiostal flap. Granulation tissue will be removed and the exposed root surfaces carefully cleaned by hand instruments, power-driven scalers (optionally with diamond-coated tips), or rotary instruments. Root anomalies such as enamel projections/pearls should be removed. If EMD is part of the regenerative strategy, it is usually applied following two minutes of root conditioning with EDTA and rinsing with sterile saline. Subsequently a bone graft/substitute can be used to fill the furcation defect. Alternatively, a GTR barrier membrane can be applied, with or without an additional defect filler (Figures 7.1 and 7.2). The barrier membrane is secured by a resorbable sling suture to cover the furcation

entrance and to promote wound and clot stabilization. In order to facilitate complete coverage of the barrier, the periosteum can be cut to allow for a coronal advancement of the flap. The flap is secured in a coronal position by a sling suture and interrupted sutures over the vertical releasing incisions (Figure 7.2), or interdental sutures in the case of a laterally extended flap (Figure 7.1). The patient is instructed to abstain from mechanical plaque removal in the surgical area for a period of up to four weeks. During this time, chlorhexidine rinses or topical gel application are used. The patient returns for monitoring of healing after one and two weeks, when sutures are removed. Interdental hygiene and mechanical plaque removal are started again after four weeks, and the personalized maintenance recall programme will be determined.

7.5 Furcation Regeneration: How to Take the Next Step?

It emerges clearly from this chapter that the main challenge for regenerating furcation defects is presented by improving the predictability in degree II FI (in particular maxillary interproximal furcations) and even more by achieving regeneration in degree III furcation defects (maxillary or mandibular). However, the previous chapter produced clinical and histological evidence for regeneration of degree III furcations in animal models, including complete closure with the formation of periodontal ligament and regrowth of the bone with GTR (Lindhe et al. 1995; Araújo et al. 1998) or GTR associated with EMD (Donos et al. 2003a, 2003b; Gkranias et al. 2012) in animal models. So how can we take the decisive step towards predictable furcation regeneration based on pre-clinical studies?

Complete flap coverage of the membrane during healing seems to be crucial, probably more than defect morphology (Lindhe et al. 1995; Araújo et al. 1997, 1998; Araújo and

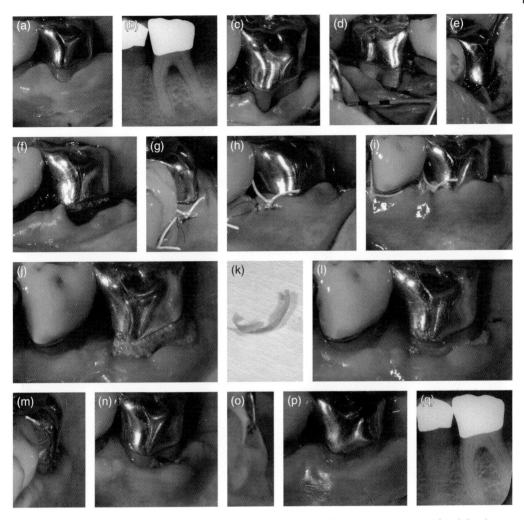

Figure 7.1 (a) Periodontal measurements at baseline, tooth no. 36 (LL6). Probing depth mesial and distal: 2 mm, furcation degree II buccally, horizontal probing: 4 mm, recession 3 mm. (b) Radiograph of tooth no.36 with visible furcation defect, adjacent bone level at forcation fornix. (c) Flap elevation: intrasulcular incision/ horizonal release, mucoperiostal flap, papillae de-epithelialized, periosteal split in the vestibule. Root surface debridement. (d) Horizontal probing bone level: 4 mm. (e, f) Placement of a bioresorbable matrix barrier (Guidor™ MSL-configuration, Sunstar Americas, Inc., Schaumburg, IL, USA) to facilitate guided tissue regeneration. Fixation of the barrier with integrated sling sutures. (g, h) Coronally advanced flap secured with sling and interrupted sutures. (i) One day after periodontal regenerative surgery. (j) Clinical view 3 weeks after surgery with matrix exposure. (k, l) Exposed matrix partially removed. (m, n) 5 weeks after surgery. (o, p) 12 months after surgery. Horizontal and vertical probing depths: 2 mm, recession 3 mm. (q) Radiograph taken 12 months after surgery. Almost complete radiographic bone fill in furcation area.

Lindhe, 1998). Unfortunately, the different anatomy and dimensions of teeth and alveolar processes in the experimental animal models reduce their external validity to human cases. Furthermore, experimentally induced furcation defects in animal models may not reproduce the chronic lesions encountered in humans. Therefore, more progress in techniques and materials is needed in order to predictably achieve in humans the same results observed in animal models, before implementing regenerative surgery as the treatment of choice for every deep furcation defect.

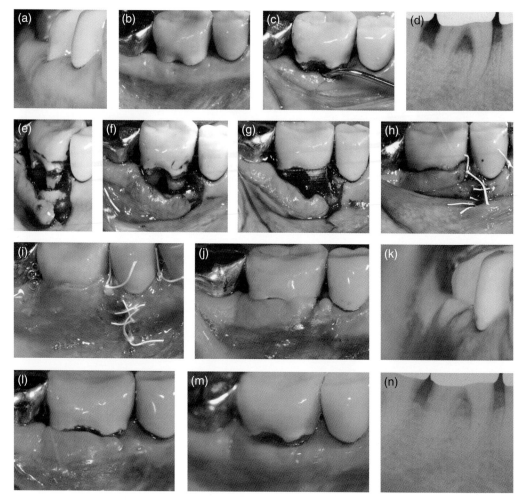

Figure 7.2 (a, b) Periodontal measurements at baseline, tooth no. 46 (LR6). Probing depth mesial and distal: 3 mm, furcation degree II. Situation 2 months after an acute abscess and mobility grade 2 treated with debridement of the accessible root surfaces and local antimicrobials. (c) Radiograph of tooth no. 46 with visible furcation defect, proximal bone loss to the level of the furcation, and a very short distal root. (d) Horizontal probing bone level: 7 mm, crown margin reduced and polished. (e, f) Debrided root surfaces. Flap design: intrasulcular incision/ vertical release mesial, mucoperiostal flap, papilla mesial de-epithelialized, periosteal split in the vestibule. The distal papilla was left intact, but mobilized and slightly elevated by a tunnelling procedure. (g) Placement of a bioresorbable matrix barrier (Guidor™ MSL-configuration, Sunstar Americas, Inc., Schaumburg, IL, USA) after application of a xenogeneic bone mineral into the furcation defect (Bio-oss collagen™, Geistlich Biomaterials, Wollhusen, Switzerland) to facilitate guided tissue regeneration. (h) Coronally advanced minimally rotated flap secured with sling and interrupted sutures. (i) Clinical view one day after periodontal regenerative surgery. (j, k) Clinical view 2 weeks after surgery. (l) Clinical view 3 months after surgery. (m) 9 months, vertical and horizontal probing depths: 2 mm. (n) 9 months, radiographic fill of the furcation defect.

Summary of Evidence

- Various regenerative approaches have shown to be effective in the treatment of degree II furcation involvement (FI) compared with access flap surgery.
- Complete furcation closure in degree II FI is not a predictable outcome
- Degree III FI cannot be improved predictably by regenerative therapy.

References

Aimetti, M., Romano, F., Pigella, E., and Piemontese, M. (2007). Clinical evaluation of the effectiveness of enamel matrix proteins and autologous bone graft in the treatment of mandibular class II furcation defects: A series of 11 patients. *International Journal of Periodontics and Restorative Dentistry* 27, 441–447.

Araújo, M.G., Berglundh, T., and Lindhe, J. (1997). On the dynamics of periodontal tissue formation in degree III furcation defects: An experimental study in dogs. *Journal of Clinical Periodontology* 24, 738–746.

Araújo, M.G., Berglundh, T., and Lindhe, J. (1998). GTR treatment of degree III furcation defects with 2 different resorbable barriers: An experimental study in dogs. *Journal of Clinical Periodontology* 25, 253–259.

Araújo, M.G., and Lindhe, J. (1998). GTR treatment of degree III furcation defects following application of enamel matrix proteins: An experimental study in dogs. *Journal of Clinical Periodontology* 25, 524–530.

Avera, J.B., Camargo, P.M., Klokkevold, P.R. et al. (1998). Guided tissue regeneration in class II furcation involved maxillary molars: A controlled study of 8 split-mouth cases. *Journal of Periodontology* 69, 1020–1026.

Avila-Ortiz, G., De Buitrago, J.G., and Reddy, M.S. (2015). Periodontal regeneration – furcation defects: A systematic review from the AAP regeneration workshop. *Journal of Periodontology* 86 (Suppl.), S108–S130.

Bajaj, P., Pradeep, A.R., Agarwal, E. et al. (2013). Comparative evaluation of autologous platelet-rich fibrin and platelet-rich plasma in the treatment of mandibular degree II furcation defects: A randomized controlled clinical trial. *Journal of Periodontal Research* 48, 573–581.

Barros, R.R.M., Oliveira, R.R., Novaes, A.B., Jr et al. (2005). Treatment of class II furcation defects with guided tissue regeneration or enamel matrix derivative proteins: A 12-month comparative clinical study. *Perio* 2, 275–284.

Becker, W., Becker, B.E., Berg, L. et al. (1988). New attachment after treatment with root isolation procedures: Report for treated class III and class II furcations and vertical osseous defects. *International Journal of Periodontics and Restorative Dentistry* 3, 2–16.

Blumenthal, N.M. (1993). A clinical comparison of collagen membranes with ePTFE membranes in the treatment of human mandibular buccal Class II furcation defects. *Journal of Periodontology* 64, 454–459.

Bouchard, P., Ouhayoun, J.-P., and Nilvéus, R.E. (1993). Expanded polytetrafluoroethylene membranes and connective tissue grafts support bone regeneration for closing mandibular class II furcations. *Journal of Periodontology* 64, 1193–1198.

Bowers, G.M., Schallhorn, R.G., McClain, P.K. et al. (2003). Factors influencing the outcome of regenerative therapy in mandibular class II furcations: Part I. *Journal of Periodontology* 74, 1255–1268.

Bremm, L.L., Sallum, A.W., Casati, M.Z. et al. (2004). Guided tissue regeneration in class II furcation defects using a resorbable polylactic acid barrier. *American Journal of Dentistry* 17, 443–446.

Caffesse, R.G., Mota, L., Quinones, C., and Morrison, E. (1997). Clinical comparison of resorbable and non-resorbable barriers for guided tissue regeneration. *Journal of Clinical Periodontology* 24, 747–752.

Camelo, M., Nevins, M.L., Schenk, R.K. et al. (2003). Periodontal regeneration in human class II furcations using purified recombinant human platelet-derived growth factor-BB (rhPDGF-BB) with bone allograft. *International Journal of Periodontics and Restorative Dentistry* 23, 213–225.

Casarin, R.C., Del Peloso, R.E., Nociti, F.H., Jr et al. (2008). A double-blind randomized clinical evaluation of enamel matrix derivative proteins for the treatment of proximal class-II furcation involvements. *Journal of Clinical Periodontology* 35, 429–437.

Casarin, R.C., Ribeiro Edel, P., Nociti, F.H. Jr et al. (2010). Enamel matrix derivative proteins for the treatment of proximal class II furcation involvements: A prospective 24-month randomized clinical trial. *Journal of Clinical Periodontology* 37, 1100–1109.

Castro, A.B., Meschi, N., Temmerman, A. et al. (2017). Regenerative potential of leucocyte- and platelet-rich fibrin. Part A: Intra-bony defects, furcation defects and periodontal plastic surgery: A systematic review and meta-analysis. *Journal of Clinical Periodontology* 44, 67–82.

Caton, J., Greenstein, G., and Zappa, U. (1994). Synthetic bioabsorbable barrier for regeneration in human periodontal defects. *Journal of Periodontology* 65, 1037–1045.

Chen, T.H., Tu, Y.K., Yen, C.C., and Lu, H.K. (2013). A systematic review and meta-analysis of guided tissue regeneration/ osseous grafting for the treatment of class II furcation defects. *Journal of Dental Science* 8, 209–224.

Chitsazi, M.T., Farahani, R.M.Z., Pourabbas, M., and Bahaeddin, N. (2007). Efficacy of open flap debridement with and without enamel matrix derivatives in the treatment of mandibular degree II furcation involvement. *Clinical Oral Investigations* 11, 385–389.

Christgau, M., Schmalz, G., Reich, E., and Wenzel, A. (1995). Clinical and radiographical split-mouth-study on resorbable versus non-resorbable GTR-membranes. *Journal of Clinical Periodontology* 22, 306–315.

Cury, P.R., Sallum, E.A., Nociti, F.H. et al. (2003). Long-term results of guided tissue regeneration therapy in the treatment of class II furcation defects: A randomised clinical trial. *Journal of Periodontology* 74, 3–9.

Del Fabbro, M., Bortolin, M., Taschieri, S., and Weinstein, R. (2011). Is platelet concentrate

advantageous for the surgical treatment of periodontal diseases? A systematic review and meta-analysis. *Journal of Periodontology* 82, 1100–1111.

Dohan Ehrenfest, D.M., Rasmusson, L., and Albrektsson, T. (2009). Classification of platelet concentrates: From pure platelet-rich plasma (P-PRP) to leucocyte- and platelet-rich fibrin (L-PRF). *Trends in Biotechnology* 27, 158–167.

Donos, N., Glavind, L., Karring, T., and Sculean, A. (2003a). Clinical evaluation of an enamel matrix derivative in the treatment of mandibular degree II furcation involvement: A 36-month case series. *International Journal of Periodontics and Restorative Dentistry* 23, 507–512.

Donos, N., Sculean, A., Glavind, L., Reich, E., and Karring, T. (2003b). Wound healing of degree III furcation involvements following guided tissue regeneration and/or Emdogain. A histologic study. *Journal of Clinical Periodontology* 30, 1061–1068.

Donos, N., Glavind, L., Karring, T., and Sculean, A. (2004). Clinical evaluation of an enamel matrix derivative and a bioresorbable membrane in the treatment of degree III mandibular furcation involvement: A series of nine patients. *International Journal of Periodontics and Restorative Dentistry* 24, 362–369.

Donos, N., Heijl, L., and Jepsen, S. (2010). Application of enamel matrix proteins in furcation defects. In: *Periodontal Regenerative Therapy* (ed. A. Sculean), 103–117. Berlin: Quintessence.

Dos Anjos, B., Novaes, A.B., Jr, Meffert, R., and Porto Barboza, E. (1998). Clinical comparison of cellulose and expanded polytetrafluoroethylene membranes in the treatment of class II furcations in mandibular molars with 6-month re-entry. *Journal of Periodontology* 69, 454–459.

Eickholz, P., and Hausmann, E. (1999). Evidence for healing of class II and III furcations 24 months after GTR therapy: Digital subtraction and clinical measurements. *Journal of Periodontology* 70, 1490–1500.

Eickholz, P., Kim, T.-S., and Holle R. (1997). Guided tissue regeneration with non-resorbable and biodegradable barriers: 6 months results. *Journal of Clinical Periodontology* 24, 92–101.

Eickholz, P., Kim, T.-S., and Holle R. (1998). Regenerative periodontal surgery with non-resorbable and biodegradable barriers: Results after 24 months. *Journal of Clinical Periodontology* 25, 666–676.

Eickholz, P., Kim, T.S., Holle, R., and Hausmann, E. (2001). Long-term results of guided tissue regeneration therapy with non-resorbable and bioabsorbable barriers. I. Class II furcations. *Journal of Periodontology* 72, 35–42.

Eickholz, P., Kim, T.-S., Steinbrenner, H. et al. (2000). Guided tissue regeneration with bioabsorbable barriers: Intrabony defects and class II furcations. *Journal of Periodontology* 71, 999–1008.

Eickholz, P., Pretzl, B., Holle, R., and Kim, T.-S. (2006). Long-term results of guided tissue regeneration therapy with non-resorbable and bioabsorbable barriers. III. Class II furcations after 10 years. *Journal of Periodontology* 77, 88–94.

Figueira, E.A., de Assis, A.O., Montenegro, S.C. et al. (2014). Long-term periodontal tissue outcome in regenerated infrabony and furcation defects: A systematic review. *Clinical Oral Investigations* 18, 1881–1892.

Flanary, D.B., Twohey, S.M., Gray, J.L. et al. (1991). The use of synthetic skin substitute as a physical barrier to enhance healing in human periodontal furcation defects: A follow up report. *Journal of Periodontology* 62, 684–689.

Garrett, S., Polson, A.M., Stoller, N.H. et al. (1997). Comparison of a bioabsorbable GTR barrier to a non-absorbable barrier in treating human class II furcation defects: A multi-center parallel design randomized single-blind trial. *Journal of Periodontology* 68, 667–675.

Gkranias, N.D., Graziani, F., Sculean, A., and Donos, N. (2012). Wound healing following regenerative procedures in furcation degree III defects: Histomorphometric outcomes. *Clinical Oral Investigation* 16, 239–249.

Gottlow, J., Nyman, S., Lindhe, J. et al. (1986). New attachment formation in the human periodontium by guided tissue regeneration: Case reports. *Journal of Clinical Periodontology* 13, 604–616.

Harris, R.J. (2002). Treatment of furcation defects with an allograft-alloplast-tetracycline composite bone graft combined with GTR: Human histologic evaluation of a case report. *International Journal of Periodontology and Restorative Dentistry* 22, 381–387.

Hoffmann, T., Richter, S., Meyle, J. et al. (2006). A randomized clinical multicentre trial comparing enamel matrix derivative and membrane treatment of buccal class II furcation involvement in mandibular molars. Part III: Patient factors and treatment outcome. *Journal of Clinical Periodontology* 33, 575–583.

Horwitz, J., Machtei, E.E., Reitmeir, P. et al. (2004). Radiographic parameters as prognostic indicators for healing of class II furcation defects. *Journal of Clinical Periodontology* 31, 105–111.

Houser, B.E., Mellonig, J.T., Brunsvold, M.A. et al. (2001). Clinical evaluation of anorganic bovine bone xenograft with a bioabsorbable collagen barrier in the treatment of molar furcation defects. *International Journal of Periodontics and Restorative Dentistry* 21, 161–169.

Hugoson, A., Ravald, N., Fornell, J. et al. (1995). Treatment of class II furcation involvements in humans with bioresorbable and nonresorbable guided tissue regeneration barriers: A randomized multi-center study. *Journal of Periodontology* 66, 624–634.

Jaiswal, R., and Deo, V. (2013). Evaluation of the effectiveness of enamel matrix derivative, bone grafts, and membrane in the treatment of mandibular class II furcation defects. *International Journal of Periodontics and Restorative Dentistry* 33, e58–e64.

Jepsen, S., Eberhard, J., Herrera, D., and Needleman, I. (2002). A systematic review of guided tissue regeneration for periodontal furcation defects: What is the effect of guided tissue regeneration compared with surgical debridement in the treatment of furcation defects? *Journal of Clinical Periodontology* 29 (Suppl. 3), 103–116.

Jepsen, S., Heinz, B., Jepsen, K. et al. (2004). A randomized clinical trial comparing enamel matrix derivative and membrane treatment of buccal Class II furcation involvement in mandibular molars. Part I: Study design and results for primary outcomes. *Journal of Periodontology* 75, 1150–1160.

Kanoriya, D., Pradeep, A.R., Garg, V., and Singhal S. (2017). Mandibular degree II furcation defects treatment with platelet-rich fibrin and 1% alendronate gel combination: A randomized controlled clinical trial. *Journal of Periodontology* 88, 250–258.

Kinaia, B.M., Steiger, J., Neely, A.L. et al. (2011). Treatment of class II molar furcation involvement: Meta-analyses of re-entry results. *Journal of Periodontology* 82, 413–428.

Koop, R., Merheb, J., and Quirynen, M. (2012). Periodontal regeneration with enamel matrix derivative in reconstructive periodontal therapy: A systematic review. *Journal of Periodontology* 83, 707–720.

Lekovic, V., Kenney, E.B., Carranza, F.A., and Martignoni, M. (1991). The use of autogenous periosteal grafts as barriers for the treatment of class II furcation involvements in lower molars. *Journal of Periodontology* 62, 775–780.

Lekovic, V., Kenney, E.B., Kovacevic, K., and Carranza, F.A. (1989). Evaluation of guided tissue regeneration in class II furcation defects: A clinical re-entry study. *Journal of Periodontology* 60, 694–698.

Lindhe, J., Pontoriero, R., Berglundh, T., and Araujo, M. (1995). The effect of flap management and bioresorbable occlusive devices in GTR treatment of degree III furcation defects: An experimental study in dogs. *Journal of Clinical Periodontology* 22, 276–283.

Luepke, P.G., Mellonig, J.T., and Brunsvold, M.A. (1997). A clinical evaluation of a bioabsorbable barrier with and without decalcified freeze-dried bone allograft in the treatment of molar furcations. *Journal of Clinical Periodontology* 24, 440–446.

Machtei, E.E. (1997). Outcome variables in the study of periodontal regeneration. *Annals of Periodontology* 2, 229–239.

Machtei, E.E., Cho, M.I., Dunford, R. et al. (1994). Clinical, microbiological, and histological factors which influence the success of regenerative periodontal therapy. *Journal of Periodontology* 65, 154–161.

Machtei, E.E., Grossi, S.G., Dunford, R. et al. (1996). Long-term stability of class II furcation defects treated with barrier membranes. *Journal of Periodontology* 67, 523–527.

Maragos, P., Bissada, N.F., Wang, R., and Cole, B.P. (2002). Comparison of three methods using calcium sulfate as a graft/barrier material for the treatment of class II mandibular molar furcation defects. *International Journal of Periodontics and Restorative Dentistry* 22, 493–501.

McGuire, M.K., and Nunn, M.E. (1996). Prognosis versus actual outcome. III. The effectiveness of clinical parameters in accurately predicting tooth survival. *Journal of Periodontology* 67, 666–674.

Mellonig, J.T., Seamons, B.C., Gray, J.L., and Towle, H.J. (1994). Clinical evaluation of guided tissue regeneration in the treatment of grade II molar furcation invasions. *International Journal of Periodontics and Restorative Dentistry* 14, 255–271.

Mellonig, J.T., Valderrama Mdel, P., and Cochran, D.L. (2009). Histological and clinical evaluation of recombinant human platelet-derived growth factor combined with beta tricalcium phosphate for the treatment of human class III furcation defects. *International Journal of Periodontics and Restorative Dentistry* 29, 169–177.

Metzler, D.G., Seamons, B.C., Mellonig, J.T. et al. (1991). Clinical evaluation of guided tissue regeneration in the treatment of maxillary class II molar furcation invasions. *Journal of Periodontology* 62, 353–360.

Meyle, J., Gonzales, J.R., Bodeker, R.H. et al. (2004). A randomized clinical trial comparing enamel matrix derivative and membrane treatment of buccal class II furcation involvement in mandibular molars. *Part II: Secondary outcomes. Journal of Periodontology* 75, 1188–1195.

Miron, R.J., Guillemette, V., Zhang, Y. et al. (2014). Enamel matrix derivative in combination with bone grafts: A review of the literature. *Quintessence International* 45, 475–487.

Miron, R.J., Sculean, A., Cochran, D.L. et al. (2016). Twenty years of enamel matrix derivative: The past, the present and the future. *Journal of Clinical Periodontology* 43, 668–683.

Mombelli, A., Zappa, U., Brägger, U., and Lang, N.P. (1996). Systemic antimicrobial treatment and guided tissue regeneration: Clinical and microbiological effects in furcation defects. *Journal of Clinical Periodontology* 23, 386–396.

Murphy, K.G., and Gunsolley, J.C. (2003). Guided tissue regeneration for the treatment of periodontal intrabony and furcation defects: A systematic review. *Annals of Periodontology* 8, 266–302.

Myhre, A.E., Lyngstadaas, S.P., Dahle, M.K. et al. (2006). Anti-inflammatory properties of enamel matrix derivative in human blood. *Journal of Periodontal Research* 41, 208–213.

Nevins, M., Camelo, M., Nevins, M.L. et al. (2003). Periodontal regeneration in humans using recombinant human platelet-derived growth factor-BB (rhPDGF-BB) and allogenic bone. *Journal of Periodontology* 74, 1282–1292.

Nibali, L., Zavattini, A., Nagata, K. et al. (2016). Tooth loss in molars with and without furcation involvement: A systematic review and meta-analysis. *Journal of Clinical Periodontology* 43, 156–166.

Nokhbehsaim, M., Deschner, B., Winter, J. et al. (2012). Anti-inflammatory effects of EMD in the presence of biomechanical loading and interleukin-1β in vitro. *Clinical Oral Investigations* 16, 275–283.

Paul, B.F., Mellonig, J.T., Towle, H.J., III, and Gray, J.L. (1992). Use of a collagen barrier to enhance healing in human periodontal furcation defects. *International Journal of Periodontics and Restorative Dentistry* 12, 123–131.

Peres, M.F.S., Ribeiro, E.D.P., Casarin, R.C.V. et al. (2013). Hydroxyapatite/β-tricalcium phosphate and enamel matrix derivative for treatment of proximal class II furcation defects: A randomized clinical trial. *Journal of Clinical Periodontology* 40, 252–259.

Pontoriero, R., and Lindhe, J. (1995a). Guided tissue regeneration in the treatment of degree II furcations in maxillary molars. *Journal of Clinical Periodontology* 22, 756–763.

Pontoriero, R., and Lindhe, J. (1995b). Guided tissue regeneration in the treatment of degree III furcation defects in maxillary molars. *Journal of Clinical Periodontology* 22, 810–812.

Pontoriero, R., Lindhe, J., Karring, T. et al. (1988). Guided tissue regeneration in degree II furcation-involved mandibular molars. *Journal of Clinical Periodontology* 15, 247–254.

Pontoriero, R., Lindhe, J., Nyman, S. et al. (1989). Guided tissue regeneration in the treatment of defects in mandibular molars: A clinical study of degree III involvements. *Journal of Clinical Periodontology* 16, 170–174.

Pradeep, A.R., Karvekar, S., Nagpal, K. et al. (2016). Rosuvastatin 1.2 mg in situ gel combined with 1:1 mixture of autologous platelet-rich fibrin and porous hydroxyapatite bone graft in surgical treatment of mandibular class II furcation defects: A randomized clinical control trial. *Journal of Periodontology* 87, 5–13.

Pradeep, A.R., Pai, S., Garg, G. et al. (2009). A randomized clinical trial of autologous platelet-rich plasma in the treatment of mandibular degree II furcation defects.

Journal of Clinical Periodontology 36, 581–588.

Prathibha, P.K., Faizuddin, M., and Pradeep, A.R. (2002). Clinical evaluation of guided tissue regeneration procedure in the treatment of grade II mandibular molar furcations. *Indian Journal of Dental Research* 13, 37–47.

Pruthi, V.K., Gelskey, S.C., and Mirbod, S.M. (2002). Furcation therapy with bioabsorbable collagen membrane: A clinical trial. *Journal of the Canadian Dental Association* 68, 610–615.

Queiroz, L.A., Santamaria, M.P., Casati, M.Z. et al. (2016). Enamel matrix derivative and/or synthetic bone substitute for the treatment of manibular class II buccal furcation defects: A 12-months randomized clinical trial. *Clinical Oral Investigations* 20, 1597–1606.

Reddy, M.S., Aichelmann-Reddy, M.E., Avila-Ortiz, G. et al. (2015). A consensus report from the AAP regeneration workshop. *Journal of Periodontology* 86 (Suppl.), S131–S133.

Reynolds, M.A., Aichelmann-Reidy, M.E., Branch-Mays, G.L., and Gunsolley, J.C. (2003). The efficacy of bone replacement grafts in the treatment of periodontal osseous defects: A systematic review. *Annals of Periodontology* 8, 227–265.

Sanz, M., Jepsen, K., Eickholz, P., and Jepsen, S. (2015). Clinical concepts for regenerative therapy in furcations. *Periodontology* 2000 68, 308–332.

Scott, T.A., Towle, H.J., Assad, D.A., and Nicoll, B.K. (1997). Comparison of bioabsorbable laminar bone membrane and non-resorbable ePTFE membrane in mandibular furcations. *Journal of Periodontology* 68, 679–686.

Sculean, A., Ausschill, T.M., Donos, N. et al. (2001). Effects of an enamel matrix protein derivative (Emdogain) on ex vivo dental plaque vitality. *Journal of Clinical Periodontology* 28, 1074–1078.

Sharma, A., and Pradeep, A.R. (2011). Autologous platelet-rich fibrin in the treatment of mandibular degree II furcation defects: A randomized clinical trial. *Journal of Periodontology* 82, 1396–1403.

Siddiqui, Z.R., Jhingram, R., Bains, V.K. et al. (2016). Comparative evaluation of platelet-rich fibrin versus beta-tri-calcium phosphate in the treatment of Grade II mandibular furcation defects using cone-beam computed tomography. *European Journal of Dentistry* 10, 496–506.

Simonpietri-C, J.J., Novaes, E.L., Jr, Batista, E.L., Jr, and Filho, E.J. (2000). Guided tissue regeneration associated with bovine-derived anorganic bone in mandibular class II furcation defects: 6 month results at re-entry. *Journal of Periodontology* 71, 904–911.

Stavropoulos, A., and Wikesjö, U.M. (2012). Growth and differentiation factors for periodontal regeneration: A review on factors with clinical testing. *Journal of Periodontal Research* 47, 545–553.

Stoller, N.H., Johnson, L.R., and Garrett, S. (2001). Periodontal regeneration of a class II furcation defect utilizing a bioabsorbable barrier in a human: A case study with histology. *Journal of Periodontology* 72, 238–242.

Suh, Y.I., Lundgren, T., Sigurdsson, T. et al. (2002). Probing bone level measurements for determination of the depths of Class II furcation defects. *Journal of Periodontology* 73, 637–642.

Troiano, G., Laino, L., Dioguardi, M. et al. (2016). Mandibular class II furcation defect treatment: Effects of the addition of platelet concentrates to open flap: A systematic review and meta-analysis of randomized cinical trials. *Journal of Periodontology* 87, 1030–1038.

Tsao, Y.-.P, Neiva, R., Al-Shammari, K. et al. (2006). Effects of a mineralized human cancellous bone allograft in regeneration of mandibular class II furcation defects. *Journal of Periodontology* 77, 416–425.

Twohey, S.M., Mellonig, J.T., Towle, H.J., and Gray, J.L. (1992). Use of a synthetic skin substitute as a physical barrier to enhance healing in human periodontal furcation defects. *International Journal of Periodontics and Restorative Dentistry* 12, 383–393.

Vernino, A.R., Wang, H.L., Rapley, J. et al. (1999). The use of biodegradable polylactic acid barrier materials in the treatment of grade II periodontal furcation defects in humans. *Part II: A multicenter investigative surgical study. International Journal of Periodontics and Restorative Dentistry* 19, 56–65.

Wallace, S.C., Gellin, R.G., Miller, M.C., and Mishkin, D.J. (1994). Guided tissue regeneration with and without decalcified freeze-dried bone in mandibular class II furcation invasions. *Journal of Periodontology* 65, 244–254.

Wang, H.L., O'Neal, R.B., Thomas, C.L. et al. (1994). Evaluation of an absorbable collagen membrane in treating class II furcation defects. *Journal of Periodontology* 65, 1029–1036.

Yukna, C.N., and Yukna, R.A. (1996). Multi-center evaluation of bioabsorbable collagen membrane for guided tissue regeneration in human class II furcations. *Journal of Periodontology* 67, 650–657.

Chapter 8

Furcation Therapy: Resective Approach and Restorative Options

Roberto Rotundo[1] and Alberto Fonzar[2]

[1] Periodontology Unit, UCL Eastman Dental Institute, London, UK
[2] Private practice, Udine, Italy

8.1 Anatomical Considerations for Treatment Planning

Furcation defects present the greatest challenges to the success of periodontal therapy, as a reduced efficacy of periodontal therapy and higher risk of tooth loss have been consistently observed in multi-rooted teeth with furcation involvement, regardless of the treatment modality employed. Regenerative therapy might be considered the ideal treatment for furcations. However, indications for regenerative periodontal therapy (discussed in Chapter 7) are still very limited. Maxillary molars with degree II interproximal furcations, as well as all degree III furcation-involved molars, are generally not suitable for regenerative therapy. Therefore, different treatment strategies (such as resective) have to be employed to eliminate or manage furcation defects.

The survival of molars with furcation involvement in longitudinal studies following different treatment procedures was discussed in Chapter 5. It is interesting to notice how a systematic review observed that the most frequent complications occurring during the follow-up period were caries in the furcation area after tunnelling procedures, and root fractures after root-resective procedures (Huynh-Ba G et al. 2009). From an anatomical point of view, the poorer prognosis of furcation-involved teeth may be due to the fact that the persistence of a defect within the inter-radicular space creates an anatomical environment that interferes with professional and domiciliary oral hygiene. Numerous morphological factors may explain the aetiology, the more severe disease progression, and the less favourable response to periodontal treatment of furcation-involved molars (De Sanctis and Murphey 2000). These factors (extensively covered in Chapter 1) are:

- Furcation access diameter.
- Root irregularities and roughness.
- Anatomical complexity of the root complex.
- Cervical enamel projections.
- Enamel pearls.
- Accessory pulp canals.

8.2 Pre-surgical Diagnosis

8.2.1 Pre-surgical Clinical Diagnosis

An accurate and precise pre-surgical diagnosis is essential in order to approach correctly patients affected by periodontal disease complicated by the invasion of molar furcation areas. Before planning the definitive

Diagnosis and Treatment of Furcation-Involved Teeth, First Edition. Edited by Luigi Nibali.
© 2018 John Wiley & Sons Ltd. Published 2018 by John Wiley & Sons Ltd.
Companion website: www.wiley.com/go/nibali/diagnosis

treatment plan, clinicians should carefully evaluate the following:

- Patient's periodontal and caries risk profile.
- Horizontal (Hamp et al. 1975) and vertical (Tarnow and Fletcher 1984) amount of periodontal tissue loss in the inter-radicular areas.
- Anatomy and morphology of the root complex: the length of the root trunk, the degree of separation, and the divergence between the roots, as well as their shape and length.
- Amount of residual attachment and probing pocket depth (PPD) of each single root.
- Access for oral hygiene procedures.
- Endodontic prognosis of each single root (endodontically treated teeth).
- Need for endodontic treatment (endodontically untreated teeth).
- Need for restorative treatment and restorative deficiencies (i.e. insufficient residual healthy tooth structure).
- Single tooth or multiple molars with furcation involvement.

This information should be obtained by carefully combining the data acquired from both clinical and radiological analysis.

8.2.2 Pre-surgical Radiological Diagnosis

It has been observed that clinical examination alone detected furcation involvement in only 3% of maxillary and 9% of mandibular molars. The combination of radiographic and clinical examinations improved detection to 65% in maxillary molars, but only 23% in mandibular molars (Ross and Thompson 1978). Parallel periapical and/or vertical bite-wing radiographs should always be taken after the clinical examination in order to confirm the information obtained through the periodontal probing (Horwitz et al. 2004). It is important to know that the bone density (especially in mandibular molars) and the superimposition of the palatal root (maxillary molars) could partially hide the root complex, and so make it difficult or impossible to confirm the defect previously detected by probing. Therefore, it appears

fundamental to combine the clinical and radiological data in order to perform an accurate diagnosis of multi-rooted affected teeth.

As discussed in Chapter 2, cone-beam computed tomography (CBCT) may improve diagnostic accuracy and optimize treatment planning in periodontal defects, particularly in maxillary molars with furcation involvement. However, the higher irradiation doses and cost–benefit ratio should be carefully analysed before using CBCT for periodontal lesions (including tooth furcation; Walter et al. 2016). The radiographic analysis should allow the clinician to evaluate the following:

- Horizontal and vertical amount of hard tissue loss in inter-radicular areas.
- Length of root trunk.
- Length, divergence, and shape of roots.
- Presence/absence of fusion between roots.
- Amount of residual support.
- Endodontic diagnosis and prognosis.
- Presence of post and core build-up restoration.
- Presence of caries in furcation-involved molars.

We should also remember that radiolucency in the inter-radicular area does not always indicate the presence of a furcation involvement. Trauma from occlusion (occlusal interferences, bruxism, clenching) with the consequent increased tooth mobility may produce vascular changes along the whole periodontal space, involving also the inter-radicular area, which leads to periodontal ligament space remodelling and bone demineralization (Svanberg and Lindhe 1973; Polson et al. 1976a, b). In such a case the radiolucency is not confirmed by the clinical examination (probing fails to detect an involvement of the furcation) and the defect usually disappears some weeks following the elimination of the occlusal overload.

8.3 Treatment of Furcation Defects

The objectives of periodontal therapy in multi-rooted teeth with furcation involvement are no different from the objective of single-rooted teeth therapy: arresting disease progression and maintaining the teeth in health and function with proper aesthetics. These goals can be met first by eliminating the microbial plaque from the surfaces of the root complex, and then by establishing an anatomy that facilitates proper self-performed plaque removal.

Treatment options for molars with furcation involvement could be divided into three different modalities:

- *Conservative procedures*: subgingival debridement, access-flap surgeries, tunnel preparation. The main aim of these procedures is to remove the residual bacterial infection and improve self-performed plaque control.
- *Regenerative procedures* (already discussed in Chapters 6 and 7): guided tissue regeneration, induced periodontal regeneration, bone grafting. The goal of these procedures is not only the removal of the residual infection, but also the elimination of the furcation defect through reconstruction of the lost inter-radicular periodontal tissues.
- *Resective procedures*: root separation, root resection, root amputation. The objective of these procedures is to eliminate the inter-radicular lesion by completely removing both the dental and osseous structures that make up the defect. The tooth and root complex morphology is deeply changed by this therapeutic modality, in order to open the furcation completely and create an area conducive to performing easier and better plaque removal.

The choice of the appropriate treatment modality for a given clinical situation depends on a wide variety of factors that should be carefully evaluated before initiating treatment:

- Degree of furcation involvement.
- Patient expectations.
- Patient compliance.
- Patient susceptibility to periodontal disease.
- Patient susceptibility to caries.
- Amount of residual attachment.

- Strategic value of the tooth.
- Root complex anatomy and morphology.
- Periodontal condition of adjacent teeth.
- Need for prosthetic rehabilitation.
- Need for endodontic treatment.
- Bone volume/quality.
- Financial considerations for the patient.

8.4 Resective Procedures and Restorative Approaches

8.4.1 Indications

Resective techniques have been developed especially for deep class II and class III furcation-involved molars to overcome these anatomical limitations by physically removing both the dental (the roof of the involved furcation) and osseous (pocket elimination) structures that make up the defect.

Several definitions for resective procedures have been proposed by different authors and therefore there is no uniformity in the terms used in the literature. According to Carnevale et al. (1995), the terms are defined as follows:

8.4.1.1 Root Separation
This indicates the sectioning of the multirooted tooth with the maintenance of all the roots (Figure 8.1). This procedure can be used for treating the following clinical situations:

- Deep class II and class III furcated molars.
- Root-trunk fracture or decay.
- Perforation of the middle of the furcation trunk.

Root separation is usually indicated in the following clinical situations:

- Mandibular molars for separating the mesial from the distal root (premolarization).
- Maxillary molars for separating the mesial root from the undivided distal and palatal roots.
- Maxillary molars for dividing the palatal root from the undivided mesial and distal roots. The separation of the three roots of a

(a)   (b)   (c)

(d)   (e)   (f)

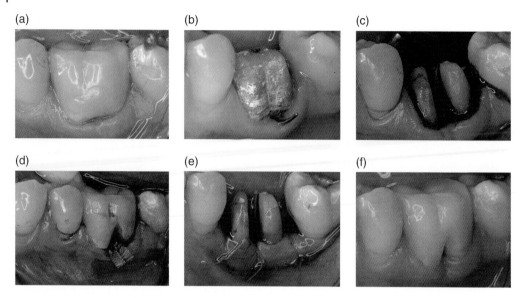

Figure 8.1 Root separation (rizotomy: sectioning of the multi-rooted tooth with the maintenance of all the roots) of a mandibular first molar affected by degree III furcation involvement (a–d), followed by an apical positioned flap (e) and final restoration (f), allowing self-performed oral hygiene.

maxillary molar should be considered quite exceptional, because the presence of all the roots would make the passage of plaque removal devices too difficult or impossible.

8.4.1.2 Root Resection

This indicates the sectioning of the multi-rooted tooth and the removal of one or two roots and the associated portion of the crown. Even if in the literature this term is often used regardless of how the crown is treated, it is opportune to distinguish it from the term 'root amputation', which refers to the removal of one root without removal of the overhanging portion of the crown. Root amputation can usually be indicated in the maxillary molars for removing the distal root, thus avoiding the need to restore the tooth with a crown in a conservative treatment plan.

The root resection procedure can be used for treating the following clinical situations:

- Deep class II and class III furcated molars with severe root proximity or a long root trunk.
- Severe bone loss affecting one or more roots of molars with and without furcation involvement.

- Root or root trunk fracture or perforation.
- Untreatable apical endodontic lesion affecting one root.
- Severe root decay or resorption.
- Severe recession or dehiscence affecting one root.

When considering root resection for treating molars with furcation involvement, the clinician has to choose between different alternatives.

Mandibular Molars

These have only one furcation and therefore there are just two possibilities (Figure 8.2):

- Resection of the mesial root.
- Resection of the distal root.

Assuming that the two roots do not present significant differences in terms of periodontal, endodontic, and restorative prognosis, the following morphological characteristics should be considered before deciding which root has to be extracted (Majzooub and Kon 1992):

- The mesial root usually presents a greater root surface, but also quite often a deep concavity, making it difficult first to properly prepare and restore it, and for the

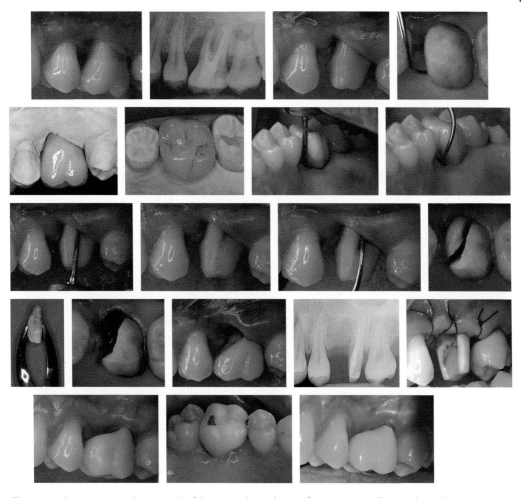

Figure 8.2 Root resection (rizectomy) of the mesio-buccal root of an upper maxillary molar, without separation of the other two roots, performed due to the severe loss of bone support caused by an endodontic-periodontal lesion. Degree III furcation involvement on the mesial and buccal furcations was present, with no distal furcation involvement. This procedure was carried out after appropriate endodontic therapy. Three months after the root resection, an apically positioned flap was performed and a provisional prosthetic crown was positioned. Three months later, a final metal-ceramic crown was cemented, with a good long-term (five years) clinical result (last image).

patient to keep clean with standard plaque-control procedures. It is important to stress the risk of producing a fenestration in the distal surface of the root, during both the tooth preparation and the endodontic treatment/retreatment of the two narrow and superficial root canals.

- The distal is a comparatively large root, with usually one wide root canal and an oval convex cross-section with a greater bulk of dentine. These characteristics make the distal root less prone to root fracture; easier to treat endodontically, to prepare, and to restore; and finally for the patient to keep clean through self-performed plaque removal.

Maxillary Molars

These have three furcations and therefore several root resection possibilities (Figure 8.3):

- Resection of the mesio-buccal root without separating the other two roots. This

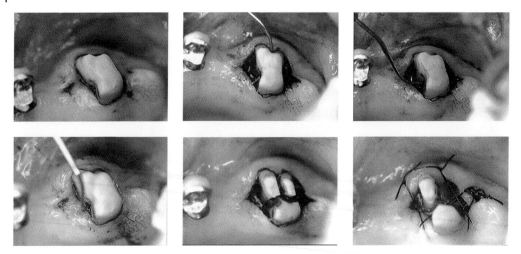

Figure 8.3 Root separation of all three roots of a maxillary upper second molar and extraction (rizectomy) of the disto-buccal root.

procedure can be performed in case of involvement of the buccal and/or mesial furcation (in such a case root separation is also possible), and when the mesio-buccal root is affected by a deep infrabony defect or an untreatable endodontic or restorative problem. After the mesio-buccal root removal, the residual root trunk shows a flat or convex mesial surface that facilitates both prosthetic procedures and self-performed plaque control.

- Resection of the disto-buccal root without separating the other two roots. This procedure can be performed in case of involvement of the buccal and/or distal furcation, and when the disto-buccal root is affected by a deep infrabony defect or by an untreatable endodontic or restorative problem. Following the extraction of the disto-buccal root, the residual root trunk often exhibits a deep distal concavity, which should be flattened during tooth preparation in order to improve the quality of the prosthetic restoration and the patient's self-performed plaque removal.
- Resection of the palatal root without separating the other two roots. This procedure can be performed in case of involvement of the mesial and/or distal furcation (in such a case root separation is also possible), or

when the palatal root is affected by a deep infrabony defect or an endodontic or restorative untreatable problem.

When all three furcations of a maxillary molar are involved, following root separation one or two roots can be extracted. In such clinical situations, if two roots are maintainable (a careful evaluation of periodontal, endodontic, and prosthetic prognosis is an essential prerequisite), the following options are possible (Figure 8.4):

- Root separation of all three roots and extraction of the disto-buccal one. The disto-buccal root is statistically the most frequently extracted (Rosenberg 1978; Ross and Thompson 1978), because it is usually the shortest with a long root trunk and therefore has a smaller amount of bone support. The anatomy and morphology of the root trunk usually make access between the divided mesial and palatal roots easy for the patient's self-performed oral hygiene.
- Root separation of all three furcations and extraction of the mesio-buccal root. This option is less frequent than the previous one, because often the disto-buccal root is too thin, and also because proper self-performed plaque removal in the distal

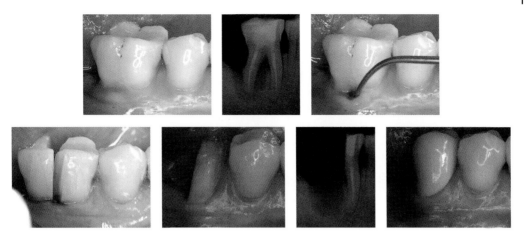

Figure 8.4 Root separation in a mandibular first molar affected by degree III furcation involvement associated with periodontal-endodontic pathology on the distal root. Distal root resection (rizectomy) was carried out, maintaining the mesial root in situ. A prosthetic metal-ceramic crown was carried out after the three-month healing period.

furcation is nearly impossible if distally the neighbouring molar is present.

- Root separation of all three furcations and extraction of the palatal root. This option is less frequent too because of the anatomy of the palatal root (large root surfaces and an oval convex cross-section with thick dentine), but also because the thickness of the palatal bone makes this root particularly stable and firm. When the clinician has to choose between the mesial and the palatal root, they should consider that the mesial root has a root surface area that is equal to or even larger than the palatal one, but it presents two or even three narrow root canals instead of the sole and wide canal of the palatal root.

8.4.2 Scientific Evidence

Ten studies (only one prospective) reporting the results of root resection with at least five-year follow-up were found in the literature (see Table 8.1). The survival rates reported in these studies range from about 60 to 100% after a mean observation period of 5–10 years.

Bergenholtz (1972) retrospectively reported the results of 45 teeth treated with root resection up to 11 years before. Out of the 20 teeth with a 5–10-year follow-up, 17 teeth were still present, 2 teeth were lost because of periodontal complications, and 1 because of root perforation, meaning a survival rate of 85%. Hamp et al. (1975) reported a survival rate of 100% after 5 years in 87 molars treated by means of root resection and/or separation. The authors attributed their success to the elimination of plaque-retentive areas in the furcations, meticulous patient oral hygiene, and regular maintenance care.

Langer et al. (1981) reported a survival rate of 62% in a 10-year retrospective evaluation of 100 molars (50 maxillary and 50 mandibular) treated with resection. The main causes of tooth loss were root fracture in 18 teeth (47.4%), periodontal complications in 10 teeth (26.3%), endodontic failures in 7 teeth (18.4%), and cement washouts leading to caries in 3 teeth (7.9%). It is interesting to point out that the ratio of maxillary to mandibular failures was approximately 2:1 and only 15.8% of the tooth loss occurred within the first five years after surgery, whereas the vast majority – that is, 55.3% of the losses – occurred between the fifth and seventh years of function. The remaining losses took place between the eighth and tenth years of observation. Buhler (1988) presented a 10-year follow-up of 28 root-resected

Table 8.1 Clinical studies on the treatment of furcation-involved molars with root separation/resection.

Author	Year	Study design	Number of teeth	Follow-up (mean)	Complications	Survival
Bergenholtz	1972	Retrospective	45	5–10 years	66.6% periodontal 33.3% root perforation	85%
Hamp et al.	1975	Retrospective	87	5 years		100%
Langer et al.	1981	Retrospective	100	10 years	47.4% root fracture 26.3% periodontal 18.4% endodontic 7.9% wash-out/caries	62%
Buhler	1988	Retrospective	28	10 years	33.3% endodontic 22.2% perio-endo 22.2% periodontal 11.1% root fracture 111% wash-out/canes	67.9%
Carnevale et al.	1991	Retrospective	488	Group I 303 teeth: 3–6 years Group II 185 teeth:7–11 years	33.3% caries 33.3% root fracture 33.3% PPD > 5mm (group II)	Group II 98.4%
Blomlof et al.	1997	Retrospective	78	5–10 years	81.3% periodontal 25% perio-endo 28.1 endodontic	5 years: 83% 10 years: 68%
Carnevale et al.	1998	Prospective	175	10years	33.3% endodontic 25% root caries 25% periodontal 16.7 root fracture	5 years: 98.9% 10 years: 93.1%
Hou et al.	1999	Retrospective	52	6.7 (5–13 years)		100%
Svardstrom & Wennstrom	2000	Retrospective	47	9.5 (8–12 years)	80% root fracture	89.4%
Dannewitz et al.	2006	Retrospective	19	~9 (~5–12 years)	Not reported	92.9%

PPD = probing pocket depth.

molars, mainly used as bridge abutments. The calculated survival rate was 67.9% and the reasons for tooth loss were as follows: endodontic failures 33.3%, combined periodontal and endodontic lesions 22.2%, periodontal reasons 22.2%, root fracture 11.1%, and loss of retention leading to secondary caries 11.1%. Curiously similar to the findings of Langer and co-workers, no tooth loss could be observed during the first four years following therapy.

Carnevale et al. (1991) published a retrospective analysis of 488 molars after tooth resection and/or separation and prosthetic reconstruction. The follow-up period was 3–6 years for 303 teeth (62%) and 7–11 years for 175 teeth (38%). Considering only the group with the longer follow-up, 3 teeth were lost (1 for caries, 1 for root fracture, and 1 for PPD > 5 mm), yielding a survival rate of 98.4%. In contrast to Langer et al. (1981) and Bühler (1998), most failures occurred early (3–6-year group) rather than later (7–11-year group). The authors attributed the high success rate to an optimal hygiene regimen and frequent maintenance recall. A more recent 10-year follow-up prospective investigation by Carnevale et al. (1998) reported the success rate of root-resective therapy in 175 molars used as abutments for single-unit crowns or fixed dental prostheses to be 98.9% after 5 years and 93% at the end of the study. Only 12 of 175 teeth (7%) were extracted, 4 for endodontic reasons, 3 for root caries, 3 for periodontal reasons, and 2 for root fracture.

Hou et al. (1999) reported a survival rate of 100% of 52 root-separated molars in a case series including 25 patients followed up for a mean observation period of 6.7 years (range 5–13 years). Svardström and Wennström (2000) reported a survival rate of 89.4% of 47 molars 8–12 years following root-resective procedures (mean observation period 9.5 years). Five teeth (10.6%) had to be extracted during the follow-up period and root fracture was the main reason for extraction (80.0%). Dannewitz et al. (2006) performed 19 root resections while treating 305 furcation-involved molars. Following a mean observation period of about 9 years, 8 resected teeth were lost, yielding a survival rate of 57.9%. The complications – that is, the reason for the tooth loss – were not reported.

It is fitting to consider that a true comparison among these studies is almost impossible: different pre-therapeutic conditions of the involved molars, no uniformity in the terminology used, different reasons for performing these procedures (periodontal? endodontic? root fracture? caries?), different techniques used in each step of both root separation and resections (endodontic treatment, tooth build-up, preparation, provisional and definitive crown morphology), different recall intervals, and smoking habits (Mullally and Linden 1996) make drawing indisputable conclusions about the efficacy of this therapeutic modality an impossible task. In spite of that, it must be pointed out that with the exception of three studies, the average survival rate of the molars treated with root separation/resection was very high (close to 90%) and comparable to that of implants inserted in the posterior areas of the mouth, and that the reasons for tooth extraction were mainly related to endodontic complications and root fractures, and not to periodontal disease recurrence.

8.4.3 Contraindications

Root-separation/resection procedures present some important anatomical and technical contraindications:

- Poor compliance with oral hygiene.
- Patients with high caries susceptibility.
- Patients with severe parafunctional habits.
- Inadequate residual attachment on the remaining roots.
- Serious discrepancies in adjacent interproximal bone level.
- Unfavourable anatomical factors (long root trunk, short divergence between roots, fused roots, presence of inter-radicular septa).
- Retained roots endodontically untreatable.

- Excessive endodontic instrumentation of retained roots.
- Severe root decay/resorption.

We should also bear in mind that these are sensitive techniques that require a careful interdisciplinary approach, a widespread knowledge of prosthodontics, endodontics, and periodontology, and an accurate evaluation of the cost–benefit ratio with respect to the treatment alternatives. The need for endodontic treatment, prosthetic rehabilitation, and periodontal surgery actually makes this therapeutic modality a demanding treatment, in terms of both economic cost and biological tissue loss.

8.4.4 Step-by-step Procedure

Considering that root separation/resection is an interdisciplinary procedure and that most of the failures reported in the literature are basically generated by reasons other than new periodontal breakdown, first careful patient selection and then precise sequencing and correct execution of each phase of the therapeutic protocol are crucial to the long-term success of the procedure. The suggested therapeutic sequence is as follows.

8.4.4.1 Patient Selection
This is the first, fundamental step of the sequence, because not all patients are equally suitable for root separation/resection. Poor patient compliance, high caries susceptibility, and limited financial resources are the most frequent factors limiting the use of this procedure. Treatment options must be presented to the patient and the potential problems should be discussed. Root separation/resection should be considered as part of an overall treatment plan aiming at complete periodontal, functional, and aesthetic rehabilitation.

8.4.4.2 Tooth Selection
As already mentioned, long root trunk, short divergences between the roots, fused roots, and presence of inter-radicular septa represent contraindications for a root-separation/resection procedure. Particular caution should be used when the multi-rooted teeth are intact, because this is an invasive procedure involving a considerable biological cost that must always be carefully evaluated.

8.4.4.3 Endodontic Treatment
Since root and/or build-up fractures have often been reported as one of the most frequent reasons for the failure of a root-separation/resection procedure, correct endodontic treatments must preserve as much tooth structure as possible at both coronal (access opening should be kept as small as possible) and radicular levels (conservative instrumentation). Excessive instrumentation of radicular canals and/or immoderate pressure during gutta-percha condensation should be avoided.

Although a vital root resection is possible without any initial post-surgical discomfort for the patient (Smukler and Tagger 1976), when the tooth to be treated is vital or the root filling is suboptimal, endodontic treatment/retreatment should be always the first procedure performed. The reasons for a preliminary root canal treatment are:

- Easier rubber dam isolation and easier access for the endodontist.
- Evaluation of tooth/root endodontic prognosis before separation/resection procedure.
- Crown build-up before separation/resection procedure.

If from a clinical and radiological point of view it is not possible to identify the root(s) to be resected with certainty, each root has to be endodontically treated/retreated. In order to avoid useless treatments and costs, when the clinical periodontal evaluation of the tooth is deeply doubtful, endodontic treatment can be exceptionally postponed until after the root separation/resection. In these cases, root canal treatment should be performed within two weeks (Smukler and Tagger 1976).

8.4.4.4 Crown Build-up

After completion of the endodontic therapy, the crown of the molar, the pulp chamber, and almost 2–3 mm of the canals apical to the furcation entrance are prepared, etched, and filled with light or chemically cured composite by using a dentine adhesive to improve the retention of the material. This step is of the outmost importance, because the replacement of the missing coronal and radicular tooth structure should provide to the abutments a complete marginal seal and proper retention and resistance for the subsequent full-coverage restoration.

8.4.4.5 Root separation/resection During Preliminary Prosthetic Preparation

Root separation/resection may be performed as part of the initial tooth preparation for the prosthetic rehabilitation ('prosthetic preparation'), when a prefabricated shell provisional restoration is relined and temporarily cemented. Performing root separation/resection prior to and not during periodontal surgery (Carnevale et al. 1981, 1997) presents several important clinical advantages:

- Accurate evaluation of the periodontal condition of the molar and thus the possibility to change the treatment plan at an early stage. In molars with furcation involvement, it is often impossible to precisely assess the inter-radicular attachment loss before root separation, and therefore no conclusive clinical decision about the prognosis of the tooth can be made prior to this procedure.
- Earlier elimination/reduction of the inter-radicular periodontal infection and earlier extraction of hopeless roots. This can enhance the healing of the infrabony lesions that might be present in the inter-radicular area at the extraction site, and therefore generate an osseous morphology more favourable for being corrected at the time of resective bone surgery.
- Creating access for plaque removal in an otherwise inaccessible area.

- Possibility of reducing tooth mobility before surgery by splinting the roots with the provisional restoration.
- If the root trunk is short and infrabony defects are not present, periodontal surgery can often be avoided.

Root separation or resection can otherwise be performed following the same technique during the periodontal surgical phase, if there is a diagnostic problem or difficult access (Carnevale et al. 1990).

Before starting with tooth preparation/resection, it is of the utmost importance to carefully probe each root and especially the furcation area in order to identify three-dimensionally the position of furcation entrances, the anatomy of the root trunk, and the potential presence of infrabony defects affecting one or more roots (Zappa et al. 1993). Considering the reduced diameter and thickness of the roots, the preparation must be as conservative as possible. For this reason, tooth structure saving a knife-edge finishing line should be preferred. Usually local anaesthesia is not necessary during the root-separation phase and therefore should not be used, because the patient's feeling of pain can help the clinician to avoid moving the bur too deeply in the tissue and therefore reducing the risk of damaging the preserved inter-radicular attachment.

In order to get access to the subgingival root surfaces with the precise root axis and to limit soft-tissue damage, a small-diameter flame-shape diamond bur can be used, and the buccal and lingual enamel prominence should be eliminated first. The access to each involved furcation (buccal and lingual in mandibular molars; buccal, mesial, and distal in the maxillary) should be initially 'marked' with vertical grooves that can be used as reference points during the root-separation/resection procedure. In every passage the flame-shape diamond bur has to be moved first forwards into the furcation and then backwards, working in both interproximal line angles of each root in order to widen the space previously created between the roots.

Once the furcation has been separated, the whole roof of the involved furcation must be eliminated and an adequate space for plaque-removal devices should be created between the roots.

It is important to remember that the distal aspect of the molar mesial root (especially the mandibular one) often presents a deep concavity. In order to avoid weakening the mesial root or creating a root fenestration, the desired distance within the distal root should be created by preparing the mesial aspect of the distal root rather than the distal of the mesial one. The mesial and distal surfaces of mesial and distal mandibular roots and the buccal and palatal surface of respectively mesio-buccal and palatal roots must be parallel to each other (if both the roots are maintained) and to the neighbouring abutments to ensure a proper insertion axis of the prosthetic rehabilitation, while the interproximal surfaces can be divergent in order to widen the space between the roots.

In order to be sure that the whole roof of the involved furcation has been eliminated, a curved periodontal probe (Nabers probe) should be moved in the apico-coronal direction to detect the potential presence of furcation lips or ledges. With the aim of facilitating provisional relining and domiciliary plaque removal in the exposed root surfaces, at the end of tooth preparation/resection, the root surfaces should be made smooth and even by using fine and extra-fine diamond burs, and the line angles of the abutment should be rounded.

8.4.4.6 Provisional Restoration

At the end of tooth separation/resection, a prefabricated shell provisional restoration is relined and temporarily cemented. In order not to disturb both soft and hard interproximal tissue healing, it is important to shorten at about the gingival level and to precisely refine the margins of the relined provisional restoration. The excess of temporary cement must be carefully removed and the patient should be taught to clean the new interproximal spaces properly with appropriate plaque-removal devices. The provisional restoration can be strengthened with specific commercially available reinforcing fibres or, in the case of long-span bridges or in patients with parafunctional habits, replaced after an impression with a custom-made metal-reinforced temporary restoration.

8.4.4.7 Periodontal Surgery

The objectives of this phase of the root-separation/resection procedure are the following:

- To eliminate possible angular bone defects around the maintained roots and recreate a positive bone architecture in order to obtain an environment favourable to good hygiene and easy dental care. Bone resection may also be performed to reduce the bucco-lingual dimension of the alveolar process in the extraction sites. Soft- and hard-tissue management and post-surgical care are the same as used for pocket elimination with resective osseous surgery.
- To facilitate both soft adaptation and domiciliary plaque removal by modifying the root contour through intrasurgical preparation of prosthetic abutments.

Following flap elevation, the maintained roots and the other non-vital abutments are newly prepared with the purpose of removing the residual plaque and calculus, improving the space between the roots, eliminating any residual undercuts, and reducing the natural anatomical concavities present on the root surfaces. As proposed by Di Febo (1985), concavities can be reduced by preparing a chamfer on only the portions of the roots that are convex, without touching the concave portions, which thereby present a knife-edge finishing line ('combined preparation').

The intra-operative preparation does not always extend to the alveolar crest. On the contrary, the operator should prepare the tooth to the level of connective tissue attachment and avoid, wherever possible, injuring intact fibres and removing healthy cementum. Following intra-surgical abutment preparation and before suturing, the temporary restoration must be relined with a self-curing acrylic resin and the margins trimmed 3 mm short of the alveolar crest so as not to disturb the healing process.

Throughout the tissue maturation period, patients are maintained on a plaque-control programme that includes professional tooth cleaning and oral hygiene instruction once a month. In order to reduce the risk of cement washout during these recall appointments, the provisional restoration should be removed and re-cemented and, where necessary, new interdental plaque-removal devices are recommended (Walter et al. 2011).

8.4.4.8 Final Prosthesis

Once the healing period is complete and before the impression for the definitive prosthesis, the endodontic, periodontal, and provisional prosthetic treatments have to be clinically and radiographically re-evaluated. If the treatments could achieve successful outcomes, the abutments can be refined and polished and the final impression can be taken, with or without extra-thin retraction cords. The design and construction of the metal framework in combination with a good crown fitting and sitting play a fundamental role in the long-term success of fixed bridges using root-separated or root-resected abutments (Carnevale et al. 1991; Newell 1991). The strength and stability of the metal framework should compensate for the structural weakness of the abutments, and for the high tooth mobility often present in severely involved periodontal cases (Wang et al. 1994). For the same mechanical reasons, occlusion should be designed and set to minimize occlusal lateral forces. Interproximal spaces should be created in order to facilitate

oral hygiene as much as possible, and the patient should be taught to use self-performed plaque-removal devices correctly. At the completion of therapy, patients are then enrolled in a personalized maintenance recall programme that generally includes three-monthly appointments.

8.5 Conclusions

The long-term prognosis of teeth with furcation involvement treated with conventional therapy demonstrates a higher frequency of tooth loss than non-furcated molars. The reduced success rate may be due to the fact that the persistence of a defect within the inter-radicular space creates an anatomical environment that interferes with oral hygiene efforts. In fact, partial gain of clinical attachment levels within the defect, although statistically or clinically significant, may not effectively improve the outcome during the maintenance phase of therapy. It is important to point out that comparative studies between the different procedures are lacking, and therefore in treatment decisions for furcation-involved molars there is no scientific evidence that a given treatment modality is superior to the others. Patient-related factors such age and health conditions, compliance, susceptibility to caries, strategic value of the tooth in relation to the overall treatment plan, functional and aesthetic demands, and, last but not least, financial resources should guide clinicians in their choice of treatment.

Summary of Evidence

An accurate and precise diagnosis is essential in order to correctly approach affected molar furcation areas. In particular, clinicians must initially evaluate all the patient- and tooth/site-related factors that are able to determine indications and contraindications for the treatment of the defects. Afterwards, this step-by-step approach should be followed:

- Endodontic treatment and tooth restoration.
- Root separation/resection.
- Provisional restoration.
- Periodontal surgery.
- Final prosthesis.

References

Bergenholtz, A. (1972). Radectomy of multi-rooted teeth. *Journal of the American Dental Association* 85, 870–875.

Blomlof, L., Jansson, L., Appelgren, R. et al. (1997). Prognosis and mortality of root resected molars. *International Journal of Periodontics and Restorative Dentistry* 17, 191–201.

Buhler, H. (1988). Evaluation of root-resected teeth: Results after 10 years. *Journal of Periodontology* 59, 805–810.

Carnevale, G., Di Febo, G., and Fuzzi, M. (1990). A retrospective analysis of the perio-prosthetic aspect of teeth re-prepared during periodontal surgery. *Journal of Clinical Periodontology* 17, 313–316.

Carnevale, G., Di Febo, G., Tonelli, M.P. et al. (1991). A retrospective analysis of the periodontal-prosthetic treatment of molars with interradicular lesions. *International Journal of Periodontics and Restorative Dentistry* 11, 189–205.

Carnevale, G., Di Febo, G., and Trebbi, L. (1981). A patient presentation: Planning a difficult case. *International Journal of Periodontics and Restorative Dentistry* 1, 50–63.

Carnevale, G., Pontoriero, R., and di Febo, G. (1998). Long-term effects of root-resective therapy in furcation-involved molars: A 10- year longitudinal study. *Journal of Clinical Periodontology* 25, 209–214.

Carnevale, G., Pontoriero, R., and Hurzeler, M. (1995). Management of furcation involvement. *Periodontology 2000* 9, 69–89.

Carnevale, G., Pontoriero, R., and Lindhe, J. (1997). Treatment of furcation-involved teeth. In: *Clinical Periodontology and Implant Dentistry*, 3rd edn (ed. J. Lindhe, T. Karring, and N.P. Lang), 682–710. Copenhagen: Munksgaard.

Dannewitz, B., Krieger, J.K., Husing, J., and Eickholz, P. (2006). Loss of molars in periodontally treated patients: A retrospective analysis five years or more after active periodontal treatment. *Journal of Clinical Periodontology* 33, 53–61.

De Sanctis, M., and Murphey K.G. (2000). The role of resective periodontal surgery in the treatment of furcation defects. *Periodontology 2000* 22, 154–168.

Di Febo, G., Carnevale, G., and Sterrantino, S.F. (1985). Treatment of case of advanced peridontitis: Clinical procedures utilizing the 'combined preparation' technique. *International Journal of Periodontics and Restorative Dentistry* 1, 52–63.

Hamp, S.E., Nyman, S., and Lindhe, J. (1975). Periodontal treatment of multirooted teeth: Results after 5 years. *Journal of Clinical Periodontology* 2, 126–135.

Horwitz, J., Machtei, E.E., Reitmeir, P. et al. (2004). Radiographic parameters as prognostic indicators for healing of class II furcation defects. *Journal of Clinical Periodontology* 31, 105–111.

Hou, G.L., Tsai, C.C., and Weisgold, A.S. (1999). Treatment of molar furcation involvement using root separation and a crown and sleeve-coping telescopic denture: A longitudinal study. *Journal of Periodontology* 70, 1098–1109.

Huynh-Ba, G., Kuonen, P., Hofer, D. et al. (2009). The effect of periodontal therapy on the survival rate and incidence of complications of multirooted teeth with furcation involvement after an observation period of at least 5 years: A systematic review. *Journal of Clinical Periodontology* 36, 164–176.

Langer, B., Stein, S.D., and Wagenberg, B. (1981). An evaluation of root resections: A ten-year study. *Journal of Periodontology* 52, 719–722.

Majzoub, Z., and Kon, S. (1992). Tooth morphology following root resection procedures in maxillary molars. *Journal of Periodontology* 63, 290–296.

Mullally, B.H., and Linden, G.J. (1996). Molar furcation involvement associated with cigarette smoking in periodontal referrals. *Journal of Clinical Periodontology* 23, 658–661.

Newell, D.H. (1991). The role of the prosthodontist in restoring root-resected molars: A study of 70 molar root resections. *Journal of Prosthetic Dentistry* 65, 7–15.

Polson, A.M., Meitner, S.W., and Zander, H.A. (1976a). Trauma and progression of marginal periodontitis in squirrel monkeys. IV Reversibility of bone loss due to trauma alone and trauma superimposed upon periodontitis. *Journal of Periodontal Research* 11, 290–298.

Polson, A.M., Meitner, S.W., and Zander, H.A. (1976b). Trauma and progression of marginal periodontitis in squirrel monkeys. III Adaption of interproximal alveolar bone to repetitive injury. *Journal of Periodontal Research* 11, 279–289.

Rosenberg, M.M. (1978). Management of osseous defects. In: *Clinical Dentistry*, vol. 3 (ed. J.W. Clark), 103. Philadelphia, PA: Harper & Row.

Ross, I.F., and Thompson, R.H., Jr (1978). A long term study of root retention in the treatment of maxillary molars with furcation involvement. *Journal of Periodontology* 49, 238–244.

Smukler, H., and Tagger, M. (1976). Vital root amputation: A clinical and histologic study. *Journal of Periodontology* 47, 324–330.

Svanberg, G., and Lindhe, J. (1973). Experimental tooth hypermobility in the dog: A methodological study. *Odontologisk Revy* 24, 269–282.

Svardstrom, G., and Wennstrom, J.L. (2000). Periodontal treatment decisions for molars: An analysis of influencing factors and long-term outcome. *Journal of Periodontology* 71, 579–585.

Tarnow, D., and Fletcher, P. (1984). Classification of the vertical component of furcation involvement. *Journal of Periodontology* 55, 283–284.

Walter. C., Schmidt, J.C., Dula, K., and Sculean, A. (2016). Cone beam computed tomography (CBCT) for diagnosis and treatment planning in periodontology: A systematic review. *Quintessence International* 47, 25–37.

Walter, C., Weiger, R., and Zitzmann, N.U. (2011). Periodontal surgery in furcation-involved maxillary molars revisited: An introduction of guidelines for comprehensive treatment. *Clinical Oral Investigations* 15, 9–20.

Wang, H.L., Burgett, F.G., Shyr, Y., and Ramfjord, S. (1994). The influence of molar furcation involvement and mobility on future clinical periodontal attachment loss. *Journal of Periodontology* 65, 25–29.

Zappa, U., Grosso, L., Simona, C. et al. (1993). Clinical furcation diagnosis and interradicular bone defects. *Journal of Periodontology* 64, 219–227.

Chapter 9

Furcation Tunnelling

Stefan G. Rüdiger

Department of Periodontology, Public Dental Service/Malmö University, Malmö, Sweden

9.1 Introduction

Furcation involvement has been shown to be associated with tooth loss during supportive periodontal therapy (Graetz et al. 2015; Dannewitz et al. 2016; see also Chapter 5). Characterized by ridges and concavities (Svärdström and Wennström 1988), the furcation area is – for patients and dental professionals alike – particularly difficult to clean. High plaque and consequently high bleeding scores are generally associated with breakdown of periodontal tissues during maintenance (Lang et al. 1990; Eickholz et al. 2008). Creating an inter-radicular space accessible for brushing between the roots at deeply involved furcation sites – a procedure referred to as 'furcation tunnelling' – will allow for regular plaque removal from the furcation area (Figure 9.1), thus reducing the bacterial challenge to the periodontal tissues and possibly the risk of disease recurrence at these sites. In this chapter, case selection, treatment procedure, and the scientific background of the long-term prognosis of molars undergoing tunnel preparation will be discussed.

9.2 Indication

The furcation tunnelling procedure should be considered at stable (no more than mobility grade I) furcation-involved molars with advanced inter-radicular bone loss (furcation involvement of at least deep grade II or grade III 'through and through'; Hamp et al. 1975) when accessibility to the furcation area for plaque removal is difficult. This is particularly the case if a deep lingual (at lower molars) or mesio-palatal (at upper molars) furcation involvement is present. If there is no bone loss at the lingual furcation (at lower molars) or the mesio-buccal furcation entrance (at upper molars), and at the same time a buccal furcation involvement grade II not exceeding half the buccal-lingual width of the molar, there might be a possibility of the patient accessing the furcation entrance with an interdental brush and thus create healthy conditions. The converse condition – that is, no bone loss at the buccal furcation entrance and a lingual involvement grade II – would speak in favour of a tunnel procedure to ensure lingual healing, as cleaning of a lingual furcation entrance is difficult to manage for the patient.

A prerequisite for the tunnelling procedure is sufficient residual bone support at all roots. As a rule of thumb, the alveolar bone support should be of equal amounts at all roots, and at least cover one-third of the root length. Bone loss should mainly be horizontal. Otherwise, root resection may be considered instead (see Chapter 8).

The accessibility of the buccal furcation entrance should already at an early stage be

Diagnosis and Treatment of Furcation-Involved Teeth, First Edition. Edited by Luigi Nibali.
© 2018 John Wiley & Sons Ltd. Published 2018 by John Wiley & Sons Ltd.
Companion website: www.wiley.com/go/nibali/diagnosis

(a)

(b)

(c)

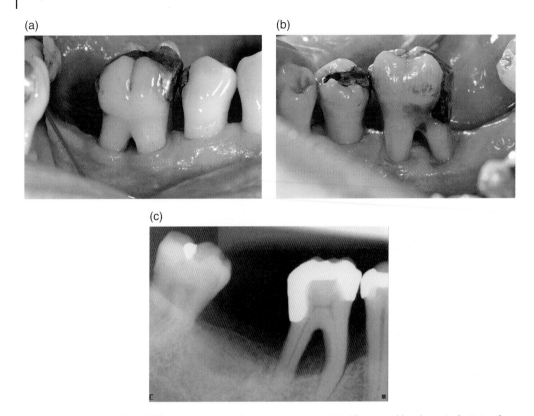

Figure 9.1 Example of a well-functioning tunnel at a maintenance visit. The tunnel has been in function for seven years. Healthy periodontal tissues are noted around the two roots from the buccal (a) and lingual (b) aspects. On the intraoral radiograph (c), the inter-radicular alveolar bone is dense, which can be taken as a sign of stable conditions.

judged clinically and radiographically. The length of the root trunk and the diameter of the furcation entrance are variables to consider. Reasonably, the length of the root trunk should not exceed 4 mm and the diameter of the furcation entrance should be at least 0.5 mm. Otherwise, it will be difficult for the patient to find the furcation entrance and insert the interdental brush into the furcation. Considering anatomical measurements, first mandibular molars would be the most suitable candidates for the tunnelling procedure, considering root trunk dimensions and the divergence angle of the roots (Chiu et al. 1991; Hou and Tsai 1997; Paolantonio et al. 1998; Kerns et al. 1999). In addition, the angle of the furcation area itself should be looked at. A narrow furcation roof would impede brushing.

Assessing the upper molars is more difficult, as the palatal root is often superimposed on the furcation area on radiographs. An eccentrically taken (especially distal eccentric) radiograph might help to project the furcation area in a mesio-buccal direction. In comparison to lower molars, upper molars more often have a longer root trunk and a narrower divergence angle between the two buccal roots. A further anatomical complication in the upper jaw is the fact that three roots create three furcation entrances. If an interdental brush is inserted into the buccal furcation entrance, the tooth anatomy would usually guide the brush to the mesio-palatal furcation entrance (Figure 9.2). Thus the distal furcation entrance, which is usually located in the middle of the distal approximal surface, would not be cleaned

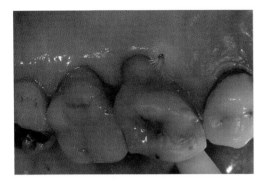

Figure 9.2 Root anatomy guides the interdental brush from the buccal to the mesio-palatal furcation entrance. When an interdental brush is inserted into the buccal furcation entrance, root anatomy will usually lead the brush to the mesial furcation entrance.

(see Section 9.6). Provided that proper case selection is carried out, the decision on tunnelling procedure can be taken intraoperatively. This bears the advantage of a more accurate furcation measurement, as calculus and in particular granulation tissue can obstruct the path for the furcation probe, thus underestimating the degree of furcation involvement.

Another factor to consider when planning for a tunnelling procedure is if prosthetic treatment will be necessary in the area. A tunnelling procedure might help avoid prosthetic treatment and thereby preserve an intact dental arch. If prosthetic treatment is inevitable, the prognosis of a furcation-tunnelled molar should be weighed thoroughly against the prognosis of the entire prosthetic construction, considering a possible loss of the furcation-tunnelled tooth. It can be noted that in one study 33 out of 156 tunnelled teeth were given a prognosis sufficient to serve as an abutment for fixed bridges (Helldén et al. 1989). Given the fact that specific anatomical prerequisites and the patient's full cooperation are required for a successful tunnelling procedure, this type of treatment is performed only occasionally. In follow-up studies of periodontal patients in specialist surroundings, 1–5% of molars (Hamp et al. 1975; Kuhrau et al. 1990;

Graetz et al. 2015; Dannewitz et al. 2016) in periodontitis patients underwent this treatment. Though deep grade II furcation involvements are often given as an indication for the tunnelling procedure in textbooks, in an actual retrospective cohort of maintenance patients in a specialist unit, the tunnelling procedure was considered only for molars with initial furcation involvement grade III (Dannewitz et al. 2016).

9.3 Patient Selection

Before introducing the tunnelling procedure as a possible treatment option, the patient's ability and attitude to brushing between roots should be assessed. If a surgical tunnel preparation has been performed and the patient is not able or willing to brush it, the purpose of the treatment will be defied and compliance could be further affected. Further on, it is advisable not to introduce interradicular cleaning as the first oral hygiene instruction procedure, but instead to concentrate on getting to know the patient by their ability at ordinary interdental brushing. As soon as the standard of oral hygiene is acceptable, brushing of a furcation entrance can be introduced as a preparatory step to a furcation preparation.

9.4 The Tunnelling Procedure: Surgical Steps

If an interdental brush can be inserted easily into the buccal furcation entrance and with only minor resistance pass through the entire furcation area, it may be worth trying to create the furcation non-surgically. This can be an advisable strategy if otherwise there is no indication for periodontal surgery. If the gingiva over the lingual furcation entrance obstructs the interdental brush from passing through an otherwise entirely accessible through-and-through furcation, lingual gingivectomy may be performed (Figure 9.3).

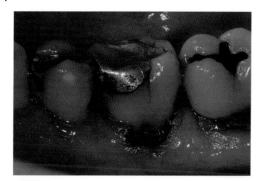

Figure 9.3 Tunnel preparation by gingivectomy. If the interdental brush – coming from the buccal furcation entrance – cannot pass a through-and-through furcation involvement at the lingual aspect due to soft-tissue obstruction, gingivectomy at the lingual aspect will create accessibility through the whole furcation.

In most cases, periodontal flap surgery should be performed to ensure good post-operative access through the whole furcation area. After local anaesthesia and elevation of a full-thickness flap, granulation tissue is removed to judge the bone level in the furcation involvement. Before flap design, careful attention should be paid to the amount of buccal ketarinized gingiva present. In cases of large amounts of keratinized gingiva, a scalloped incision can be performed by the furcation entrance, followed by the removal of the secondary flap after intrasulcular incisions, to expose the furcation area. Otherwise, in cases with a limited amount of keratinized gingiva, intrasulcular incisions with no paramarginal incisions are preferred, in order to preserve the keratinized tissues and facilitate tissue handling. In this case, a full split-thickness flap can be executed, if possible associated with lateral buccal relieving incisions, to then apically reposition the flap by periosteal suturing (Friedman 1962) to expose the furcation area. These two different options are illustrated in Figure 9.4.

A straight periodontal probe, or alternatively a sterile interdental brush (e.g. size yellow 0.7; TePe, Malmö, Sweden) can be used to test accessibility. If bone must be removed to ensure accessibility for the interdental brush, a round bur or Waerhaug diamond can be used. The bur should preferably first be inserted from the furcation entrance that is more involved. As soon as the operator has an idea of the direction, further osteoplasty is performed stepwise from both furcation entrances. The furcation entrances should be free of any bone ridges, which have to be removed, thus ensuring full accessibility to the furcation (Figure 9.5).

The ideal distance from the fornix to the bone crest to allow for interfurcation cleaning should be around 5–6 mm, which is the diameter of a size 7 interdental brush (3 mm) plus 2–3 mm needed for the dento-gingival junction, and to allow for possible rebound of gingival tissues inside the furcation. However, no specific studies have investigated this aspect. The advantage of the Waerhaug diamond is that its torpedo-like form allows the bur to find its way through the furcation, whereas such tactility is not achieved with a round bur. Oscillating techniques (e.g. piezoelectric instruments) can also be applied for gentle ostectomy/osteoplasty, particularly in the inner furcation area. After scaling and root planing, the flaps are repositioned by sutures, ensuring bone coverage. Interproximal single interrupted or vertical mattress sutures may be used. Sutures anchoring the flap to the periosteum need to be performed in case of an apically repositioned flap. At lower molars, a suture can be placed through the furcation. In the upper jaw, root anatomy makes the furcation more difficult to access for interdental cleaning, and exposure of the furcation entrances by trimming the periodontal flap can be advisable (Figure 9.6). Periodontal dressing can be applied to avoid granulation tissue growing in the furcation area. Thus, the furcation tunnel will be void of granulation tissue and already accessible to an interdental brush at suture removal. It is important to remember that the periodontal dressing should only be placed into the furcation entrance and not through the whole furcation area, as it can be painful for the patient when the dressing is

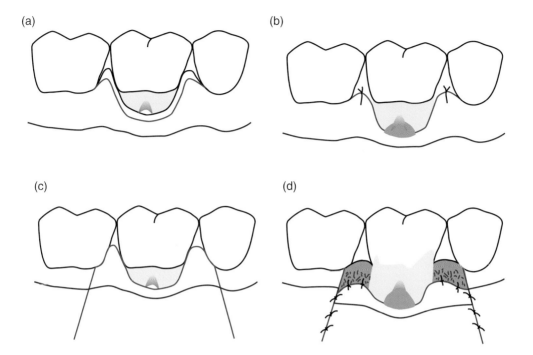

Figure 9.4 Different approaches for tunnelling surgery needed according to the amount of keratinized gingiva (KG). In a case of an adequate amount of KG (a), scalloped incisions can be performed to expose the furcation area for self-performed cleaning (b). In a case of a reduced amount of KG (c), an apically repositioned flap is performed in order to preserve the KG while still exposing the furcation area for self-performed cleaning (d).

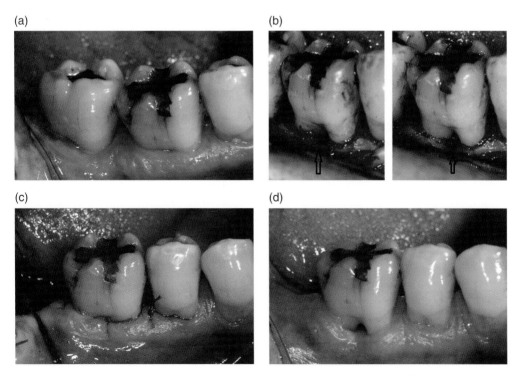

Figure 9.5 Osteoplasty during tunnel operation and suturing through the furcation. A furcation entrance can be obstructed by soft tissue (a) and bone ridges (b). A positive bone architecture has to be created by intrasurgical osteoplasty (see arrows) to secure easy insertion of the interdental brush through the furcation. Good soft-tissue adaptation can be achieved in the furcation entrances by placing a suture through the furcation (c), ensuring good healing (d).

(a)

(b)

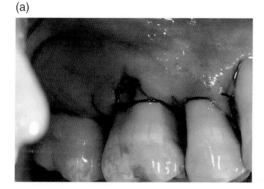
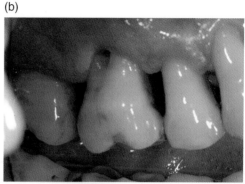

Figure 9.6 At upper molars, root anatomy does often not form a straight pathway from the buccal to the mesial furcation entrance (in contrast to the furcation at lower molars). In such a case, it is more advisable to open the furcation by trimming the flaps, to leave the furcation entrances to heal openly (a), and not to place sutures, which after healing ensures good accessibility for the patient (b).

removed from the inner part of the furcation. In such cases, brushing in the furcation might even not be possible at suture removal due to tenderness in the inner part of the furcation.

To a greater extent than ordinary flap surgery, periodontal surgery for tunnel preparation involves a certain ambivalence between leaving the surgical area to heal by secondary intention and the general intention of periodontists to achieve primary healing (which means that areas, such as the furcation entrance, that it is crucial to clean at an early stage should be covered by tissue). Post-operative follow-up of the latter needs to concentrate on training the patient to find the furcation entrance, whereas in the case of secondary healing the patient has to be encouraged to dare to brush the furcation area despite postoperative tenderness. This dilemma can only be solved for each patient individually. As already pointed out, the patient's attitude towards oral hygiene has to be known to the therapist before the treatment decision for a tunnelling procedure should be taken.

9.5 Postoperative Follow-Up and Oral Hygiene in the Furcation

At suture removal 7–10 days after the surgery, the tissues in the furcation area are often still too tender to allow for through-and-through brushing. At this time point in healing, there may not be epithelial coverage of the intraoperatively exposed bone, which will be the cause of tenderness on touching. The focus for the first post-operative oral hygiene instruction should be on the correct horizontal insertion of the interdental brush into the furcation entrance. The direct instruction to the patient should be to 'insert the brush as far as possible.' Ideally, the patient should be seen for post-operative follow-up four and eight weeks after surgery. At four weeks, it should be tested whether the brush can be inserted over the middle of the furcation area, possibly to the lingual furcation entrance. An interdental brush should preferably be used in its original straight shape, but if necessary it can be bent to prevent the brush getting stuck in the lingual gingival tissues, which tend to grow in a coronal direction during the healing process. The patient should be instructed to feel the tip of the brush on the inside to ensure that it has been inserted the whole way through (Figure 9.7). If tissue regrowth is too extensive, an additional gingivectomy can be advisable. Good oral hygiene can be revealed anatomically by good adaptation of the gingiva in the furcation entrances (Figure 9.8).

From a psychological point of view, it is important that all personnel involved should truly believe in the concept of the tunnelling procedure. Otherwise, the patient will not learn to brush the furcation tunnel. Especially for a referral clinic, this aspect is important, as

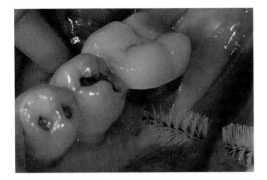

Figure 9.7 Meticulous oral hygiene instruction. It is necessary to thoroughly explain to the patient the technique of brushing a furcation tunnel. One crucial piece of information is to point out that the interdental brush has to be inserted through the whole furcation tunnel. The patient should feel the tip of the brush with the tongue.

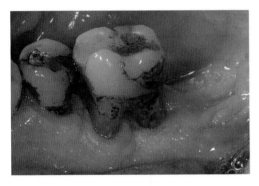

Figure 9.8 Gingival topography reveals the patient's capability to brush the tunnel. Excellent oral hygiene after furcation tunnelling is often revealed by the inter-radicular gingiva showing the path of the interdental brush through the tunnel furcation. Good adaption of the gingiva to the root surface is seen.

keeping patients with a furcation tunnel for a prolonged maintenance phase can be considered to ensure a good long-time prognosis.

In some cases it may be necessary to instruct the patient to brush the furcation from the palatal or lingual aspect to get the best brushing result. This technique requires extensive training exercises with the patient.

In one study, patients were asked about their experience and brushing habits as far as the furcation tunnel was concerned (Helldén et al. 1989). The majority (92%) did not experience discomfort in relation to the furcation tunnel; 70% of patients said it was easy to brush the furcation tunnel, 80% used an interdental brush, and 27% an interspace brush in addition to a common toothbrush (see also Chapter 13).

9.6 Types of Teeth

For lower molars, the brushing procedure is straightforward. There is one way in and one way out, and usually the interdental brush can easily be inserted through the whole furcation. The trifurcation of upper molars makes matters more complicated. In most cases, the root anatomy guides an interdental brush from the buccal furcation entrance to the mesial furcation entrance, which is in most cases located in the mesio-palatal line angle. Often the pathway through the furcation does not allow a straight brush to be inserted. Thus, the patient must be instructed to bend the brush to get it through the whole furcation. Alternatively, the patient can be instructed to insert the brush from the lingual aspect.

The distal furcation entrance of upper molars is located in the middle of the approximal space. The distal furcation entrance is not accessible for brushing as long as the neighbouring distal tooth is in place. It can be argued that ordinary interdental brushing would result in some cleaning of the furcation entrance, since the bristles would open as the interdental brush is moved through the interdental space. This might be an explanation for why upper molars with a functioning tunnel from the buccal to the mesial furcation entrance can be kept over a prolonged period of time, despite the fact that the distal furcation entrance might not always be accessible for direct brushing. When the neighbouring posterior tooth is missing and the patient's dexterity is well developed, a functioning double tunnel may be created (Figure 9.9). Double tunnels are not often mentioned in the literature. Helldén et al. (1989) reported double tunnels performed on 33 maxillary molars; however, they did not specify the treatment outcome for this type of tunnelling. Two contralateral double tunnels had in a case report been

(a)   (b)

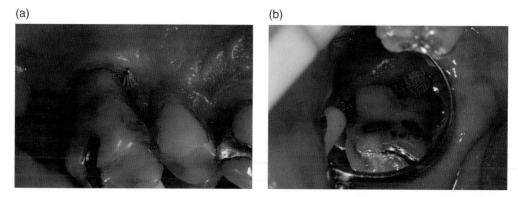

Figure 9.9 In rare cases, double tunnels can be created. In this case, the distal furcation entrance was reached through the buccal entrance (a). The patient had learned to access both the mesial and the distal entrance through the buccal entrance (b).

proven to remain in stable condition over a period of two years of maintenance therapy (Rüdiger 2001).

Furcation tunnels in second molars are more difficult to reach for the patient in both the upper and lower jaws. Firstly, traction of the corner of the mouth in combination with the more posterior positioning of second molars impedes correct positioning of the interdental brush into the furcation entrance. Secondly, the diverging angle of the roots (buccal roots for the upper jaw) of second is smaller than that of first molars, and the root trunk is usually longer of second than of third molars (Kerns et al. 1999).

In the literature, one case of a furcation tunnel of a first upper premolar is mentioned. However, no details were given on how this furcation tunnelling worked in terms of oral hygiene, and if this tunnelled premolar was among the tunnelled teeth that had to be extracted (Hamp et al. 1975). As both furcation entrances of first upper premolars are situated in the approximal spaces, the furcation entrances are difficult to reach if the tooth is not rotated and no neighbouring teeth are missing. Further on, the majority of maxillary first premolars (63%) have fused roots, and of those having furcated roots only 10% had the bifurcation in the cervical third of the root lengths; that is, possibly accessible

for brushing (Joseph et al. 1996; see also Chapter 1). Thus, the position of the maxillary first premolar in the dental arch and its root anatomy do not favour the possibility of using furcation tunnel procedures in first upper premolars. During 15 years of clinical work at a referral clinic for periodontology, the author has only once come across the opportunity to introduce the brushing procedure in a through-and-through furcation involvement in an upper first premolar. The second premolar was missing and the first premolar was rotated to such a degree that the insertion of an interdental brush through the furcation was possible. The bone loss had reached the apical third of the roots (Figure 9.10). Initially an improvement was noted, but when the patient came back for a three-month follow-up, the bone loss to the apices was noted and the tooth had to be extracted.

9.7 Pulp Reaction

The tunnelling procedure exposes considerable root surface areas. A pulp reaction might be expected, as accessory root canals are frequently found in the furcation area of multi-rooted teeth (Lowman et al. 1973; Vertucci and Williams 1974; Niemann et al.

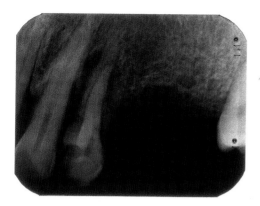

Figure 9.10 Upper left first premolar with mesial bone loss reaching the apical third of the root was chosen for furcation tunnelling. Clinically, at the mesial aspect over the furcation entrance, there was a pronounced swelling corresponding to the radio-juxtaradicular translucency. Though good compliance with interdental brushing was achieved, the progression of periodontitis could not be arrested. The tooth lost stability only a few months later and had to be extracted.

1993; Zuza et al. 2006). However, only a minority (10%) of the accessory canals in the furcation are real communications connecting the pulpal chamber with the periodontium; the majority are blind canals with an opening to either side and ending in the dentine (Zuza et al. 2006). Further on, pulpal necrosis only occurs when the main apical foramina are involved, even if a pulpal inflammation can be seen at accessory canals (Langeland et al. 1974). These anatomical and histological findings corroborate clinical observation that endodontic complications were not reported as a major complication after furcation tunnelling (see Table 9.1).

9.8 Caries after Furcation Tunnelling

Molars subjected to furcation tunnelling were reported to be at risk for root caries in the furcation area. The prevalence of root caries in the furcation ranges from 4.4 to 57.1% (see Table 9.1). Considering that root caries after periodontal treatment in general has been reported to occur with a prevalence of 82–90% after 10 years of maintenance therapy (Ravald and Hamp 1981; Reiker et al. 1999), caries at furcation-tunnelled teeth is not to be seen as an unusual finding. Caries in the furcation tunnel is often difficult to detect clinically and – when clinically manifest – is beyond restorative dentistry's therapeutic range, thus extraction may become inevitable (Figures 9.11 and 9.12).

9.9 Maintenance Phase

A crucial point during the maintenance phase is the time when the patient is discharged from the periodontal practice. The introduction and instruction of the referring clinic are indicative of continuous good prognosis of the furcation-tunnelled tooth. A general recommendation is periodontal supportive therapy every third month. Reminding the patient of the furcation tunnel is an important psychological aspect for this type of patient. It has been shown that tunnelled molars can be kept over several years of supportive periodontal therapy (see Table 9.1). Caries was given as a main reason for tooth loss during maintenance. There are indications of a prognostic breaking point at 10 years of maintenance, when the percentage of tooth loss notably increases (Dannewitz et al. 2006, 2016). In several studies (see Table 9.1), fluoride prophylaxis is recommended to prevent the development of caries lesions in the furcation tunnel. In two studies (Topoll and Lange 1987; Eickholz et al. 1991), patients not complying with this recommendation were over-represented among patients losing the tunnelled tooth. Large studies are needed to draw conclusions and provide guidelines on long-term survival of tunnelled molars.

Table 9.1 Summary of follow-up studies of multi-rooted teeth subjected to furcation tunnel preparation.

Author/Year	Sample n	Follow-up years (mean ± SD/range)	Type of study	No. of teeth	Types of tunnelled teeth	Supportive periodontal therapy (SPT); flouride application	Extracted tunnelled teeth/all re-examined tunnelled teeth (%)	Reason for extraction
Hamp et al. 1975	100	5	Prospective follow-up of multi-rooted teeth	310 multi-rooted teeth, 7 (2.3%) of which tunnelled	6 lower first molars, 1 upper first premolar	3–6 months	3/7 = 42.9%	Caries
Topoll and Lange 1987	28	1–8; mean 3.4	Retrospective follow-up of tunnelled molars	34 tunnelled molars	32 lower molars, 2 upper molars after resection of the palatal root	3–4 months; 14 patients complied with recommendation of fluoride prophylaxis (gel application)	No extractions reported	–
Helldén et al. 1989	107	0.8–8.9; mean 3.1	Retrospective follow-up of tunnelled molars; 102/107 of patients and 149/156 of tunnelled molars were reexamined	156 tunnelled molars	52 lower molars, 91 upper molars, 33 of which had 'double' tunnels	3–6 months; all patients were advised to use fluoride dentrifice, also directly in the tunnel, and to rinse with 0.025% fluoride solution	10/149 = 6.7%	6/10 teeth because of caries; other reasons not specified
Kuhrau et al. 1990	59	4–8; mean 5.8	Retrospective follow-up of molars under SPT	275 molars, 14 (5.1%) of which tunnelled	14 lower molars	Regular SPT; intervals not specified	2/14 = 14.3%	Caries
Eickholz et al. 1991	56	1–5; mean 2.0	Retrospective follow-up of tunnelled lower molars under SPT; 49/56 of patients and 68/76 of tunnelled molars were reexamined	76 tunnelled lower molars	76 lower molars	3 months; 39 patients complied with recommendation to brush a concentrated fluoride gel into the tunnel	5/68 = 7.4%	Not specified
Little et al. 1995	18	5.8 ± 0.83	Prospective follow-up of tunnelled molars	18 tunnelled molars	13 lower, 5 upper molars	3 months;	2/18 = 11.1%	Caries

Feres et al. 2006	18	2–10	Retrospective follow-up of tunnelled molars under SPT	30 tunnelled molars	Not specified	3–6-month interval professional prophylaxis, fluoride gel application inside the tunnels; and oral hygiene instructions	No extractions reported	
Kaltschmitt et al. 2006	41	1–13	Retrospective follow-up of tunnelled molars under SPT	56 tunnelled molars	6 upper, 50 lower molars	SPT to varying degrees	8/56 = 14.3%; 7 lower molars, 1 upper molar	Not specified
Dannewitz et al. 2006	71	8.9; 5.2–12.2	Retrospective follow-up of molars under SPT	505 molars, 14 (2.3%) of which tunnelled	1 upper, 13 lower molars	3-, 6-, 12-month intervals according to individual risk; on average 1.9 ± 0.6 visits/year	1/14 = 7.1%	Not specified
Dannewitz et al. 2016	136*	13.2 ± 2.8	Retrospective follow-up of molars under SPT	1015 molars, 14 (1.4%) of which tunnelled	1 upper, 13 lower molars	3-, 6-, 12-month intervals according to individual risk; on average 1.8 ± 0.5 visits/year	5/14 = 35.7%	Not specified

SD = standard deviation.

*37 of which already were reported on by Dannewitz et al. 2006.

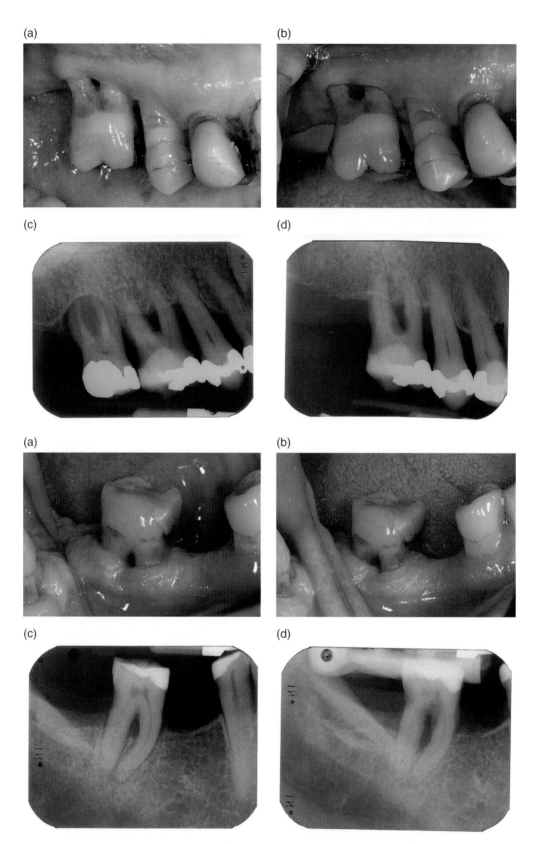

Figures 9.11 and 9.12 Development of caries in furcation tunnels. In these two cases, caries developed within the furcation area – before caries developed (a) and (c); with the established lesions (b) and (d). Caries development was associated with inadequate oral hygiene during supportive periodontal therapy. The lesions may be easily missed by mere clinical examination. Radiographs should therefore be taken during supportive periodontal therapy to detect caries development at an early stage.

Summary of Evidence

- The tunnelling procedure is a treatment method applicable in approximately 1–5% of all molar teeth in patients referred for the treatment of periodontal disease.
- The best candidates for the tunnelling procedure are lower first molars.

- After periodontal treatment, the majority of tunnelled molars can successfully be kept in maintenance care over many years. The prognosis declines after a decade.
- Caries is the most frequent complication leading to loss of tunnelled molars during maintenance.

References

Chiu, B.M., Zee, K.Y., Corbet, E.F., and Holmgrcn, C.J. (1991). Periodontal implications of furcation entrance dimensions in Chinese first permanent molars. *Journal of Periodontology* 62, 308–311.

Dannewitz, B., Krieger, J.K., Hüsing, J., and Eickholz, P. (2006). Loss of molars in periodontally treated patients: A retrospective analysis five years or more after active periodontal treatment. *Journal of Clinical Periodontolology* 33, 53–61.

Dannewitz, B., Zeidler, A., Hüsing, J. et al. (2016). Loss of molars in periodontally treated patients: Results 10 years and more after active periodontal therapy. *Journal of Clinical Periodontolology* 43, 53–62.

Eickholz, P., Kaltschmitt, J., Berbig, J. et al. (2008). Tooth loss after active periodontal therapy. 1: Patient-related factors for risk, prognosis, and quality of outcome. *Journal of Clinical Periodontolology* 43, 165–174.

Eickholz, P., Topoll, H.H., Hucke, H.P., and Lange, D.E. (1991). Postoperative Befunde nach Tunnelierung furkationsbeteiligter Unterkiefermolaren (Grad III) [Postsurgical findings after tunnel preparation in mandibular molars with class III furcation involvement]. *Deutsche Zahnärztliche Zeitschrift* 45, 356–357.

Feres, M., Araujo, M.W., Figueiredo, L.C., and Oppermann, R.V. (2006). Clinical evaluation of tunnelled molars: A retrospective study. *Journal of the International Academy of Periodontology* 8, 96–103.

Friedman, N. (1962). Mucogingival surgery: The apically repositioned flap. *Journal of Periodontolology* 33, 328–340.

Graetz, C., Schützhold, S., Plaumann, A. et al. (2015). Prognostic factors for the loss of molars: An 18-years retrospective cohort study. *Journal of Clinical Periodontolology* 42, 943–950.

Hamp, S.-E., Nyman, S., and Lindhe, J. (1975). Periodontal treatment of multirooted teeth: Results after 5 years. *Journal of Clinical Periodontology* 2, 126–135.

Helldén, L.B., Elliot, A., Steffensen, B., and Steffensen, J.E.M. (1989). Prognosis of tunnel preparations in treatment of class III furcations: A follow-up study. *Journal of Periodontology* 60, 182–187.

Hou, G.L., and Tsai, C.C. (1997). Types and dimensions of root trunk correlating with diagnosis of molar furcation involvements. *Journal of Clinical Periodontology* 24, 129–135.

Joseph, I., Varma, B.R., and Bhat, K.M. (1996). Clinical significance of furcation anatomy of the maxillary first premolar: A biometric study on extracted teeth. *Journal of Periodontology* 67, 386–389.

Kaltschmitt, J., Radek, M., Dannewitz, B., and Eickholz, P. (2006). Success of tunnel preparations in molars with class III furcation involvement. *Journal of Clinical Periodontology* 33 (7), 116.

Kerns, D.G., Greenwell, H., Wittwer, J.W. et al. (1999). Root trunk dimensions of 5 different tooth types. *International Journal of*

Periodontics and Restorative Dentistry 19, 83–91.

Kuhrau, N., Kocher, T., and Plagmann, H.C. (1990). Parodontalbehandlung furkationsbefallener Zähne: Mit oder ohne Radektomie? [Periodontal treatment of furcally involved teeth: With or without root resection?]. *Deutsche Zahnärztliche Zeitschrift* 45, 455–457.

Lang, N.P., Adler, R., Joss, A., and Nyman, S. (1990). Absence of bleeding on probing: An indicator of periodontal stability. *Journal of Clinical Periodontology* 17, 714–721.

Langeland, K., Rodrigues, H., and Dowden, W. (1974). Periodontal disease, bacteria, and pulpal histopathology. *Oral Surgery, Oral Medicine, Oral Pathology* 37, 257–270.

Little, L.A., Beck, F.M., Bagci, B., and Horton, J.E. (1995). Lack of furcal bone loss following the tunnelling procedure. *Journal of Clinical Periodontology* 22, 637–641.

Lowman, J.V., Burke R.S., and Pelleu G.B. (1973). Patent accessory canals: Incidence in molar furcation region. *Oral Surgery, Oral Medicine, Oral Pathology* 36, 580–584.

Niemann, R.W., Dickinson, G.L., Jackson, C.R. et al. (1993). Dye ingress in molars: Furcation to chamber floor. *Journal of Endodontics* 19, 293–296.

Paolantonio, M., di Placido, G., Scarano, A., and Piattelli, A. (1998). Molar root furcation: Morphometric and morphologic analysis. *International Journal of Periodontics and Restorative Dentistry* 18, 489–501.

Ravald, N., and Hamp, S.-E. (1981). Prediction of root surface caries in patients treated for advanced periodontal disease. *Journal of Clinical Periodontology* 8, 400–414.

Reiker, J., van der Velden, U., Barendregt, D.S., and Loos, B.G. (1999). A cross-sectional study into the prevalence of root caries in periodontal maintenance patients. *Journal of Clinical Periodontology* 26, 26–32.

Rüdiger, S.G. (2001). Mandibular and maxillary furcation tunnel preparations: Literature review and a case report. *Journal of Clinical Periodontology* 28, 1–8.

Svärdström, G., and Wennström, J.L. (1988). Furcation topography of the maxillary and the mandibular first molars. *Journal of Clinical Periodontology* 15, 271–275.

Topoll, H.H., and Lange, D.E. (1987). Die Tunnelierung mehrwurzliger Zähne: Ergebnisse 8 Jahre post operationem. [Tunnel preparation of multirooted teeth: Results 8 years after surgery]. *Deutsche Zahnärztliche Zeitschrift* 42, 445–449.

Vertucci, F.J., and Williams, R.G. (1974). Furcation canals in the human mandibular first molar. *Oral Surgery, Oral Medicine, Oral Pathology* 38, 308–314.

Zuza, E.P., Toledo, B.E., Hetem, S. et al. (2006). Prevalence of different types of accessory canals in the furcation area of third molars. *Journal of Clinical Periodontology* 77, 1755–1761.

Chapter 10

Innovative and Adjunctive Furcation Therapy: Evidence of Success and Future Perspective

Luigi Nibali and Elena Calciolari

Centre for Immunobiology and Regenerative Medicine, Centre for Oral Clinical Research, Institute of Dentistry, Barts and the London School of Medicine and Dentistry, Queen Mary University of London (QMUL), London, UK

10.1 Introduction

This book's journey has taken the reader through the anatomy of molars with furcation involvement (FI) and the challenges facing the clinician engaging in periodontal treatment of such molars. Recent technological advances have led to the birth of several techniques and devices which can help in the treatment of molars with FI. The aim of this chapter is to review what has changed in the treatment of furcation-involved teeth in recent years, to present the evidence for the efficacy of these new therapeutic modalities, and to predict possible future treatment avenues. A major improvement in periodontal non-surgical treatment, including the treatment of furcation defects, has been achieved with the introduction of mini-curettes and slim-line ultrasonic inserts, which have been covered in Chapter 3. Other treatments, which we could consider 'alternative' to the 'traditional' treatments described so far, are described in what follows.

10.2 Periodontal Endoscope

In an attempt to overcome the limitations of traditional closed-root instrumentation and to give the clinician the possibility of visually debriding root surfaces, periodontal endoscopy was proposed nearly 20 years ago (Ozawa et al. 1999). The periodontal endoscope has been specifically designed to explore and visualize periodontal pockets in patients with periodontitis. The advantage of this instrument is the subgingival visualization of the root surface at high magnification (24× to 48×; Kwan 2005). When combined with the use of micro ultrasonic instruments, endoscopic debridement can be accomplished in a more accurate, conservative, and minimally invasive way (Geisinger et al. 2007), thus potentially reducing the need for surgical intervention. Molars with FI, due to their difficult access for debridement, may represent optimal candidates for this technology. However, when comparing 35 pairs of multi-rooted teeth that received either endoscopy-aided scaling and root planing (SRP) or traditional SRP, Michaud and co-workers (2007) did not find a significant difference in calculus deposit removal between the two groups, as assessed on digital images taken with a stereomicroscope. The same conclusions were reported by a more recent randomized split-mouth study, where one quadrant underwent traditional SRP and another quadrant underwent SRP with the help of the periodontal endoscope (Blue et al. 2013). Nevertheless, a significant decrease in periodontal outcomes of inflammation (namely

Diagnosis and Treatment of Furcation-Involved Teeth, First Edition. Edited by Luigi Nibali.
© 2018 John Wiley & Sons Ltd. Published 2018 by John Wiley & Sons Ltd.
Companion website: www.wiley.com/go/nibali/diagnosis

bleeding on probing, BOP, and gingival index, GI) was observed in the endoscopy-aided SRP group compared to the SRP group.

Although endoscopy may be an attractive option, especially for sites that have not responded to traditional non-surgical treatment and for patients where surgery is contraindicated, the use of the periodontal endoscope may be difficult in narrow furcations, or in curved roots, root proximity, and in the presence of overhanging restorations, as that may hinder the access for the endoscope and the instruments (Kwan 2005). Furthermore, we should not forget that, apart from the high cost, the use of endoscopic instrumentation can be difficult to master, it requires dedicated training, and it is associated with a steep learning curve.

10.3   Laser Therapy

In the past two decades, the use of lasers in the treatment of periodontal disease has attracted increasing interest. The word 'laser' is an acronym for 'light amplification by stimulated emission of radiation' and it broadly refers to any device that emits light, is spatially coherent, and is collimated. Lasers can be classified according to their active medium (gas lasers and solid lasers), tissue applicability (hard-tissue and soft-tissue lasers), range of wavelength, and risk associated with their application (Verma et al. 2012). Dental laser wavelengths are typically located within the near, mid, and far infrared portions of the electromagnetic spectrum (EMS; Lomke, 2009).

In periodontal therapy, different lasers have been proposed for removal of pocket epithelium (Borrajo et al. 2004; Saglam et al. 2014; Ustun et al. 2014), removal of subgingival calculus deposits (Eberhard et al. 2003; Schwarz et al., 2003; Lopes et al. 2010), reduction of bacterial load (Moritz et al. 1998; Yaneva et al. 2014), root surface decontamination (Barone et al. 2002), and enhancement of periodontal regeneration (Dogan et al. 2016; Taniguchi et al. 2016).

The current evidence supporting the adjunctive use of dental lasers (mainly the diode or the Nd:YAG) is of poor quality and insufficient to warrant their use in the treatment of chronic or aggressive periodontitis or in periodontal maintenance therapy (Cobb 2016). In fact, since the 2011 statement from the American Academy of Periodontology that the use of dental lasers as monotherapy or in addition to non-surgical periodontal instrumentation did not provide any tangible advantage in terms of subgingival debridement, reduction of subgingival bacterial levels, and root debridement (American Academy of Periodontology 2011), very little has changed. Recent meta-analyses have claimed short-term (six months) benefits of the use of the Nd:YAG or diode lasers in conjunction with non-surgical periodontal therapy in terms of probing pocket depth (PPD) and BOP reductions compared with mechanical debridement alone (Roncati and Gariffo 2014; Sgolastra et al. 2014). However, they also highlighted the poor quality of the available studies and the need for long-term, well-designed, parallel, independent randomized controlled trials (RCTs) with sufficient statistical power and appropriate laser settings in order to be able to draw more robust conclusions.

Besides the limited scientific evidence, current limitations on the use of lasers to treat molars with FI include the often high cost of the devices (which makes it difficult to justify their use to the patient), the need for additional education/training of the practitioner (this includes education on the different properties associated with the different wavelengths, as well as some fundamentals of physics), and the need to implement safety measures. In addition, and probably most importantly, there is a lack of evidence on the best setting to use for each different laser in terms of wavelength, energy density, power output, frequency/duration of irradiation, distance between the cells, and the laser spot/probe.

To the best of our knowledge, there is only a limited number of studies that have specifically considered laser treatment in molars with FI, and the results are in line with those reported for other periodontally involved teeth. In a double-blind RCT, de Andrade et al. (2008) compared clinical and microbiological parameters of 17 patients with class II furcation lesions treated either with SRP, or with SRP followed by pulsed Nd:YAG laser treatment. The results showed that the adjunctive laser promoted a significant higher reduction in the total bacteria colony-forming units (CFU) immediately after the treatment, but after six weeks no significant differences were detected between the two groups. Furthermore, no significant differences in terms of periodontal clinical parameters between baseline and six weeks after treatment were found between the two groups. In a more recent split-mouth study, an erbium, chromium: yttrium-scandium-gallium-garnet (Er,Cr:YSGG) laser was used in association with SRP in molars with degree II or III furcation involvement (Ge et al. 2017). A significantly higher reduction of PPD and BOP was observed at six and twelve weeks in the laser-treated group compared to the control group (SRP only). The visual analogue scale (VAS) pain score was also significantly lower when the laser was applied.

An attractive additional laser-based treatment modality is the so-called phototherapy, photomodulation, or low-level laser therapy (LLLT), which employs lasers at a low dose with the aims of alleviating pain or inflammation, inducing immunomodulation, and promoting wound healing and tissue regeneration (Anders et al. 2015). Recent evidence suggests that LLLT is able to enhance osteoblastic proliferation and differentiation (Amid et al. 2014), increase gene expression of collagen and vascular endothelial growth factor in fibroblastic cells (Martignago et al. 2015), promote the production of nucleic acid (Saperia et al. 1986), and increase mitochondrial respiratory chain and adenosine triphosphate (ATP) synthesis (Agrawal et al. 2014). Future studies are needed to explore the potential benefits of adding LLLT to, for instance, periodontal regenerative treatment,

also in furcation-involved molars. Another application of phototherapy in periodontology is antimicrobial photodynamic therapy, which combines LLLT and a photosensitizer with the aim of destroying pathogens in the pocket with reactive oxygen species, and this will be discussed in more detail in the next section.

10.4 Photodynamic Therapy

The rationale behind photodynamic therapy (PDT) comes from the need to obtain antimicrobial effects without the risk of causing the onset of microbial resistance. With PDT, bacteria are sensitized using a dye (photosensitizer) coming into contact with their membrane, and are then destroyed following irradiation with light of the correct energy and wavelength. More specifically, a laser light is used to activate the dye molecules to reach a high energy triplet state, which reacts with oxygen to create singlet oxygen, which in turn destroys the bacterial membrane. Toluidine blue (TBO) and methylene blue (MB) are used as dyes, due to their ideal properties of low toxicity, cationic charge for attachment to Gram- membranes, red light absorption, rapid transition from 'singlet' to 'triplet' state, long maintenance of 'triplet' state, and high production of photoproduct (Atieh 2010; Soukos and Goodson 2011; Gursoy et al. 2013).

Although the original concept of PDT is already over 100 years old, only in recent years has it reached clinical applications in various fields of medicine, including oncology, dermatology, and dentistry (Konopka and Goslinski 2007). Its characteristics make PDT potentially suitable for the treatment of periodontitis, either in the non-surgical or surgical phase, with the aim of boosting the antimicrobial effects of mechanical plaque removal without the risk of causing microbial resistance (Andrade et al. 2013; Sgolastra et al. 2013a, b; Souza et al. 2016). Studies have shown that photo-inactivation of pathogenic bacteria harvested from periodontal pockets is possible in vitro by using TBO and a 635 nm laser activation (Qin et al. 2008). Despite some promising animal models and clinical studies, a systematic review and meta-analysis of seven RCTs using PDT as an adjunct or alternative to subgingival debridement showed no significant clinical benefits, with reduction in some bacteria in some studies (*Porphyromonas gingivalis*) but not in others, and no consistent adverse events reported (Sgolastra et al. 2013a). The same group performed a new systematic review that included both RCTs and parallel-design studies (Sgolastra et al. 2013b). After removing outlier studies, the meta-analysis indicated a significant positive effect in terms of PPD reduction (0.19, 95% confidence interval [CI] 0.007–0.31, p = 0.002) and CAL gain (0.37, 95% CI 0.26–0.47, p < 0.0001) at three months. However, the clinical significance of these data is limited and no differences were observed at six months. Remarkably, subgroup analysis revealed that studies adopting a time of application of 60 seconds showed a higher and significant PPD reduction and CAL gain.

Owing to the difficult access for mechanical debridement, furcation defects represent an ideal scenario where PDT could be helpful during initial therapy, surgical therapy, or maintenance in order to reduce bacterial load and promote healing. An advantage of PDT includes the possibility to apply it topically into a periodontal pocket, thus avoiding overdose and reducing the probability of side effects and microflora disturbance in other sites of the oral cavity (which are instead associated with systemic antimicrobials; Wainwright 1998; Hamblin and Hasan 2004). Figure 10.1 shows a case of furcation involvement treated with PDT.

De Almeida and co-workers (2008) histometrically assessed the influence of PDT on bone loss in furcation areas of rats with experimentally induced periodontitis. The PDT group demonstrated less bone loss compared to the control group, the group treated only with topical MB, and the group treated only with LLLT at 7 days ($1.986 \pm 0.417 \, mm^2$). At 15 days, the PDT ($1.641 \pm 0.115 \, mm^2$) and MB groups ($1.991 \pm 0.294 \, mm^2$) demonstrated

(a) (b)

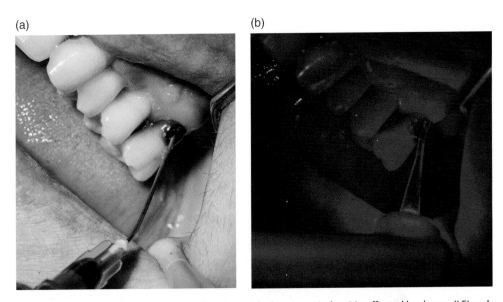

Figure 10.1 Upper left first molar (UL6) of patient with chronic periodontitis, affected by degree II FI and treated with photodynamic therapy, following non-surgical furcation debridement with ultrasonic devices. (a) Application of dye (methylene blue) inside the furcation area; (b) activation of the dye by photodynamic therapy light.

less bone loss compared to the control $(4.062 \pm 0.416 \, mm^2)$ and LLLT $(2.641 \pm 0.849 \, mm^2)$ groups.

To the best of our knowledge, only a few RCTs have evaluated PDT specifically in molars with FI. A double-blind RCT evaluated PDT for the treatment of class II furcations in patients with chronic periodontitis (Luchesi et al. 2013); 21 patients who underwent SRP with the adjunct of the photosensitizer only (control) and 16 patients who underwent SRP followed by PDT (test) completed the six-month follow-up. While PDT was able to reduce gingival crevicular fluid (GCF) levels of inflammatory mediators and the concentration of *P. gingivalis* and *Tannerella forsythia* at six months, no significant differences in terms of CAL and PPD were detected between the two groups at either three or six months. Nevertheless, when interpreting these results we need to consider that the study lacked a true negative control group, as the presence of the photosensitizer dye may have optimized the results of the control group. Moreover, this study used a single PDT application as an adjunct to SRP, while it is plausible that repeated PDT applications would have resulted in more positive outcomes (Lulic et al. 2009). In a split-mouth RCT, Andrade et al. (2013) collected data on 14 patients with bilateral lower molars with class III furcation lesions scheduled for extraction. In the control side traditional SRP was performed, while in the test side SRP was followed by a session of PDT. At 45 days post initial therapy, the class III furcation lesions were surgically accessed, and flap surgery with SRP and flap surgery with SRP + PDT was performed in the control and test group, respectively. At 21 days post surgery, the newly formed granulation tissue was collected, and real-time polymerase chain reaction (PCR) showed a significant up-regulation of the TIMP-, 2/MMP-2, and OPG/RANKL mRNA ratios in the test group, thus suggesting a role for PDT in positively modulating extracellular matrix and bone remodelling.

10.5 Air-polishing Devices

Since in periodontally compromised teeth root surfaces are subjected to continuous abrasive instrumentation during lifelong periodontal maintenance therapy, debridement techniques that are at the same time effective and minimally invasive should be aimed at. Keeping this in mind, air-polishing devices might represent a valid alternative to mechanical instrumentation. Air-abrasive technology has been applied in the dental field for more than 60 years (reviewed by Petersilka 2011). The idea is to use an abrasive powder that is introduced into a stream of compressed air to clean and polish the tooth surface by removing the deposits attached to it or by smoothing their texture. This abrasive process depends on the properties of the particles applied (shape, geometrical form, hardness) and on the pressure of the air and water used (Petersilka 2011).

Sodium bicarbonate–based air polishing has been successfully applied for supragingival plaque and stain removal since the 1980s (Berkstein et al. 1987; Barnes et al. 1990). However, the use of sodium bicarbonate on cement and dentine is not advisable, as significant tissue removal may occur (Atkinson et al. 1984; Horning et al. 1987; Petersilka et al. 2003a). Furthermore, this type of air-polishing device may cause reversible soft-tissue irritation and damage, such as epithelial erosions with exposure of the underlying connective tissue (Hunter et al. 1989; Kontturi-Narhi et al. 1989; Kozlovsky et al. 2005). To overcome these limitations and minimize the hard- and soft-tissue trauma, glycine powder air-polishing devices have been introduced. Several clinical trials have evaluated the efficacy of this air-polishing system for subgingival biofilm removal with positive results, but no study distinguished between single- and multi-rooted teeth. In a randomized split-mouth controlled study in patients receiving supportive periodontal therapy, the use of glycine powder was more effective in reducing the number of CFU in comparison to hand instrumentation with curettes in pockets of 3–5 mm (Petersilka et al. 2003b, c). Another split-mouth controlled study did not find significant differences at a microbiological level between SRP and subgingival air polishing; however, the use of glycine-based air polishing was perceived as less painful/uncomfortable by the patients and less time consuming by the operator (Moene et al. 2010). While only shallow pockets (up to 5 mm) were included in these studies, a more recent study from Flemmig and co-workers (2012) considered pockets from 4 to 9 mm. Their results showed that glycine air polish is more effective in removing the subgingival biofilm, and may induce a beneficial shift of the oral microbiota (lower total viable bacterial count) compared to traditional SRP.

In conclusion, air-polishing devices might represent a valid alternative to mechanical instrumentation, for both periodontal treatment and periodontal maintenance therapy. The use of glycine powder air polishing seems well tolerated by the patient and no severe adverse events have been reported. However, a few cases of air emphysema (all successfully healed) have been reported (Finlayson and Stevens 1988; Fruhauf et al. 2005) and the patient needs to be informed about this rare complication. New air-polishing powders, such as erythritol-based powders (Hagi et al. 2013, 2015), are now under investigations and future randomized trials will have to confirm their efficacy. Further studies on molars with FI are advisable to test the efficacy of this technique specifically for multi-rooted teeth.

10.6 Local Antimicrobials

Given the microbial aetiology of periodontitis, antimicrobial adjuncts to mechanical debridement could be considered a valid treatment option for periodontal treatment. Bearing in mind that mechanical subgingival biofilm disruption with ultrasonic inserts and curettes is essential for the healing of periodontal pockets (Badersten et al. 1984), the additional use of antimicrobial agents

directly in the site could lead to a further reduction in microbial load and a better healing of the lesion. Local antimicrobials could be used as topical applications, for sustained release (drug delivered in effective concentrations for less than 24 hours) or controlled delivery (drug delivered in effective concentrations for more than 24 hours), within different delivery systems (Herrera et al. 2012; Jepsen and Jepsen 2016). The use of antiseptics (including chlorhexidine, sodium hypochlorite, and povidone-iodine) and antibiotics (including tetracyclines and metronidazole) has been reported in the periodontal literature and several agents are available on the market. Systematic reviews show that when local antibiotics are used as adjuncts to subgingival debridement, short-term improvement in clinical parameters measured as PPD reductions and CAL gain can be achieved (Hanes and Purvis 2003; Bonito et al. 2005; Matesanz-Perez et al. 2013). No studies with long-term data on periodontal stability or tooth loss are available.

As repeatedly observed before, difficulty in accessing the furcation area for debridement and the potentially high microbial load inside the furcation lesions make FI potentially amenable to the adjunctive use of local antimicrobials. However, what is the evidence for the role of local antimicrobials specifically for the healing and maintenance of FI molars? Tonetti and co-workers (1998) included 127 patients with class II mandibular furcation with BOP in SPT in a randomized multicentre controlled trial. All subjects received SRP and oral hygiene instructions, while tests also had tetracycline fibres applied inside the furcation defects. Subjects were followed up to six months, when periodontal clinical measurements were taken for the last time before the end of the study. The authors observed that, despite increased reductions in BOP and PPD in the test group at three months (compared to controls), no differences between groups were observed at six months. Consistent results were observed in a separate study on 32 patients with chronic periodontitis, who received initial pocket/root debridement by ultrasonic instrumentation, followed by random assignment to further treatment by ultrasonic instrumentation with or without adjunctive local application of an 8.8% doxycycline gel in residual defects (Tomasi and Wennstrom 2011). Clinical examinations were repeated three and nine months after retreatment. The retreatment including the local antibiotic resulted in 'closure' of 50% of degree I furcation sites, compared to 29% for sites treated with mechanical debridement only (p > 0.05), and in a reduction in depth of degree II furcation sites of 17% in the test and 11% in the control group (p > 0.05). No differences for the outcome variable 'furcation improvement' were detected between the two groups, suggesting that improvement in molar FI after non-surgical periodontal therapy was not enhanced by adjunctive locally applied doxycycline (Tomasi and Wennstrom 2011).

The use of povidone-iodine as an adjunct to SRP in the treatment of class II furcations has been investigated in two RCTs, but only limited (Ribeiro Edel et al. 2010) or no additional clinical benefits (Del Peloso Ribeiro et al. 2006) resulted from the use of this antiseptic. In a randomized parallel-arm controlled study, the clinical efficacy of subgingival ultrasonic instrumentation irrigated with essential oils (EOs) was compared with chlorhexidine (CHX) or distilled water (control) in 45 patients with class II FI (Yilmaz and Bayindir 2012). When comparing the test groups (EOs and CHX) to the control group, no significant differences in the improvement of periodontal clinical parameters were reported at one and three months after treatment, with the exception of BOP, which was significantly reduced in the EOs group compared to the CHX and control groups at both one and three months. Figure 10.2 shows a case of a maxillary molar furcation lesion treated with local antibiotics.

10.7 Systemic Antimicrobials

Systemic antibiotics have been proposed since the 1970s as adjuncts for the treatment of periodontitis, initially mainly for early-onset forms, thanks to their effect on the subgingival microbiota. Baer and Socransky (1979) followed up patients with 'periodontosis' (what we would now classify as aggressive periodontitis, AgP), treated with oral hygiene instructions, non-surgical, and surgical approaches associated with adjunctive systemic antibiotics, and concluded that antibiotics such as tetracyclines and penicillin could be a helpful adjunct to patient management, including full-thickness flaps and curettage. Later, metronidazole was introduced in periodontal therapy for its effect on *Aggregatibacter actinomyecetemcomitans* (then known as *Actinobacillus actinomycetemcomitans*; Saxen and Asikainen 1993). Interest in the use of adjunctive systemic antibiotics increased with the evidence from laboratory studies, showing that the rate of metronidazole uptake by *A. actinomyecetemcomitans* bacterial cells simultaneously incubated with amoxicillin was higher than the uptake in cells incubated with metronidazole alone (Pavicic et al. 1995). Hence, several papers were published suggesting improved clinical outcomes (PPD reductions and CAL gains) when the amoxicillin–metronidazole 'cocktail' was used as an adjunct to SRP (van Winkelhoff et al. 1992; Winkel et al. 2001). While several randomized placebo-controlled trials on the adjunctive use of amoxicillin and metronidazole flourished, several other antibiotics or combinations of them were introduced as adjuncts to periodontal therapy, for both chronic and aggressive periodontitis.

Most original papers and systematic reviews only report short-term data (e.g. six months or twelve months), making it difficult to understand possible long-term benefits. Systematic reviews tend to agree that systemic antibiotics used as adjuncts to SRP provide clinical improvements (PPD reductions, CAL gain) compared with SRP alone or SRP and placebo. These clinical improvements range from 0.3 to 0.5 additional PPD reductions and 0.2 to 0.4 mm additional CAL gain (as full-mouth average), and seem to be more pronounced in AgP cases (Herrera et al. 2002, 2012; Sgolastra et al. 2012a, b; Buset et al. 2015). Studies venturing into

(a)

(b)

(c)

(e)

(d)

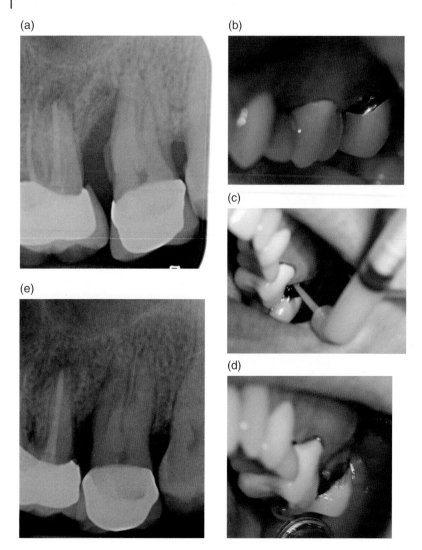

Figure 10.2 Application of local antibiotic after non-surgical debridement in degree II mesial furcation lesion of a maxillary second molar, associated with mesial intrabony defect (10 mm probing pocket depth) and extensive presence of subgingival deposits. (a) Periapical radiograph; (b) clinical photograph; (c) antibiotic application from the mesio-buccal aspect of the pocket associated with the furcation defect; (d) antibiotic overflowing from the pocket; (e) radiographic re-evaluation six months after treatment, showing bone fill with reduction in the intrabony defect depth (now 6 mm probing pocket depth and degree I furcation involvement).

longer-term follow-ups show conflicting evidence. A study on 506 patients with moderate to severe periodontitis observed reductions in attachment loss favouring the test group (adjunctive amoxicillin and metronidazole) for up to 27 months of follow-up (Harks et al. 2015). A prospective study with 13-year follow-up using 250 mg tetracycline hydrochloride (HCl) four times a day for three weeks adjunctive to SRP found that short-term benefits seemed to disappear with time (Ramberg et al. 2001). A recent systematic review highlighted that the clinical benefits of adjunctive systemic antibiotics seem to diminish over time, from the three-month follow-up to the one-year follow-up

(Keestra et al. 2015). Hence, doubts persist about the long-term effect of antibiotics used as adjunctive therapy.

Furthermore, adverse events and risk of developing antibiotic resistance should be an important concern when deciding whether to use adjunctive antibiotic therapy. Generally, deep pockets seem to benefit more from an adjunctive antibiotic regime, as the antibiotic could be of more help in sites where the effectiveness of mechanical debridement is more limited (Guerrero et al. 2005). For the same reasons, it can be supposed that teeth affected by FI could benefit from adjunctive systemic antibiotics. However, no study seems to have specifically tested this hypothesis. To the best of our knowledge, only a subanalysis of data from a large clinical trial has tried to answer the question of whether systemic amoxicillin and metronidazole adjunctively to mechanical debridement might significantly improve periodontal clinical parameters at molar and premolar furcation sites (Eickholz et al. 2016). Although PPD reduction and CAL gain at furcation sites were noticeably improved after antibiotic therapy compared with placebo, no difference in the change of furcation degrees between the treatments could be detected.

10.8 Probiotics

When considering the pathogenesis of periodontitis, it is well accepted that this disease requires the presence of a susceptible host together with the presence of pathogenic bacteria (Socransky and Haffajee 1992). Periodontitis is thought to be the result of a dysbiotic process, characterized by a shift in the composition of the normal subgingival biofilm towards a more pathogenic one (Hajishengallis and Lamont 2012). Therefore, there has been growing interest in the possibility of using probiotics with the aim of shifting the oral microbiota equilibrium back to a condition of oral health.

Probiotics are defined as 'living microorganisms which, when administered in adequate amounts, confer a health benefit for the host' (FAO/WHO 2001). The most common probiotics belong to two main genera, *Lactobacillus* and *Bifidobacterium.* The suggested mechanisms of action of probiotics in the oral cavity include a modulation of the host immune-inflammatory response, a direct inhibition of periodontopathogenic bacteria via the production of antimicrobial substances (such as lactic acid, hydrogen peroxide, and bacteriocin-like substances), and an indirect effect originating from competitive exclusion systems, so that by competing for the same niches and nutrients, 'good' bacteria can reduce the chances of pathogens replicating and adhering to tooth surfaces (Laleman and Teughels 2015). However, three systematic reviews have been recently published to evaluate the overall efficacy of probiotic therapy in the treatment of periodontally compromised teeth. Matsubara and co-workers (2016) included 12 RCTs (both split mouth and parallel designed) and concluded that the use of oral probiotics alone or associated with SRP is well tolerated (no adverse effects reported) and is associated with an overall tendency for improved clinical parameters and reduced levels of periodontal pathogens. Martin-Cabezas and co-workers (2016) included only RCTs comparing SRP alone (or associated with placebo) to SRP associated with assumption of *Lactobacillus reuteri* in the quality assessment. Meta-analysis showed a statistically significant CAL gain (-0.42 mm, $p = 0.002$) and BOP reduction (-14.66, $p = 0.003$) for SRP associated with the probiotic treatment versus SRP alone in the short term. Furthermore, when stratifying for pocket depth, the use of probiotics was significantly beneficial in moderate (-0.18, $p = 0.001$) and deep (-0.67, $p < 0.001$) pockets. Finally, Gruner and co-workers (2016) included RCTs broadly evaluating the efficacy of any form of probiotic therapy for the management of caries and periodontitis.

The meta-analysis reported that probiotics significantly reduced BOP (standardized mean difference, SMD: -1.15; 95% CI -1.68/-0.62), PPD (SMD: -0.86, 95% CI -1.55/-0.17), and gingival index (SMD: -0.86; 95% CI -1.52/-0.20), but did not affect plaque index or CAL. Unfortunately, specific studies investigating this treatment modality in furcation lesions are missing.

Although clinical data look promising, the heterogeneity of the available studies in terms of population included (experimental gingivitis patients, healthy patients, patients with chronic periodontitis, patients with aggressive periodontitis), parameters evaluated (microbiological parameters in plaque or saliva, plaque index, PPD, CAL, etc.), protocol adopted (probiotics as monotherapy vs probiotics after SRP), and probiotics employed do not allow robust conclusions to be drawn. Further research is needed to demonstrate the efficacy of certain probiotic strains in oral health, as well as their desired concentration and vehicle.

10.9   Surgical Innovations

Periodontal surgical techniques have gradually striven to become less and less invasive, in order to reduce morbidity and patient discomfort. The development of minimally invasive surgical periodontal techniques includes the use of microsurgical instruments and magnification, and it is based on the principle of preserving as much of the soft tissue as possible (Harrel 1999). Incisions, flap elevation, and suturing techniques have been modified by a series of papilla-preservation techniques (Takei et al. 1985; Cortellini et al. 1995, 1999) and, more recently, by minimally invasive surgical therapy (Cortellini and Tonetti 2007, 2009; Trombelli et al. 2009), moving from double flaps to single flaps. These techniques are aimed mainly at the treatment of intrabony defects, and have been shown to yield favourable clinical results with reduced tissue trauma compared

with traditional surgical techniques. Remarkably, recent RCTs show that, when a good stabilization of the blood clot in the surgical area is achieved, the use of grafting materials may not add any additional benefits in intrabony defects (Trombelli et al. 2010; Cortellini and Tonetti 2011; Ribeiro et al. 2011; Mishra et al. 2013). The same principles of reduction of surgical flap, minimizing trauma, and stimulating the formation of a stable blood clot could be implemented for surgical approaches to furcations. However, these techniques are explicitly not indicated for furcation lesions (Cortellini and Tonetti 2007), and there seems to be a lack of specific innovative surgical techniques for the treatment of furcation-involved molars.

10.10   Furcation 'Filling'

Some researchers have attempted closure of the furcation lesion with the use of restorative materials (e.g. ionomeric cement or calcium hydroxiapatite cement). This defies the principles of periodontal regeneration and of maintenance of reduced microbial load in the furcation region discussed in this book. Not surprisingly, such therapy has encountered failure, with worsening in periodontal clinical measurements and high risk of tooth loss (Anderegg and Metzler 2000; Fowler and Breault 2001; Rupprecht et al. 2001). This stresses once more the importance of allowing plaque removal, either self-performed or professional or both, inside the furcation lesion when regeneration of the furcation lesion is not feasible.

Conclusion

Researchers and clinicians are striving to identify more efficient ways for the successful treatment of periodontitis, and specifically of molars with furcation involvement. Keeping in mind the uncontested importance of oral hygiene instructions and subgingival debridement, new technologies could soon provide a helping hand for the treatment of complex cases. Tools to improve the efficacy of intrafurcation biofilm removal, to reduce the treatment time, and to improve the patient's perceived comfort, such as periodontal endoscope, lasers and air-powder devices, or antimicrobial agents (local or systemic antibiotics, photodynamic therapy)

and probiotics have been tested as adjuncts for the treatment and long-term maintenance of furcation lesions. Sadly, the evidence for their efficacy in the clinical outcomes of furcation treatment is still lacking, despite some initial promising results. Future well-designed studies are warranted to shed light on the additional benefits associated with these new treatment modalities.

Summary of Evidence

- The treatment of molars with furcation involvement desperately needs new methods to improve clinical efficacy, patient comfort, and long-term outcomes.
- Antimicrobial adjuncts (local antibiotics, photodynamic therapy) and probiotics and technology for improved biofilm removal (periodontal endoscope, lasers, and air-powder devices) are being tested,

with the potential of being used for the treatment of specific furcation cases.
- Clinical efficacy, costs, and learning curves for these potential adjuncts still need to be systematically assessed before they can potentially be routinely implemented in the treatment of molars with furcation involvement.

References

Agrawal, T., Gupta, G.K., Rai, V. et al. (2014). Pre-conditioning with low-level laser (light) therapy: Light before the storm. *Dose Response* 12, 619–649. doi:10.2203/dose-response.14-032.Agrawal.

American Academy of Periodontology (2011). American Academy of Periodontology statement on the efficacy of lasers in the non-surgical treatment of inflammatory periodontal disease. *Journal of Periodontology* 82, 513–514. doi:10.1902/jop.2011.114001.

Amid, R., Kadkhodazadeh, M., Ahsaie, M.G., and Hakakzadeh, A. (2014). Effect of low level laser therapy on proliferation and differentiation of the cells contributing in bone regeneration. *Journal of Lasers in Medical Science* 5, 163–170.

Anderegg, C.R., and Metzler, D.G. (2000). Retention of multi-rooted teeth with class III furcation lesions utilizing resins: Report of 17 cases. *Journal of Periodontology* 71, 1043–1047. doi:10.1902/jop.2000.71.6.1043.

Anders, J.J., Lanzafame, R.J., and Arany, P.R. (2015). Low-level light/laser therapy versus photobiomodulation therapy. *Photomedicine and Laser Surgery* 33, 183–184. doi:10.1089/pho.2015.9848.

Andrade, P.F., Garlet, G.P., Silva, J.S. et al. (2013). Adjunct effect of the antimicrobial photodynamic therapy to an association of non-surgical and surgical periodontal treatment in modulation of gene expression: A human study. *Journal of Photochemistry and Photobiology B* 126, 119–125. doi:10.1016/j.jphotobiol.2013.06.012.

Atieh, M.A. (2010). Photodynamic therapy as an adjunctive treatment for chronic periodontitis: A meta-analysis. *Lasers in Medical Science* 25, 605–613. doi:10.1007/s10103-009-0744-6.

Atkinson, D.R., Cobb, C.M., and Killoy, W.J. (1984). The effect of an air-powder abrasive system on in vitro root surfaces. *Journal of Periodontology* 55, 13–18. doi:10.1902/jop.1984.55.1.13.

Badersten, A., Nilveus, R., and Egelberg, J. (1984) Effect of nonsurgical periodontal therapy. II. Severely advanced periodontitis. *Journal of Clinical Periodontology* 11, 63°76.

Baer, P.N., and Socransky, S.S. (1979). Periodontosis: Case report with long-term follow-up. *Periodontal Case Reports* 1, 1–6.

Barnes, C.M., Russell, C.M., Gerbo, L.R. et al. (1990). Effects of an air-powder polishing system on orthodontically bracketed and banded teeth. *American Journal of Orthodontics and Dentofacial Orthopedics* 97, 74–81. doi:10.1016/S0889-5406(05)81712-3.

Barone, A., Covani, U., Crespi, R., and Romanos, G.E. (2002). Root surface morphological changes after focused versus defocused CO2 laser irradiation: A scanning electron microscopy analysis. *Journal of Periodontology* 73, 370–373. doi:10.1902/jop.2002.73.4.370.

Berkstein, S., Reiff, R.L., McKinney, J.F., and Killoy, W.J. (1987). Supragingival root surface removal during maintenance procedures utilizing an air-powder abrasive system or hand scaling: An in vitro study. *Journal of Periodontology* 58, 327–330. doi:10.1902/jop.1987.58.5.327.

Blue, C.M., Lenton, P., Lunos, S. et al. (2013). A pilot study comparing the outcome of scaling/root planing with and without Perioscope technology. *Journal of Dental Hygiene* 87, 152–157.

Bonito, A.J., Lux, L., and Lohr, K.N. (2005). Impact of local adjuncts to scaling and root planing in periodontal disease therapy: A systematic review. *Journal of Periodontology* 76, 1227–1236. doi:10.1902/jop.2005.76.8.1227.

Borrajo, J.L., Varela, L.G., Castro, G.L. et al. (2004). Diode laser (980 nm) as adjunct to scaling and root planing. *Photomedicine and Laser Surgery* 22, 509–512. doi:10.1089/pho.2004.22.509.

Buset, S.L., Zitzmann, N.U., Weiger, R., and Walter, C. (2015). Non-surgical periodontal therapy supplemented with systemically administered azithromycin: A systematic review of RCTs. *Clinical Oral Investigations* 19, 1763–1775. doi:10.1007/s00784-015-1499-z.

Cobb, C.M. (2016). Is there clinical benefit from using a diode or Nd:YAG laser in the treatment of periodontitis? *Journal of Periodontology* 87, 1117–1131. doi:10.1902/jop.2016.160134.

Cortellini, P., Prato, G.P., and Tonetti, M.S. (1995). The modified papilla preservation technique: A new surgical approach for interproximal regenerative procedures. *Journal of Periodontology* 66, 261–266. doi:10.1902/jop.1995.66.4.261.

Cortellini, P., Prato, G.P., and Tonetti, M.S. (1999). The simplified papilla preservation flap: A novel surgical approach for the management of soft tissues in regenerative procedures. *International Journal of Periodontics and Restorative Dentistry* 19, 589–599.

Cortellini, P., and Tonetti, M.S. (2007). A minimally invasive surgical technique with an enamel matrix derivative in the regenerative treatment of intra-bony defects: A novel approach to limit morbidity. *Journal of Clinical Periodontology* 34, 87–93. doi:10.1111/j.1600-051X.2006.01020.x.

Cortellini, P., and Tonetti, M.S. (2009). Improved wound stability with a modified minimally invasive surgical technique in the regenerative treatment of isolated interdental intrabony defects. *Journal of Clinical Periodontology* 36, 157–163. doi:10.1111/j.1600-051X.2008.01352.x.

Cortellini, P., and Tonetti, M.S. (2011). Clinical and radiographic outcomes of the modified minimally invasive surgical technique with and without regenerative materials: A randomized-controlled trial in intra-bony defects. *Journal of Clinical Periodontology* 38, 365–373. doi:10.1111/j.1600-051X.2011.01705.x.

de Almeida, J.M., Theodoro, L.H., Bosco, A.F. et al. (2008). In vivo effect of photodynamic therapy on periodontal bone loss in dental furcations. *Journal of Periodontology* 79, 1081–1088. doi:10.1902/jop.2008.070456.

de Andrade, A.K., Feist, I.S., Pannuti, C.M. et al. (2008). Nd:YAG laser clinical assisted in class II furcation treatment. *Lasers in Medical Science* 23, 341–347. doi:10.1007/s10103-007-0482-6.

Del Peloso Ribeiro, E., Bittencourt, S., Ambrosano, G.M. et al. (2006). Povidone-iodine used as an adjunct to non-surgical treatment of furcation involvements. *Journal of Periodontology* 77, 211–217. doi:10.1902/jop.2006.050095.

Dogan, G.E., Aksoy, H., Demir, T. et al. (2016). Clinical and biochemical comparison of guided tissue regeneration versus guided tissue regeneration plus low-level laser therapy in the treatment of class II furcation defects: A clinical study. *Journal of Cosmetic Laser Therapy* 18, 98–104. doi:10.3109/14764172.2015.1114637.

Eberhard, J., Ehlers, H., Falk, W. et al. (2003). Efficacy of subgingival calculus removal with Er:YAG laser compared to mechanical debridement: An in situ study. *Journal of Clinical Periodontology* 30, 511–518.

Eickholz, P., Nickles, K., Koch, R. et al. (2016). Is furcation involvement affected by adjunctive systemic amoxicillin plus metronidazole? A clinical trials exploratory subanalysis. *Journal of Clinical Periodontology* 43, 839–848. doi:10.1111/jcpe.12594.

FAO/WHO (2001). *Report of joint FAO/WHO expert consultation on evaluation of health and nutritional properties of probiotics in food including powder milk with live lactic acid bacteria*. Cordoba: Food and Agriculture Organization/World Health Organization.

Finlayson, R.S., and Stevens, F.D. (1988). Subcutaneous facial emphysema secondary to use of the Cavi-Jet. *Journal of Periodontology* 59, 315–317. doi:10.1902/jop.1988.59.5.315.

Flemmig, T.F., Arushanov, D., Daubert, D. et al. (2012). Randomized controlled trial assessing efficacy and safety of glycine powder air polishing in moderate-to-deep periodontal pockets. *Journal of Periodontology* 83, 444–452. doi:10.1902/jop.2011.110367.

Fowler, E.B., and Breault, L.G. (2001). Failure of resin ionomers in the retention of multi-rooted teeth with Class III furcation involvement: A rebuttal case report. *Journal of Periodontology* 72, 1084–1091. doi:10.1902/jop.2001.72.8.1084.

Fruhauf, J., Weinke, R., Pilger, U. et al. (2005). Soft tissue cervicofacial emphysema after dental treatment: Report of 2 cases with emphasis on the differential diagnosis of angioedema. *Archives of Dermatology* 141, 1437–1440. doi:10.1001/archderm.141.11.1437.

Ge, L., Zhang, Y., and Shu, R. (2017). Er,Cr:YSGG laser application for the treatment of periodontal furcation involvements. *Photomedicine and Laser Surgery* 35, 92–97. doi:10.1089/pho.2016.4145.

Geisinger, M.L., Mealey, B.L., Schoolfield, J., and Mellonig, J.T. (2007). The effectiveness of subgingival scaling and root planing: An evaluation of therapy with and without the use of the periodontal endoscope. *Journal of Periodontology* 78, 22–28. doi:10.1902/jop.2007.060186.

Gruner, D., Paris, S., and Schwendicke, F. (2016). Probiotics for managing caries and periodontitis: Systematic review and meta-analysis. *Journal of Dentistry* 48, 16–25. doi:10.1016/j.jdent.2016.03.002.

Guerrero, A., Griffiths, G.S., Nibali, L. et al. (2005). Adjunctive benefits of systemic amoxicillin and metronidazole in non-surgical treatment of generalized aggressive periodontitis: A randomized placebo-controlled clinical trial. *Journal of Clinical Periodontology* 32, 1096–1107. doi:10.1111/j.1600-051X.2005.00814.x.

Gursoy, H., Ozcakir-Tomruk, C., Tanalp, J., and Yilmaz, S. (2013). Photodynamic therapy in dentistry: A literature review. *Clinical Oral Investigations* 17, 1113–1125. doi:10.1007/s00784-012-0845-7.

Hagi, T.T., Hofmanner, P., Eick, S. et al. (2015). The effects of erythritol air-polishing powder on microbiologic and clinical outcomes during supportive periodontal therapy: Six-month results of a randomized controlled clinical trial. *Quintessence International* 46, 31–41. doi:10.3290/j.qi.a32817.

Hagi, T.T., Hofmanner, P., Salvi, G.E. et al. (2013). Clinical outcomes following subgingival application of a novel erythritol powder by means of air polishing in supportive periodontal therapy: A randomized, controlled clinical study. *Quintessence International* 44, 753°761. doi:10.3290/j.qi.a30606.

Hajishengallis, G., and Lamont, R.J. (2012). Beyond the red complex and into more complexity: The polymicrobial synergy and dysbiosis (PSD) model of periodontal disease etiology. *Molecular Oral Microbiology* 27, 409–419. doi:10.1111/j.2041-1014.2012.00663.x.

Hamblin, M.R., and Hasan, T. (2004). Photodynamic therapy: A new antimicrobial approach to infectious disease? *Photochemical and Photobiological Sciences* 3, 436–450. doi:10.1039/b311900a.

Hanes, P.J., and Purvis, J.P. (2003). Local anti-infective therapy: Pharmacological agents. A systematic review. *Annals of Periodontology* 8, 79–98. doi:10.1902/annals.2003.8.1.79.

Harks, I., Koch, R., Eickholz, P. et al. (2015). Is progression of periodontitis relevantly influenced by systemic antibiotics? A clinical randomized trial. *Journal of Clinical Periodontology* 42, 832–842. doi:10.1111/jcpe.12441.

Harrel, S.K. (1999). A minimally invasive surgical approach for periodontal regeneration: Surgical technique and observations. *Journal of Periodontology* 70, 1547–1557. doi:10.1902/jop.1999.70.12.1547.

Herrera, D., Matesanz, P., Bascones-Martinez, A., and Sanz, M. (2012). Local and systemic antimicrobial therapy in periodontics. *Journal of Evidence Based Dental Practice* 12, 50–60. doi:10.1016/S1532-3382(12)70013-1.

Herrera, D., Sanz, M., Jepsen, S. et al. (2002). A systematic review on the effect of systemic antimicrobials as an adjunct to scaling and root planing in periodontitis patients. *Journal of Clinical Periodontology* 29 (Suppl. 3), 136–159; discussion 160–162.

Horning, G.M., Cobb, C.M., and Killoy, W.J. (1987). Effect of an air-powder abrasive system on root surfaces in periodontal surgery. *Journal of Clinical Periodontology* 14, 213–220.

Hunter, K.M., Holborow, D.W., Kardos, T.B. et al. (1989). Bacteraemia and tissue damage resulting from air polishing. *British Dental Journal* 167, 275–278.

Jepsen, K., and Jepsen, S. (2016). Antibiotics/antimicrobials: Systemic and local administration in the therapy of mild to moderately advanced periodontitis. *Periodontology* 2000 71, 82–112. doi:10.1111/prd.12121.

Keestra, J.A., Grosjean, I., Coucke, W. et al. (2015). Non-surgical periodontal therapy with systemic antibiotics in patients with untreated chronic periodontitis: A systematic review and meta-analysis. *Journal of Periodontal Research* 50, 294–314. doi:10.1111/jre.12221.

Konopka, K., and Goslinski, T. (2007). Photodynamic therapy in dentistry. *Journal of Dental Research* 86, 694–707.

Kontturi-Narhi, V., Markkanen, S., and Markkanen, H. (1989). The gingival effects of dental airpolishing as evaluated by scanning electron microscopy. *Journal of Periodontology* 60, 19–22. doi:10.1902/jop.1989.60.1.19.

Kozlovsky, A., Artzi, Z., Nemcovsky, C.E., and Hirshberg, A. (2005). Effect of air-polishing devices on the gingiva: Histologic study in the canine. *Journal of Clinical Periodontology* 32, 329–334. doi:10.1111/j.1600-051X.2005.00678.x.

Kwan, J.Y. (2005). Enhanced periodontal debridement with the use of micro ultrasonic, periodontal endoscopy. *Journal of the California Dental Association* 33, 241–248.

Laleman, I., and Teughels, W. (2015). Probiotics in the dental practice: A review. *Quintessence International* 46, 255–264. doi:10.3290/j.qi.a33182.

Lomke, M.A. (2009). Clinical applications of dental lasers. *General Dentistry* 57, 47–59.

Lopes, B.M., Theodoro, L.H., Melo, R.F. et al. (2010). Clinical and microbiologic follow-up evaluations after non-surgical periodontal treatment with erbium:YAG laser and scaling and root planing. *Journal of Periodontology* 81, 682–691. doi:10.1902/jop.2010.090300.

Luchesi, V.H., Pimentel, S.P., Kolbe, M.F. et al. (2013). Photodynamic therapy in the treatment of class II furcation: A randomized controlled clinical trial. *Journal of Clinical Periodontology* 40, 781–788. doi:10.1111/jcpe.12121.

Lulic, M., Leiggener Gorog, I., Salvi, G.E. et al. (2009). One-year outcomes of repeated adjunctive photodynamic therapy during periodontal maintenance: A proof-of-principle randomized-controlled clinical trial. *Journal of Clinical Periodontology* 36, 661–666. doi:10.1111/j.1600-051X.2009.01432.x.

Martignago, C.C., Oliveira, R.F., Pires-Oliveira, D.A. et al. (2015). Effect of low-level laser therapy on the gene expression of collagen and vascular endothelial growth factor in a culture of fibroblast cells in mice. *Lasers in Medical Science* 30, 203–208. doi:10.1007/s10103-014-1644-y.

Martin-Cabezas, R., Davideau, J.L., Tenenbaum, H., and Huck, O. (2016). Clinical efficacy of probiotics as an adjunctive therapy to non-surgical periodontal treatment of chronic periodontitis: A systematic review and meta-analysis. *Journal of Clinical Periodontology* 43, 520–530. doi:10.1111/jcpe.12545.

Matesanz-Perez, P., Garcia-Gargallo, M., Figuero, E. et al. (2013). A systematic review on the effects of local antimicrobials as adjuncts to subgingival debridement, compared with subgingival debridement alone, in the treatment of chronic periodontitis. *Journal of Clinical Periodontology* 40, 227–241. doi:10.1111/jcpe.12026.

Matsubara, V.H., Bandara, H.M., Ishikawa, K.H. et al. (2016). The role of probiotic bacteria in managing periodontal disease: A systematic review. *Expert Revies of Anti Infection Therapy* 14, 643–655. doi:10.1080/14787210.2016.1194198.

Michaud, R.M., Schoolfield, J., Mellonig, J.T., and Mealey, B.L. (2007). The efficacy of subgingival calculus removal with endoscopy-aided scaling and root planing: A study on multirooted teeth. *Journal of Periodontology* 78, 2238–2245. doi:10.1902/jop.2007.070251.

Mishra, A., Avula, H., Pathakota, K.R., and Avula, J. (2013). Efficacy of modified minimally invasive surgical technique in the treatment of human intrabony defects with or without use of rhPDGF-BB gel: A randomized controlled trial. *Journal of Clinical Periodontology* 40, 172–179. doi:10.1111/jcpe.12030.

Moene, R., Decaillet, F., Andersen, E., and Mombelli, A. (2010). Subgingival plaque removal using a new air-polishing device. *Journal of Periodontology* 81, 79–88. doi:10.1902/jop.2009.090394.

Moritz, A., Schoop, U., Goharkhay, K. et al. (1998). Treatment of periodontal pockets with a diode laser. *Lasers in Surgical Medicine* 22, 302–311.

Ozawa, T., Tsuchida, M., Yamazaki, Y. et al. (1999). Clinical application of a fiberscope for periodontal lesions: Case reports. *Quintessence International* 30, 615–622.

Pavicic, M.J., van Winkelhoff, A.J., Pavivic-Temming, Y.A., and de Graaff, J. (1995). Metronidazole susceptibility factors in Actinobacillus actinomycetemcomitans. *Journal of Antimicrobial Chemotherapy* 35, 263–269.

Petersilka, G.J. (2011). Subgingival air-polishing in the treatment of periodontal biofilm infections. *Periodontology 2000* 55, 124–142. doi:10.1111/j.1600-0757.2010.00342.x.

Petersilka, G.J., Bell, M., Mehl, A. et al. (2003a). Root defects following air polishing. *Journal of Clinical Periodontology* 30, 165–170.

Petersilka, G.J., Steinmann, D., Haberlein, I. et al. (2003b). Subgingival plaque removal in buccal and lingual sites using a novel low abrasive air-polishing powder. *Journal of Clinical Periodontology* 30, 328–333.

Qin, Y., Luan, X., Bi, L. et al. (2008). Toluidine blue-mediated photoinactivation of periodontal pathogens from supragingival plaques. *Lasers in Medical Science* 23, 49–54. doi:10.1007/s10103-007-0454-x.

Ramberg, P., Rosling, B., Serino, G. et al. (2001). The long-term effect of systemic tetracycline used as an adjunct to non-surgical treatment of advanced periodontitis. *Journal of Clinical Periodontology* 28, 446–452.

Ribeiro, F.V., Casarin, R.C., Junior, F.H. et al. (2011). The role of enamel matrix derivative protein in minimally invasive surgery in treating intrabony defects in single-rooted teeth: A randomized clinical trial. *Journal of Periodontology* 82, 522–532. doi:10.1902/jop.2010.100454.

Ribeiro Edel, P., Bittencourt, S., Sallum, E.A. et al. (2010). Non-surgical instrumentation associated with povidone-iodine in the treatment of interproximal furcation involvements. *Journal of Applied Oral Science* 18, 599–606.

Roncati, M., and Gariffo, A. (2014). Systematic review of the adjunctive use of diode and Nd:YAG lasers for nonsurgical periodontal instrumentation. *Photomedicine and Laser Surgery* 32, 186–197. doi:10.1089/pho.2013.3695.

Rupprecht, R.D., Horning, G.M., and Towle, H.J., III (2001). A clinical evaluation of hydroxyapatite cement in the treatment of Class III furcation defects. *Journal of Periodontology* 72, 1443–1450. doi:10.1902/jop.2001.72.10.1443.

Saglam, M., Kantarci, A., Dundar, N., and Hakki, S.S. (2014). Clinical and biochemical effects of diode laser as an adjunct to nonsurgical treatment of chronic periodontitis: A randomized, controlled clinical trial. *Lasers in Medical Science* 29, 37–46. doi:10.1007/s10103-012-1230-0.

Saperia, D., Glassberg, E., Lyons, R.F. et al. (1986). Demonstration of elevated type I and type III procollagen mRNA levels in cutaneous wounds treated with helium-neon laser: Proposed mechanism for enhanced wound healing. *Biochemistry and Biophysics Reserch Communications* 138, 1123–1128.

Saxen, L., and Asikainen, S. (1993). Metronidazole in the treatment of localized juvenile periodontitis. *Journal of Clinical Periodontology* 20, 166–171.

Schwarz, F., Sculean, A., Berakdar, M. et al. (2003). In vivo and in vitro effects of an Er:YAG laser, a GaAlAs diode laser, and scaling and root planing on periodontally diseased root surfaces: A comparative histologic study. *Lasers in Surgery and Medicine* 32, 359–366. doi:10.1002/lsm.10179.

Sgolastra, F., Gatto, R., Petrucci, A., and Monaco, A. (2012a). Effectiveness of systemic amoxicillin/metronidazole as adjunctive therapy to scaling and root planing in the treatment of chronic periodontitis: A systematic review and meta-analysis. *Journal of Periodontology* 83, 1257–1269. doi:10.1902/jop.2012.110625.

Sgolastra, F., Petrucci, A., Gatto, R., and Monaco, A. (2012b). Effectiveness of systemic amoxicillin/metronidazole as an adjunctive therapy to full-mouth scaling and root planing in the treatment of aggressive periodontitis: A systematic review and meta-analysis. *Journal of Periodontology* 83, 731–743. doi:10.1902/jop.2011.110432.

Sgolastra, F., Petrucci, A., Gatto, R. et al. (2013a). Photodynamic therapy in the treatment of chronic periodontitis: A systematic review and meta-analysis. *Lasers in Medical Science* 28, 669–682. doi:10.1007/s10103-011-1002-2.

Sgolastra, F., Petrucci, A., Severino, M. et al. (2013b). Adjunctive photodynamic therapy to non-surgical treatment of chronic periodontitis: A systematic review and meta-analysis. *Journal of Clinical Periodontology* 40, 514–526. doi:10.1111/jcpe.12094.

Sgolastra, F., Severino, M., Petrucci, A. et al. (2014). Nd:YAG laser as an adjunctive treatment to nonsurgical periodontal therapy: A meta-analysis. *Lasers in Medical Science* 29, 887–895. doi:10.1007/s10103-013-1293-6.

Socransky, S.S., and Haffajee, A.D. (1992). The bacterial etiology of destructive periodontal disease: Current concepts. *Journal of Periodontology* 63, 322–331. doi:10.1902/jop.1992.63.4s.322.

Soukos, N.S., and Goodson, J.M. (2011). Photodynamic therapy in the control of oral biofilms. *Periodontology 2000* 55, 143–166. doi:10.1111/j.1600-0757.2010.00346.x.

Souza, E., Medeiros, A.C., Gurgel, B.C., and Sarmento, C. (2016). Antimicrobial photodynamic therapy in the treatment of aggressive periodontitis: A systematic review and meta-analysis. *Lasers in Medical Science* 31, 187–196. doi:10.1007/s10103-015-1836-0.

Takei, H.H., Han, T.J., Carranza, F.A., Jr et al. (1985). Flap technique for periodontal bone implants: Papilla preservation technique. *Journal of Periodontology* 56, 204–210. doi:10.1902/jop.1985.56.4.204.

Taniguchi, Y., Aoki, A., Sakai, K. et al. (2016). A novel surgical procedure for Er:YAG laser-assisted periodontal regenerative therapy: Case series. *International Journal of Periodontics and Restorative Dentistry* 36, 507–515. doi:10.11607/prd.2515.

Tomasi, C., and Wennstrom, J.L. (2011). Locally delivered doxycycline as an adjunct to mechanical debridement at retreatment of periodontal pockets: Outcome at furcation sites. *Journal of Periodontology* 82, 210–218. doi:10.1902/jop.2010.100308.

Tonetti, M.S., Cortellini, P., Carnevale, G. et al. (1998). A controlled multicenter study of adjunctive use of tetracycline periodontal fibers in mandibular class II furcations with persistent bleeding. *Journal of Clinical Periodontology* 25, 728–736.

Trombelli, L., Farina, R., Franceschetti, G., and Calura, G. (2009). Single-flap approach with buccal access in periodontal reconstructive procedures. *Journal of Periodontology* 80, 353–360. doi:10.1902/jop.2009.080420.

Trombelli, L., Simonelli, A., Pramstraller, M. et al. (2010). Single flap approach with and without guided tissue regeneration and a hydroxyapatite biomaterial in the management of intraosseous periodontal defects. *Journal of Periodontology* 81, 1256–1263. doi:10.1902/jop.2010.100113.

Ustun, K., Erciyas, K., Sezer, U. et al. (2014). Clinical and biochemical effects of 810 nm diode laser as an adjunct to periodontal therapy: A randomized split-mouth clinical trial. *Photomedicine and Laser Surgery* 32, 61–66. doi:10.1089/pho.2013.3506.

van Winkelhoff, A.J., Tijhof, C.J., and de Graaff, J. (1992). Microbiological and clinical results of metronidazole plus amoxicillin therapy in *Actinobacillus actinomycetemcomitans*-associated periodontitis. *Journal of Periodontology* 63, 52–57. doi:10.1902/jop.1992.63.1.52.

Verma, S.K., Maheshwari, S., Singh, R.K., and Chaudhari, P.K. (2012). Laser in dentistry: An innovative tool in modern dental practice. *National Journal of Maxillofacial Surgery* 3, 124–132. doi:10.4103/0975-5950.111342.

Wainwright, M. (1998). Photodynamic antimicrobial chemotherapy (PACT). *Journal of Antimicrobial Chemotherapy* 42, 13–28.

Winkel, E.G., Van Winkelhoff, A.J., Timmerman, M.F. et al. (2001). Amoxicillin plus metronidazole in the treatment of adult periodontitis patients: A double-blind placebo-controlled study. *Journal of Clinical Periodontology* 28, 296–305.

Yaneva, B., Firkova, E., Karaslavova, E., and Romanos, G.E. (2014). Bactericidal effects of using a fiber-less Er:YAG laser system for treatment of moderate chronic periodontitis: Preliminary results. *Quintessence International* 45, 489–497. doi:10.3290/j.qi.a31803.

Yilmaz, H.G., and Bayindir, H. (2012). Clinical evaluation of chlorhexidine and essential oils for adjunctive effects in ultrasonic instrumentation of furcation involvements: A randomized controlled clinical trial. *International Journal of Dental Hygiene* 10, 113–117. doi:10.1111/j.1601-5037.2011.00538.x.

Chapter 11

Furcation: Why Bother? Treat the Tooth or Extract and Place an Implant?

Nikos Mardas[1] and Stephen Barter[2]

[1] Centre for Immunobiology and Regenerative Medicine, Centre for Oral Clinical Research, Institute of Dentistry, Barts and the London School of Medicine and Dentistry, Queen Mary University of London (QMUL), London, UK
[2] Private practice, Eastbourne, UK

11.1 Implants vs Periodontal Multi-rooted Teeth: What is the Clinical Problem?

Previous chapters have unequivocally shown that in periodontal patients, the posterior maxilla and mandible are often those areas that are the worst affected in terms of severity of periodontal disease and ultimately tooth loss (Hirschfeld and Wasserman 1978; McFall, 1982; McGuire and Nunn 1996), and that furcation defects are a well-established local risk factor for both attachment and tooth loss. The predictability of either regenerative (Avila-Ortiz 2015) or resective (Langer et al. 1981; Carnevale et al. 1991; Blomlöf et al. 1997) surgical management of teeth with furcation involvement (FI) is variable, and is dependent on a number of local (related to furcation anatomy) and systemic factors. Besides the therapeutic advances in the management of furcation defects, periodontal treatment success rates are higher in single-rooted teeth (Wang et al. 1994), making it easier to predict their prognosis in comparison to multi-rooted teeth (McGuire 1991).

Therefore, patient-related factors, treatment cost, and the dentist's clinical experience and training often influence the decision on whether to treat or extract a multi-rooted tooth with a furcation defect (Zitzmann et al. 2011; Donos et al. 2012).

The difficulty in assessing the prognosis of teeth with bone loss beyond the root furcation following periodontal treatment and the increased popularity of dental implants have shifted the decision from treating these teeth towards replacing them with implants. In other words, why bother with treating difficult-to-treat molars with FI, when we could extract them and replace them with implants? The concept of extracting teeth with FI with questionable prognosis and substituting them with dental implants is mainly based on the following clinical assumptions:

- The lower predictability of furcation treatment in relation to the high morbidity, time, and cost of such treatments, which usually involve complex periodontal surgery, endodontic and restorative components, and the need for lengthy supportive periodontal therapy.
- The higher long-term survival rates of implant-supported restorations (Moraschini et al. 2015), which, besides their higher cost, can make them a better restorative solution in terms of cost versus benefit (Brägger et al. 2005; Bouchard et al. 2009).
- The potentially superior functional and aesthetic outcomes of implant-supported

Diagnosis and Treatment of Furcation-Involved Teeth, First Edition. Edited by Luigi Nibali.
© 2018 John Wiley & Sons Ltd. Published 2018 by John Wiley & Sons Ltd.
Companion website: www.wiley.com/go/nibali/diagnosis

restorations over the surgical management of teeth with FI, which may result in increased tooth mobility, root hypersensitivity, and gingival recession.

- An early, 'strategic' extraction will prevent further bone loss and thereby facilitate implant treatment that may otherwise be difficult considering the anatomical limitations that are usually present in the posterior maxilla and mandible (Kao 2008).

All these assumptions could be strongly debated in the light of clinical evidence. Although reported implant survival rates are high, they may not surpass the longevity of periodontally compromised teeth (Donos et al. 2012), especially in the posterior maxilla, where a variety of local factors (quality and quantity of bone, proximity to anatomical structures, and need for grafting) may result in reduced implant survival rates (Drago 1992; Becker et al. 1999; Graziani et al. 2004, Pjetursson et al. 2008). When implants are placed in patients with a history of periodontal disease, they are associated with a higher incidence of biological complications (peri-implantitis), characterized by a similar pathogenesis and systemic risk factors (e.g. smoking, diabetes) to periodontal disease.

Consequently, implants in 'periodontal patients' present lower success and probably lower survival rates than implants placed in periodontally healthy patients (Donos et al 2012; Sousa et al. 2016a). Severe forms of periodontal disease, which commonly result in posterior teeth with advanced furcation defects, are associated with higher rates of implant loss (Sousa et al. 2016a) and increased peri-implant bone loss around implants placed to substitute teeth with FI (Hardt et al. 2002). In the only comparative study available to date, Fugazzotto (2001) reported similar success rates of implants (97%) and root-resected molars (96.8%) after 0–13 years of function. Furthermore, more recent cost-effectiveness studies have shown that the cost of periodontal therapy is relatively lower than the cost and maintenance of implants or bridgework (Pretzl et al. 2009; Fardal et al. 2013). This is of course related to the additional consideration of the higher rate of technical complications associated with implant-borne prostheses (Brägger et al., 2005; Albrektsson et al. 2012). This will be discussed in more detail in Chapter 12. Finally, we cannot base our decision on patient preferences or aesthetic outcomes, since studies comparing aesthetic or patient-based outcomes following periodontal treatment for retention of teeth with FI or dental implants do not exist (Lang et al. 2012).

Based on this evidence, we could claim that dental implants are not a substitute for furcation-involved teeth, but rather a solution for restoring a lost molar when the treatment to maintain teeth has failed or is not indicated. Therefore, different considerations should be involved in the decision-making process for each clinical approach, and it cannot simply be about 'keeping bone for an implant' by removing the tooth early. These considerations include the following:

- The strategic role of the furcation-involved tooth in the overall restorative treatment plan.
- The predictability of the periodontal furcation treatment following an estimation of:
  - Local factors such as the extent of FI, the residual attachment levels, presence of caries, endodontic complications, and restorative problems.
  - Systemic factors such as smoking, diabetes, or specific medication that may influence the longevity of periodontal teeth (but potentially also of implants).
  - The patient's compliance in maintaining a high level of oral hygiene and in following an intensive supportive periodontal therapy programme.
- The predictability of an implant-supported restoration following an estimation of:
  - Residual bone quantity in relation to anatomical limitations and the complexity of any bone augmentation procedures necessary to overcome these limitations.

- Systemic factors that may influence the longevity of implants or compromise the results of bone augmentation.
- Patient compliance and their ability to undergo the necessary surgical and restorative procedures.
- Patient's expectations in terms of aesthetics, function, duration, and type of treatment.
- A detailed cost–benefit analysis that should be presented to the patient and include initial and maintenance therapies, as well as the cost for the management of complications for each clinical approach.

When the decision to extract a tooth with FI is taken, the clinical issues with placing an implant are largely centred on whether sufficient residual alveolar bone remains for the placement of an implant of adequate length without the need for bone augmentation. There are different anatomical considerations in each arch and conditions may have significant variance, even between different sites in the same patient. These are described later in the chapter, as are the subquestions regarding what constitutes 'sufficient' alveolar bone height and implant length.

11.2 Anatomical Considerations for implant Placement in the Posterior Maxilla and Mandible

11.2.1 Bone 'Quality'

Leckholm and Zarb (1985) classified the concept of bone 'quality' into four subtypes depending on the ratio of cortical to cancellous bone, and since then other classifications of bone quality have been proposed. However, bone quality is not only determined by the density of the cortical and cancellous components. It is characterized by a combination of factors, such as the degree of vascularity and cellular vitality, the quality of the collagen content and mineral crystal size, plus accumulated microscopic damage and rate of bone turnover.

It is often assumed that the posterior maxilla has 'poor' bone quality, based on thinner cortical plates and a less dense trabecular structure, with increasing adipose content towards the maxillary tuberosity region giving a lower bone 'density'. Some authors suggest that implant placement in type 4 bone is associated with an increased failure rate (Goiato et al. 2014). However, higher rates of implant failure have also been reported in dense mandibular bone (van Steenberghe et al. 2003).

Bone density in the posterior mandible can also be variable. When alveolar ridge width reduces following tooth loss, the cortical plates may become closer together, leaving a smaller trabecular space between them. Conversely, a medullary compartment with sparse trabeculation may be found, even in the presence of thick cortical plates, and achieving primary implant stability may be difficult.

The lower vascularity of bone with a smaller trabecular compartment may result in decreased oxygen tension in the bone and a reduction in vital osteocytes, with a consequent effect on bone healing and osseo-integration (van Steenberghe et al. 2003). However, there are publications that show little variation in implant survival rates in 'poor'- or 'good'-quality bone, particularly if the implants have a micro-roughened surface (Stanford 2010).

It is possible that a significant confounding factor is the operator, in that it may be more difficult to achieve adequate primary implant stability in soft bone. On the contrary, osteotomy preparation may be more challenging in dense bone, and without careful technique, sharp drills, and adequate cooling, the bone may be overheated, causing local necrosis and rapid loss of initial mechanical implant stability, before the biological stability achieved by new bone formation has reached a sufficient state (Bashutski et al. 2009).

Excessive insertion torque of an implant placed in dense bone may also cause 'compression necrosis' (Chrcanovic and Custódio 2009), with damage to the microvascular system and trabecular structure beyond the physiological capacity of bone repair. Similar mechanisms have been described in orthopaedic surgery (Winwood et al. 2006).

Similar criticism has been applied to the use of osteotomes in the posterior maxilla to 'improve' bone density by condensation rather than drilling in soft bone (Blanco et al. 2008). Compressing bone in this way does not increase bone density, but may lead to a need for increased bone remodelling due to trabecular damage that cannot be fully realized due to microvascular damage.

In conclusion, besides bone quality there are considerable site- and patient-specific variables that, together with operator experience and skill, can have a significant impact on the outcome of implant placement.

11.2.2 Bone Loss and Implant Positioning

It is an accepted fact that resorption and remodelling of the alveolar process takes place following the extraction of a tooth. The relative volumes of alveolar and basal bone loss will be subject to variation between different individuals and even between different sites in the same individual, and will affect the possibility of implant placement with or without bone augmentation. When a molar tooth with periodontal disease-related bone loss to or beyond the root furcations is extracted, a greater degree of pre-extraction alveolar bone loss will have occurred, resulting in an even bigger osseous defect (Figure 11.1).

Alveolar ridge preservation is a treatment concept that could potentially reduce the post-extraction ridge dimensional changes (MacBeth et al. 2017), decrease the clinical need for additional ridge augmentation during implant placement, and consequently facilitate implant placement (Mardas et al. 2015). These potential advantages, however, may not directly apply to the molar regions, and the clinician should base their decision on the accurate diagnosis of all local and patient-related factors (i.e. tooth location, reason for extraction, treatment duration, healing time, cost–benefit, and patient expectations and preferences).

Post-extraction alveolar resorption occurs in an apico-lingual direction, moving the crest of the ridge medially and reducing the available vertical height of bone (Cawood

(a)   (b)

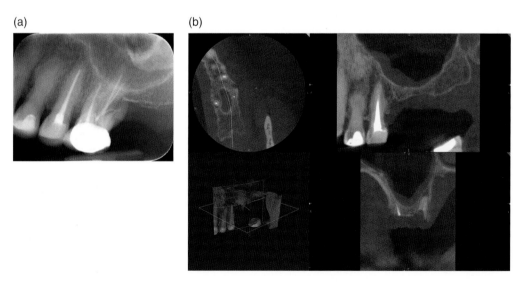

Figure 11.1 (a) Left maxillary first molar affected by endodontic-periodontal pathology. (b) Computed tomography (CT) scan taken after extraction, showing reduction of vertical height, as well as root residuals.

and Howell 1988). The former may lead to a tendency to place the implant too medially in the bony ridge; the latter may create a tendency to place the implant at a deeper vertical position than adjacent teeth in bounded saddles, or complicate implant placement due to the proximity of important anatomical structures.

It is no longer acceptable merely to place the implant into the available bone volume and attempt to restore this 'as well as possible' once the implant is integrated. According to the principle of 'restoration-driven implant placement', the implant should be installed in the correct position for the intended restoration. Therefore, whatever the intended restorative outcome is, the optimal implant position should be planned at the outset. Furthermore, the ongoing maintenance of peri-implant tissue health should be an essential part of the pre-operative planning, especially in patients who are clearly susceptible to periodontal disease and therefore at a greater risk of biological complications. The pre-operative implant restorative plan should be based on the following factors:

- The restoration being in the appropriate position for a balanced occlusion.
- The possibility of placing the implant such that it emerges through attached mucosa.
- The avoidance of lateral overhangs of the restoration such as ridge-lap, either of the implant-supported crown or caused by pink-coloured gingivae imitating extensions of veneering material. These create stagnation areas, and may impede effective oral hygiene by the patient and access for peri-implant probing for the clinician.
- The avoidance of a significant vertical difference between the bone crest of an adjacent tooth and the implant/abutment interface, which may otherwise result in a deep soft-tissue pseudo-pocket around the implant, again creating a stagnation area.
- Even in the posterior region, aesthetics may still be an issue. Maxillary molar-to-molar smiles are common, particularly in females,

and orthodontic treatment with premolar extractions may result in mesial movement of molar teeth, making the region more visible. While it may not be possible to avoid a longer implant crown than adjacent teeth, 'filling' the buccal corridor with the correct crown contour may be of aesthetic and functional importance.

Bone loss renders certain anatomical structures more superficial and this may create problems for implant placement. In the maxillary molar regions, the main issue is the degree of pneumatization of the maxillary antra; in the mandible, the position of the inferior alveolar nerve and submandibular fossa are the relevant considerations. In clinical practice these anatomical limitations are usually managed with bone-augmentation procedures or reduced-length implants.

11.3 Implant Placement in the Mandibular Molar Region

Loss of vertical height of bone in the posterior mandible may occur following extraction of mandibular multi-rooted teeth. As this process occurs, the residual crest of bone becomes closer to the mandibular canal. Depending on individual site anatomy, this can commonly render the inferior alveolar nerve so superficial that implant placement can be difficult, or inadvisable.

Damage to the inferior alveolar nerve in the mandibular canal may occur by compression, penetration, or transection of the canal, with either surgical drills or the implant itself. As the nerve exits the canal, there is also a risk of iatrogenic damage during flap preparation, elevation, or retraction.

Careful pre-surgical investigation is essential, taking into consideration that there is a considerable degree of variation in the course of the inferior alveolar nerve, including bifid canals, multiple canals, and multiple mental foramina (Carter and Keen 1971; Naitoh et al. 2009).

Damage to the inferior alveolar nerve can take many forms, with all but the most minor carrying a significant risk of irreversible neuropathy (Seddon 1942). Consequent altered sensation, often accompanied by neuropathic pain, can cause a lifelong reduction in quality of life and significant psychological difficulties (Lam et al. 2003).

It is important to realize that nerve damage can occur even without actual penetration of the canal, via a compression injury (neurapraxia) being compounded by inflammatory oedema within the canal, or bleeding that, as a consequence of the neurotoxicity of haemoglobin, causes further neural damage (Regan and Rogers 2003). Prompt and appropriate action must be taken in the event of actual or suspected damage; early intervention can reduce the risk of lifetime impact (Renton and Yilmaz 2012).

In cases of multiple tooth loss and extended edentulous spaces, more advanced vertical bone loss will also render the submandibular space more superficial. Within this space are branches of blood vessels, which, if damaged by inadvertent perforation of the lingual mandibular cortex, can cause significant haemorrhage. In rare cases the airway may be compromised to a life-threatening degree (Niamtu 2001; Dubois et al. 2010).

Accurate pre-surgical clinical and radiological investigation is therefore paramount, and an adequate safety margin must be maintained between the osteotomy preparation and important anatomical features.

11.3.1 Bone Augmentation for Implant Placement in the Mandibular Molar Region

When there is inadequate vertical height of bone over the inferior dental canal for the safe placement of dental implants, short-arch or non-implant-supported restoration is undoubtedly the most predictable option, and should always be considered rather than risking iatrogenic nerve damage.

The options available to the clinician for implant placement in resorbed mandibular molar sites are:

- Horizontal augmentation (where vertical height is not an issue).
- Vertical augmentation.
- Use of shorter implants.

The technique of inferior alveolar nerve lateralization will not be discussed, as this is neither a technique that is commonly used due to a significant complication rate, nor for which there is a large body of clinical and scientific documentation.

Vertical bone-augmentation techniques have been described for many years, including onlay grafting and distraction osteogenesis. However, the ability of these techniques to predictably regenerate the desired vertical bone volume is limited, both by anatomical and biological demands as well as the due to practical difficulties often encountered by the operator (Rocchietta et al. 2008).

It is difficult to determine the efficacy of different techniques due to the usual factors: few studies, wide variation in techniques and materials, and a lack of appropriate measurements, even in such basic matters as pre- and post-augmentation bone levels (Keestra et al. 2016).

A similar criticism can be applied to lateral bone augmentation (Esposito et al. 2009). Consequently, it is valid considering the alternative of short or reduced-diameter implants.

11.4 Bone Augmentation for Implant Placement in the Maxillary Molar Region

The options available to the clinician for implant placement in resorbed maxillary molar sites are:

- Horizontal augmentation (where vertical height is not an issue).
- Subantral augmentation via a lateral antrostomy (classic 'sinus lift').

- Subantral augmentation via implant oste-otomy (variously called 'osteotome technique', 'sinus tap', and other monikers).
- Use of shorter implants.

11.4.1 Horizontal Bone Augmentation

The concept of horizontal (lateral) bone augmentation is well documented (Donos et al. 2008; Chappuis et al. 2017), with predictable outcomes provided that the basic tenets of guided bone regeneration are observed:

- Space maintenance and form shaping.
- Blood clot stabilization.
- Effective compartmentalization of the graft (prevention of soft-tissue invasion).
- Adequate vascular and cell supply.

For the first and second requirements to be satisfied, the graft material and the membrane have to possess sufficient rigidity to preserve the form of the graft and eliminate micro-motion. This could be achieved in three-walled defects that can adequately contain a particulate graft, or when a block of augmentation material or a semirigid and reinforced membrane is used in cases of non-space-containing defects.

It is widely recognized that barrier membrane function is an essential component in the achievement of a predictable outcome, particularly when using particulate grafts.

Any free graft has to have an adequate cell and vascular supply to be viable. This is largely derived from adequate adjacent healthy bone. One therefore has to exercise caution when considering the simultaneous placement of an implant, which has the potential to form a barrier between the host bone and the graft material, depending on defect morphology.

11.4.2 Sinus Lift

The sinus lift technique was first described using a lateral antrostomy in 1980 by Boyne and James, and has since proved to be a safe and predictable procedure, with no lasting effect on maxillary sinus health and function (Timmenga et al. 2003). The general principle is that access to the antrum is created via an osseous window and the Schneiderian membrane is elevated intact, creating a subantral space into which a biocompatible scaffold can be inserted to conduct new bone growth, providing an adequate bed for implant placement. As with any surgical procedure there is the potential for complications; consequently, any surgeon performing the procedure should be properly trained and experienced, and able to deal with intra- and post-operative complications.

The main complication leading to chronic rhino-sinus symptoms is the perforation of the Schneiderian membrane, with the potential escape of graft materials into the sinus. Loss of graft compartmentalization may result in an inflammatory reaction, the loss of patency of the ostium (van den Bergh et al. 2000; Wiltfang et al. 2000; Doud Galli et al. 2001), a compromised mucociliary transport system, and ultimately a potential need for graft removal with endoscopic sinus surgery. The reported incidence of membrane perforation is from 10% to over 50% of cases (Timmenga et al. 1997; Block et al. 1998; Schwartz-Arad et al. 2004; Pikos 2008; Pjetursson et al. 2008). There are many authors who suggest that, up to a certain size, repair of the ruptured sinus lining with a collagen membrane is possible (Becker et al. 2008); others question the efficacy of this technique (Aimetti et al. 2001).

Even without membrane perforation, there is a certain incidence of post-operative chronic sinusitis in patients predisposed to rhino-sinus disease (Timmenga et al. 1997). An accurate medical history with relevant questions is therefore important in patient assessment.

There is evidence that certain osteoconductive bone grafts, like deproteinized bovine bone mineral, can provide a bone-formation outcome as reliable as autogenous bone, which removes the need for a donor site and simplifies the overall procedure considerably (Handschel et al. 2009; Kim et al. 2009). It seems that covering the antrostomy with a barrier membrane after graft placement tends to result in a better implant prognosis (Jensen and Terheyden 2009), perhaps because to achieve the optimal restorative position, the implant tends to be placed as buccally as possible and the use of membranes appears to have a significant impact on the amount of soft-tissue invasion into the lateral aspect of the graft (Choi et al. 2009).

However, subantral augmentation does not replace the alveolar bone; it provides a different volume of bone to facilitate implant placement. Depending on the degree of lateral bone loss, implants placed into this bone bed may not be closely related to the positions of the missing teeth. Some clinicians suggest that for implant placement to be appropriate for a fixed reconstruction, lateral augmentation will also be required (Chiapasco and Zaniboni 2009). Lateral bone grafting in such a situation will not always be practical, particularly if there are adjacent teeth with bone loss: reconstruction of any vertical component of bone loss will be technically difficult and unpredictable.

Implant survival rates are variously quoted as being equal to (61.7–100%, average 91.8%; Wallace and Froum 2003) or slightly more variable (73–100% for non- augmented sinuses, 36–100% for augmented sinuses on a patient basis; 75–100% for both non-augmented and augmented sites on an implant basis; Graziani et al. 2004) than those reported in the unaugmented posterior maxilla, suggesting that variables such as implant type and operator experience are important factors.

11.4.3 Osteotome-mediated Sinus Floor Elevation

This technique was first described by Summers (1998) and has since seen several iterations of modifications, in a desire to simplify the process of subantral augmentation. The basic theory is that the floor of the antrum is elevated blindly, via the implant osteotomy, without perforating the Schneiderian membrane. Most of the reports detailing this technique were performed in

situations of significant residual alveolar ridge height (rAH). When a perforation of the Schneiderian membrane was suspected, the implant was placed without any bone grafts to reduce the risk of sinusitis presented by graft particles escaping into the sinus; something that did not influence the implant-related outcomes.

A significant determinant of implant success using the osteotome technique is the height of the rAH (Toffler 2004). As rAH decreases, the need for greater graft height increases. This means a greater degree of membrane elevation, which may result in an increased rate of Schneiderian membrane perforation (Nkenke et al. 2002; Velloso 2006). However, with this 'blind' approach it is not possible to reliably detect membrane perforations (Ferrigno et al. 2006; Ardekian et al. 2006). Other risks associated with the osteotome technique include benign paroxysmal positional vertigo (Iida et al. 2000; Kaplan et al. 2003; Di Girolamo et al. 2005; Chiarella et al. 2008; Kim et al. 2010) and loss of the implant into the sinus where simultaneous implant placement is attempted (Galindo et al. 2005; Chiapasco et al. 2009), or even several years after implant placement (Udea and Kaneda 1992; Iida et al. 2000).

Even if a reasonable degree of augmentation material can be inserted via the implant osteotomy without membrane perforation, bone growth is known to be incremental from the bony walls, since the vascular and osteoblastic cell supply derives primarily from there (Jensen et al. 1998). It has been shown that there is significant remodelling of grafts placed using the osteotome technique, and that actual bone gain is limited to small amounts of additional bone on the walls of the implant, with little bone at the apex after 12 months (Brägger et al. 2004; Leblebicioglu et al. 2005). Furthermore, occlusal load in the posterior maxilla is primarily borne by the cortical plates and dissipated to the palatal bone and zygomatic process (Gross and Nissan 2001; Gross et al. 2001; Yacoub et al. 2002). The degree of bone contact on the implant is of course determined by available rAH, and also by the amount of graft; however, if that graft is not in contact with the walls of the sinus, contribution to load-bearing capacity is insignificant (Tepper et al. 2002). The quality of regenerated bone is also important in reducing the stress in the native bone, which could otherwise lead to crestal bone resorption (Fanascu et al. 2003).

This has raised questions of whether there is a critical height of bone at which there is an advantage of the osteotome technique over the lateral window approach in terms of implant survival. In a meta-regression analysis of the two approaches, it was noted that there was a correlation between bone height and implant survival, with an rAH of 4 mm, in the lateral window approach. There was no correlation with the osteotome approach, but the rAH and implant survival rate were highly variable in the included studies, with many different techniques being used (Chao et al. 2010).

Besides the technique's extensive use, the 'evidence' supporting the osteotome-mediated sinus floor elevation has a significant degree of heterogeneity and drawing meaningful conclusions is difficult (Tan et al. 2008). Similar outcomes in terms of implant survival can be achieved with short implants, and some authors have suggested that there may not be any harm in placing an implant that penetrates the antral floor (Brånemark et al. 1984; Pierreisnard et al. 2003).

Given the increased morbidity and overall treatment time scale associated with the lateral window approach to sinus floor augmentation, and the doubt surrounding the value of the osteotome technique, it is highly relevant to question the need for such additional surgery if it can be avoided. An example of osteotome-mediated sinus elevation and implant placement is provided in Figure 11.2.

(a)

(b)

(c)

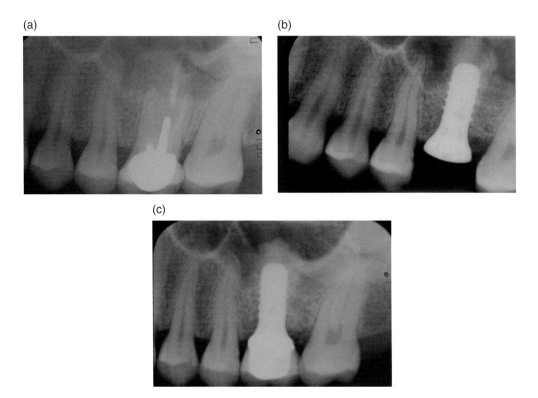

Figure 11.2 (a) Left maxillary first molar affected by root fracture. (b) Implant placement was carried out three months after extraction, with the use of osteotome-mediated sinus elevation associated with bone grafts. (c) An implant-supported crown was placed three months later.

11.5 Short Implants

Dental implants with an infrabony length of $\leq 8\,mm$ have been defined as short (Renouard and Nisand 2006), although 'ultra-short' implants are considered to be those with lengths $\leq 6\,mm$ (Deporter 2013). Short implants have been suggested as an alternative to bone augmentation procedures in the maxillary and mandibular posterior segments, where the residual post-extraction bone volume is limited by anatomical structures (maxillary sinus, mandibular canal), but there is sufficient alveolar ridge width to allow the use of standard implant diameters of $\geq 3.75\,mm$. Short implants offer a less invasive treatment approach for patients who are not able to undergo more complex bone-augmentation procedures, thereby minimizing complication rates, morbidity, cost, and duration of treatment (Nisand and Renouard 2014; Thoma et al. 2015). On the other hand, short implants will usually present a higher crown-to-implant ratio, especially in cases with increased interarch distance that may lead to unfavourable loading conditions and more technical complications (Quaranta et al. 2014). It remains uncertain whether a high crown-to-implant ratio may lead to excessive crestal bone loss and implant failure (Garaicoa-Pazmino et al. 2014). Various modifications in implant design, surface technology, and different implant insertion methods have been suggested to address these issues (Deporter 2013). Finally, the clinical implications of peri-implantitis on implant prognosis may be more pronounced in the case of shorter implants compared to longer implants.

Systematic reviews present comparable mid-term survival rates between short and longer implants with moderate rough surfaces (Annibali et al. 2012; Atieh et al. 2012). Most of the reported failures were predominantly early, with superior survival rates in the mandible. However, short implants with a reduced diameter ($<3.75\,mm$) may have higher failure rates (up to 10%) after 3–5 years in function (das Neves et al. 2006). For ultra-short implants the available data are limited. One study showed that 6 mm long implants had an average survival rate of 93.7% following an observation period of at least one year after placement (Srinivasan et al. 2014).

Short implants could be considered as a valid treatment alternative to sinus floor augmentation for the restoration of maxillary molars, provided that the residual height of the alveolar ridge is $\geq 5\,mm$. The 16–18-month survival rate for short implants was similar to that of long implants placed in augmented sinuses (99% vs 99.5%; Thoma et al. 2015). The complication rate was significantly higher in patients receiving sinus augmentation. Membrane perforation (Figure 11.3) was the most common complication, although this did not seem to compromise implant survival.

Short implants may also be considered as an alternative to simultaneous or staged vertical bone augmentation in the posterior mandible when the residual height of the alveolar ridge is $\geq 5\,mm$. Felice et al. (2014) reported similar survival rates but fewer complications and peri-implant crestal bone loss with 6.6 mm short implants placed in posterior maxilla in comparison to vertical augmentation after five years of loading. A recent systematic review based on only four randomized controlled trials, mainly by the same group, concluded that similar survival rates (95.1% vs 96.2%) and maintenance of crestal bone level should be expected after both procedures in the short term (Nisand et al. 2015). The complication rate was again higher with vertical augmentation, where temporary nerve paraesthesia was observed in 56% of cases, in contrast to only 17% when short implants were used. Graft fracture, inability to place long implants, and soft-tissue dehiscence were other observed complications.

Besides the encouraging short-term results in terms of survival rates, long-term data on short implants as an alternative to sinus or vertical bone augmentation are still lacking, and it remains unclear to what extent the

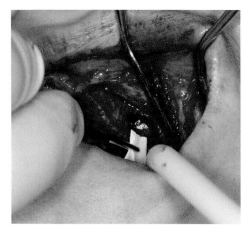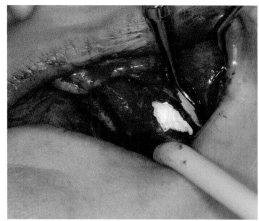

Figure 11.3 Sinus membrane perforation occurred during lateral window sinus elevation approach and repaired with the use of a resorbable membrane.

type of prosthetic restoration (single or splinted crowns, cantilevers) may influence bone levels or implant survival. For this reason, it has been recommended that short implants should be used only if bone quality is favourable, and that immediate loading and non-working side occlusal interferences are avoided.

11.6 Implant Biological Complications

Several longitudinal studies report implant survival rates ranging from 92.8 to 97.1% over a period up to 10 years (Albrektsson and Donos 2012; Srinivasan et al. 2014), supporting the use of dental implants as a valid treatment option for the replacement of missing teeth. However, implant failures remain a possibility. Failures can be divided into biological (early or primary, and late or secondary), mechanical, technical, iatrogenic, and those related to inadequate patient adaptation (Heitz-Mayfield et al. 2014).

The biological complications (and specifically peri-implantitis) are usually the most difficult to manage. Peri-implantitis is a site- and patient-specific, chronic infection that is initiated by polymicrobial dysbiotic biofilms (Edmiston et al. 2015; Hajishengallis 2015).

The disease affects both soft and hard tissues around osseo-integrated implants, leading to bone loss and the formation of a peri-implant pocket (Zitzmann and Berglundh 2008). The prevalence of peri-implantitis was reported to be of the order of 10% of implants and 20% of patients (circa 5–10-year follow-up after implant placement; Mombelli et al. 2012), and from 1 to 47% (estimated weighted mean [EWM] 22%, 95% confidence interval [CI] 14–30%; Derks and Tomasi 2015). However, the prevalence of peri-implantitis was 39.3% at a patient level in patients with a history of periodontitis (Marrone et al. 2013), and lower survival and success rates were observed in these patients when compared to periodontally healthy individuals (Sousa et al. 2016). In addition, the severity and type of periodontal disease appear to exert a negative effect on the rate of biological complications with dental implants (Mengel et al. 2007; Gatti et al. 2008; De Boever et al. 2009; Levin et al. 2011; Roccuzzo et al. 2014).

Other risk indicators strongly associated with peri-implantitis are smoking, excess cement, poor oral hygiene, and lack of supportive periodontal therapy (Renvert and Quirynen 2015), whereas there is limited evidence regarding the association between diabetes, alcohol consumption, and peri-implant diseases, with conflicting and limited evidence for the association with peri-implant diseases and absence of keratinized mucosa, genetic traits, implant surface characteristics, time of loading, and the position of the implant within the arch (Heitz-Mayfield 2008; Dereka et al. 2012; Renvert and Polyzois 2015).

The therapy of peri-implantitis is mainly directed at the disruption and removal of the biofilm, the resolution of inflammation, and ultimately the arrest of disease progression (Heitz-Mayfield and Mombelli 2014). Suggested therapies are based on well-established clinical protocols used for the treatment of periodontitis, including various combinations of mechanical and non-mechanical debridement methods with or without surgical access, and the use of adjunctive therapies such as antibiotics, antiseptics, and laser treatments (Lindhe and Meyle 2008). While the elimination of the bacterial pathogens and their remnants is vital for clinically stable outcomes, implant surface topography, the initial severity of disease, and defect morphology may influence the outcome of non-surgical and surgical therapies (Schwarz et al. 2006, 2010; Sousa et al. 2016). Although there is evidence that some non-surgical methods for implant surface decontamination may be effective at reducing the bacterial load, non-surgical treatment is insufficient to treat peri-implantitis and does not lead to satisfactory clinical outcomes (Renvert et al. 2008, 2009). A meta-analysis of treatment outcomes has identified the main surgical procedures that are predominantly performed: access-flap debridement; surgical resection; regeneration with bone grafts; and guided tissue regeneration (Chan et al. 2014). In the latter case, the outcomes of regenerative therapy are reported to vary the most. For this reason, several clinicians often suggest implant explantation as the only predictable approach for managing advanced peri-implantitis, and advocate that prevention is the most effective way to manage biological complications around implants.

Summary of Evidence

- Dental implants are not an alternative to periodontal treatment of furcation-involved teeth, but rather a restorative solution when any other treatment to maintain them in the dentition has failed or is not indicated.
- Loss or extraction of furcation-involved teeth usually results in extensive bone loss that may complicate implant placement: in the maxilla due to sinus pneumatization and in the mandible due to the position of the inferior alveolar nerve and submandibular fossa. In clinical practice these anatomical limitations are usually managed with extensive bone augmentation procedures that increase the complexity, cost, and sometimes the treatment time and risk of complications.
- Short implants could be an alternative to extensive vertical bone-augmentation procedures; however, their use has not been adequately evaluated in the long term.
- Biological complications and especially peri-implantitis are quite common in patients with a history of periodontal disease. This risk should be extensively presented and discussed with the patient before the extraction of teeth with furcation involvement and their replacement with dental implants, acknowledging at the same time the limitations of current peri-implantitis treatment modalities.

References

Aimetti, M., Romagnoli, R., Ricci, G., and Massei G. (2001). Maxillary sinus elevation: The effect of macrolacerations and microlacerations of the sinus membrane as determined by endoscopy. *International Journal of Periodontics and Restorative Dentistry* 21, 581–589.

Albrektsson, T., Donos, N., and Working Group 1 (2012). Implant survival and complications: The third EAO consensus conference 2012. *Clinical Oral Implants Research* 23 (Suppl. 6), 63–65.

Annibali, S., Cristalli, M.P., Dell'Aquila, D. et al. (2012). Short dental implants: A systematic review. *Journal of Dental Research* 91, 25–32.

Ardekian, L., Oved-Peleg, E., Mactei, E.E., and Peled, M. (2006). The clinical significance of sinus membrane perforation during augmentation of the maxillary sinus. *Journal of Oral and Maxillofacial Surgery* 64, 277–282.

Atieh, M.A., Zadeh, H., Stanford, C.M., and Cooper, L.F. (2012). Survival of short dental implants for treatment of posterior partial edentulism: A systematic review. *International Journal of Oral and Maxillofacial Implants* 27, 1323–1331.

Avila-Ortiz, G., De Buitrago, J.G., and Reddy, M.S. (2015). Periodontal regeneration – furcation defects: A systematic review from the AAP Regeneration Workshop. *Journal of Periodontology* 86 (Suppl. 2), S108–S130. doi: 10.1902/jop.2015.130677.

Bashutski, J.D., D'Silva, N.J., Wang, H.L. (2009). Implant compression necrosis: Current understanding and case report. *Journal of Periodontology* 80, 700–704. doi:10.1902/jop.2009.080581.

Becker, S.T., Terheyden, H., Steinriede, A. et al. (2008). Prospective observation of 41 peforations of the Schneiderian membrane during sinus floor elevation. *Clinical Oral Implants Research* 19, 1285–1289.

Becker, W., Becker, B.E., Alsuwyed, A., and Al-Mubarak, S. (1999). Long-term evaluation of 282 implants in maxillary and mandibular molar positions: A prospective study. *Journal of Periodontology* 70, 896–901.

Blanco, J., Suárez, J., Novio, S. et al. (2008). Histomorphometric assessment in human cadavers of the peri-implant bone density in maxillary tuberosity following implant placement using osteotome and conventional techniques. *Clinical Oral Implants Research* 19, 505–510.

Block, M., Kent, J., Kallukaran, F. et al. (1998). Bone maintenance 5 to 10 years after sinus grafting. *Journal of Oral and Maxillofacial Surgery* 56, 706–714.

Blomlöf, L., Jansson, L., Appelgren, R. et al. (1997). Prognosis and mortality of root-resected molars. *International Journal of Periodontics and Restorative Dentistry* 17, 190–201.

Bouchard, P., Renouard, F., Bourgeois, D. et al. (2009). Cost-effectiveness modeling of dental implant vs. bridge. *Clinical Oral Implants Research* 20, 583–587.

Boyne, P.J., and James, R.A. (1980). Grafting of the maxillary sinus floor with autogenous marrow and bone. *Journal of Oral Surgery* 38, 613–616.

Brägger, U., Gerber, C., Joss, A. et al. (2004). Patterns of tissue remodelling after placement of ITI dental implants using an osteotome technique: A longitudinal radiographic case cohort study. *Clinical Oral Implants Research* 15, 158–166.

Brägger, U., Krenander, P., and Lang, N.P. (2005). Economic aspects of single-tooth replacement. *Clinical Oral Implants Research* 16, 335–341.

Brånemark, P.-I., Adell, R., Albrektsson, T. et al. (1984). An experimental and clinical study of osseointegrated implants penetrating the nasal cavity and maxillary sinus. *Journal of Oral and Maxillofacial Surgery* 42, 497–505.

Carnevale, G., Di Febo, G., Tonelli, M.P. et al. (1991). A retrospective analysis of the periodontal-prosthetic treatment of molars with interradicular lesions. *International Journal of Periodontics and Restorative Dentistry* 11, 189–205.

Carter, R.B., and Keen, E.N. (1971). The intramandibular course of the inferior alveolar nerve. *Journal of Anatomy* 108, 433–440.

Cawood, J.I., and Howell, R.A. (1988). A classification of the edentulous jaws. *International Journal of Oral and Maxillofacial Surgery* 17, 232–236.

Chan, H.-L., Lin, G.-H., Suarez, F. et al. (2014). Surgical management of peri-implantitis: A systematic review and meta-analysis of treatment outcomes. *Journal of Periodontology* 85, 1027–1041.

Chao, Y.L., Chen, H.H., Mei, C.C. et al. (2010). Meta-regression analysis of the initial bone height for predicting implant survival rates of two sinus elevation procedures. *Journal of Clinical Periodontology* 37, 456–465.

Chappuis, V., Cavusoglu, Y., Buser, D., and von Arx, T. (2017). Lateral ridge augmentation using autogenous block grafts and guided bone regeneration: A 10-year prospective case series study. *Clinical Implant Dentistry and Related Research* 19, 85–96.

Chiapasco, M., Felisati, G., Maccari, A. et al. (2009). The management of complications following displacement of oral implants in the paranasal sinuses: A multicenter clinical report and proposed treatment protocols. *International Journal of Oral and Maxillofacial Surgery* 38, 1273–1278.

Chiapasco, M., and Zaniboni, M. (2009). Methods to treat the edentulous posterior maxilla: Implants with sinus grafting. *Journal of Oral and Maxillofacial Surgery*, 67, 867–871.

Chiarella, G., Leopardi, G., De Fazio, L. et al. (2008). Benign paroxysmal positional vertigo after dental surgery. *European Archives of Oto-Rhino-Laryngology* 265, 119–122.

Choi, K., Kan, J.Y.K., Boyne, P.J. et al. (2009). The effects of resorbable membrane on human maxillary sinus graft: A pilot study. *International Journal of Oral and Maxillofacial Implants* 24, 73–80.

Chrcanovic, B.R., and Custódio, A.L. (2009). Mandibular fractures associated with endosteal implants. *Oral and Maxillofacial Surgery* 13, 231–238. doi:10.1007/s10006-009-0171-7.

das Neves, F.D., Fones, D., Bernardes, S.R. et al. (2006). Short implants: An analysis of longitudinal studies. *International Journal of Oral and Maxillofacial Implants* 21, 86–93.

De Boever, A.L., Quirynen, M., Coucke, W. et al. (2009). Clinical and radiographic study of implant treatment outcome in periodontally susceptible and non-susceptible patients: A prospective long-term study. *Clinical Oral Implants Research* 20, 1341–1350.

Deporter D. (2013). Short dental implants: What works and what doesn't? A literature interpretation. *International Journal of Periodontics and Restorative Dentistry* 33, 457–464.

Dereka, X., Mardas, N., Chin, S. et al. (2012). A systematic review on the association between genetic predisposition and dental implant biological complications. *Clinical Oral Implants Research* 23, 775–788.

Derks, J., and Tomasi, C. (2015). Peri-implant health and disease: A systematic review of current epidemiology. *Journal of Clinical Periodontology* 42 (Suppl. 16), S158–S171.

Di Girolamo, M., Napolitano, B., Arullani, C.A. et al. (2005). Paroxysmal positional vertigo as a complication of osteotome sinus floor elevation. *European Archives of Oto-Rhino-Laryngology* 262, 631–633.

Donos, N., Laurell, L., and Mardas, N. (2012). Hierarchical decisions on teeth vs. implants in the periodontitis-susceptible patient: The modern dilemma. *Periodontology 2000* 59, 89–110.

Donos, N., Mardas, N., and Chadha, V. (2008). Clinical outcomes of implants following lateral bone augmentation: Systematic assessment of available options (barrier membranes, bone grafts, split osteotomy). *Journal of Clinical Periodontology* 35, 173–120.

Doud Galli, S.K., Lebowitz, R.A., Giacchi, R.J. et al. (2001). Chronic sinusitis complicating sinus lift surgery. *American Journal of Rhinology* 15, 181–186.

Drago, C.J. (1992). Rates of osseointegration of dental implants with regard to anatomical location. *Journal of Prosthodontics* 1, 29–31.

Dubois, L., de Lange, J., Baas, E., and Van Ingen, J. (2010). Excessive bleeding in the floor of the mouth after endosseous implant placement: A report of two cases. *International Journal of Oral and Maxillofacial Surgery* 39, 412–415.

Edmiston, C.E., McBain, A.J., Roberts, C., and Leaper, D. (2015). Clinical and microbiological aspects of biofilm-associated surgical site infections. *Advances in Experimental Medicine and Biology* 830, 47–67.

Esposito, M., Grusovin, M.G., Felice, P. et al. (2009). The efficacy of horizontal and vertical bone augmentation procedures for dental implants: A Cochrane systematic review. *European Journal of Oral Implantology* 2, 167–184.

Fanuscu, M.I., Iida, K., Caputo, A.A., and Nishimura, R.D. (2003). Load transfer by an implant in a sinus-grafted maxillary model. *International Journal of Oral and Maxillofacial Implants* 18, 667–674.

Fardal, Ø., and Grytten, J. (2013). A comparison of teeth and implants during maintenance therapy in terms of the number of disease-free years and costs: An in vivo internal control study. *Journal of Clinical Periodontology* 40, 645–651.

Felice, P., Cannizzaro, G., Barausse, C. et al. (2014). Short implants versus longer implants in vertically augmented posterior mandibles: A randomised controlled trial with 5-year after loading follow-up. *European Journal of Oral Implantology* 7, 359–369.

Fugazzotto, P.A. (2001). A comparison of the success of root resected molars and molar position implants in function in a private practice: Results of up to 15-plus years. *Journal of Periodontology* 72, 1113–1123.

Galindo, P., Sánchez-Fernández, E., Avila, G. et al. (2005). Migration of implants into the maxillary sinus: Two clinical cases. *International Journal of Oral and Maxillofacial Implants* 20, 291–285.

Garaicoa-Pazmino, C., Suarez-Lopez del Amo, F., Monje, A. et al. (2014). Influence of crown/implant ratio on marginal bone loss: A systematic review. *Journal of Periodontology* 85, 1214–1221.

Gatti, C., Gatti, F., Chiapasco, M., and Esposito, M. (2008). Outcome of dental implants in partially edentulous patients with and without a history of periodontitis: A 5-year interim analysis of a cohort study. *European Journal of Oral Implantation* 1, 45–51.

Goiato, M.C., dos Santos, D.M., Santiago, J.F. Jr et al. (2014). Longevity of dental implants in type IV bone: A systematic review. *International Journal of Oral and Maxillofacial Surgery* 43, 1108–1116. doi:10.1016/j.ijom.2014.02.016.

Graziani, F., Donos, N., Needleman, I. et al. (2004). Comparison of implant survival following sinus floor augmentation procedures with implants placed in pristine posterior maxillary bone: A systematic review. *Clinical and Oral Implants* 15, 677–682.

Gross, M.D., and Nissan, J. (2001). Stress distribution around maxillary implants in anatomic photoelastic models of varying geometry. Part II. *Journal of Prosthetic Dentistry* 85, 450–454.

Gross, M.D., Nissan, J., and Samuel, R. (2001). Stress distribution around maxillary implants in anatomic photoelastic models of varying geometry. Part I. *Journal of Prosthetic Dentistry* 85, 442–449.

Hajishengallis, G. (2015). Periodontitis: From microbial immune subversion to systemic inflammation. *Nature Reviews: Immunology* 15, 30–44.

Handschel, J., Simonowska, M., Naujoks, C. et al. (2009). A histomorphometric meta-analysis of sinus elevation with various grafting materials. *Head & Face Medicine* 5, 12.

Hardt, C.R.E., Gröndahl, K., Lekholm, U., and Wennström, J.L. (2002). Outcome of implant therapy in relation to experienced loss of periodontal bone support. *Clinical Oral Implants Research* 13, 488–494.

Heitz-Mayfield, L.J. (2008). Peri-implant diseases: Diagnosis and risk indicators. *Journal of Clinical Periodontology* 35 (Suppl. 8), 292–304.

Heitz-Mayfield, L.J.A., and Mombelli, A. (2014). The therapy of peri-implantitis: A systematic review. *International Journal of Oral and Maxillofacial Implants* 29, 325–345.

Heitz-Mayfield, L.J., Needleman, I., Salvi, G.E., and Pjetursson, B.E. (2014). Consensus statements and clinical recommendations for prevention and management of biologic and technical implant complications. *International Journal of Oral and Maxillofacial Implants* 29 (Suppl.), 346–350.

Hirschfeld, A., and Wasserman, B. (1978). A long-term survey of tooth loss in 600 treated periodontal patients. *Journal of Periodontology* 49, 225–237.

Iida, S., Tanaka, N., Kogo, M., and Matsuya, T. (2000). Migration of a dental implant into the maxillary sinus: A case report. *International Journal of Oral and Maxillofacial Surgery* 29, 358–359.

Jensen, O.T., Shulman, L.B., Block, M.S., and Iacono, V.J. (1998). Report of the Sinus Consensus Conference of 1996. *International Journal of Oral and Maxillofacial Implants* 13 (Suppl.), 11–45.

Jensen, S.S., and Terheyden, H. (2009). Bone augmentation procedures in localized defects in the alveolar ridge: Clinical results with different bone grafts and bone-substitute materials. *International Journal of Oral and Maxillofacial Implants* 24, 218–236.

Kao, R.T. (2008). Strategic extraction: A paradigm shift that is changing our profession. *Journal of Periodontology* 79, 971–977.

Kaplan, D.M., Attal, U., and Kraus, M. (2003). Bilateral benign paroxysmal positional vertigo following a tooth implantation. *Journal of Laryngology and Otology* 117, 312–313.

Keestra, J.A.J., Barry, O., de Jong, L., and Wahl, G. (2016). Long-term effects of vertical bone augmentation: A systematic review. *Journal of Applied Oral Science* 24, 3–17.

Kim, M.S., Lee, J.K., Chang, B.S., and Um, H.S. (2010). Benign paroxysmal positional vertigo as a complication of sinus floor elevation. *Journal of Periodontology and Implant Science* 40, 86–89.

Kim, Y.K., Yun, P.Y., Kim, S.G., and Lim, S.C. (2009). Analysis of the healing process in sinus bone grafting using various grafting materials. *Oral Surgery, Oral Medicine, Oral Pathology, Oral Radiology, Endodontology* 107, 204–211.

Lam, N.P., Donoff, R.B., Kaban, L.B., and Dodson, T.B. (2003). Patient satisfaction after trigeminal nerve repair. *Oral Surgery, Oral Medicine, Oral Pathology, Oral Radiology, Endodontology* 95, 538–543.

Lang, N.P., Zitzmann, N.U.; Working Group 3 of the VIII European Workshop on Periodontology (2012). Clinical research in implant dentistry: Evaluation of implant-supported restorations, aesthetic and patient-reported outcomes. *Journal of Clinical Periodontology* 39, 133–138.

Langer, B., Stein, S.D., and Wagenberg, B. (1981). An evaluation of root resections: A ten-year study. *Journal of Periodontology* 52, 719–722.

Leblebicioglu, B., Ersanli, S., Karabuda, C. et al. (2005). Radiographic evaluation of dental implants placed using an osteotome technique. *Journal of Periodontology* 76, 385–390.

Lekholm, U., and Zarb, G.A. (1985). Patient selection and preparation. In: *Tissue Integrated Prostheses: Osseointegration in Clinical Dentistry* (ed. P.I. Branemark, G.A. Zarb, and T. Albrektsson), 199–209. Chicago, IL: Quintessence.

Levin, L., Ofec, R., Grossmann, Y., and Anner, R. (2011). Periodontal disease as a risk for dental implant failure over time: A long-term historical cohort study. *Journal of Clinical Periodontology* 38, 732–737.

Lindhe, J., and Meyle, J.; Group D of European Workshop on Periodontology (2008). Peri-implant diseases: Consensus Report of the Sixth European Workshop on Periodontology. *Journal of Clinical Periodontology* 35 (Suppl. 8), 282–285. doi:10.1111/j.1600-051X.2008.01283.x.

MacBeth, N., Trullenque-Eriksson, A., Donos, N., and Mardas, N. (2017). Hard and soft tissue changes following alveolar ridge preservation: A systematic review. *Clinical Oral Implants Research* 28, 982–1004.

Mardas, N., Trullenque-Eriksson, A., MacBeth, N. et al. (2015). Does ridge preservation following tooth extraction improve implant treatment outcomes: A systematic review. Group 4: Therapeutic concepts & methods. *Clinical Oral Implants Research* 26 (Suppl. 11), 180–201.

Marrone, A., Lasserre, J., Bercy, P., and Brecx, M.C. (2013). Prevalence and risk factors for peri-implant disease in Belgian adults. *Clinical Oral Implants Research* 24, 934–940.

McFall, W.T., Jr (1982). Tooth loss in 100 treated patients with periodontal disease: A long-term study. *Journal of Periodontology* 53: 539–549.

McGuire, M.K. (1991). Prognosis versus actual outcome: A long-term survey of 100 treated periodontal patients under maintenance care. *Journal of Periodontology* 62, 51–58.

McGuire, M.K., and Nunn, M.E. (1996). Prognosis versus actual outcome. *III. The effectiveness of clinical parameters in accurately predicting tooth survival. Journal of Periodontology* 67, 66–74.

Mengel, R., Behle, M., and Flores-de-Jacoby, L. (2007). Osseointegrated implants in subjects treated for generalized aggressive periodontitis: 10-year results of a prospective, long-term cohort study. *Journal of Periodontology* 78, 2229–2237.

Mombelli, A., Müller, N., and Cionca, N. (2012). The epidemiology of peri-implantitis. *Clinical Oral Implants Research* 23 (Suppl. 6), 67–76.

Moraschini, V., Poubel, L.A., Ferreira, V.F., and Barboza Edos, S. (2015). Evaluation of survival and success rates of dental implants reported in longitudinal studies with a follow-up period of at least 10 years: A systematic review. *International Journal of Oral and Maxillofacial Surgery* 44, 377–388.

Naitoh, M., Hiraiwa, Y., Aimiya, H. et al. (2009). Accessory mental foramen assessment using cone-beam computed tomography. *Oral Surgery, Oral Medicine, Oral Pathology, Oral Radiology, Endodontology* 107, 289–294.

Niamtu, J., III (2001). Near-fatal airway obstruction after routine implant placement. *Oral Surgery, Oral Medicine, Oral Pathology, Oral Radiology, Endodontology* 92, 597–600.

Nisand, D., Picard, N., and Rocchietta, I. (2015). Short implants compared to implants in vertically augmented bone: A systematic review. *Clinical Oral Implants Research* 26 (Suppl. 11), 170–179. doi:10.1111/clr.12632.

Nisand, D., and Renouard, F. (2014). Short implant in limited bone volume. *Periodontology 2000* 66, 72–96.

Nkenke, E., Schlegel, A., Schultze-Mosgau, S. et al. (2002). The endoscopically controlled osteotome sinus floor elevation: A preliminary prospective study. *International Journal of Oral and Maxillofacial Implants* 17, 557–566.

Pierrisnard, L., Renouard, F., Renault, P., and Barquins, M. (2003). Influence of implant length and bicortical anchorage on implant stress distribution. *Clinical Implant Dentistry and Related Research* 5, 254–262.

Pikos, M.A. (2008). Maxillary sinus membrane repair: Update on technique for large and complete perforations. *Implant Dentistry* 17, 24–31.

Pjetursson, B.E., Tan, W.C., Zwahlen, M., and Lang, N.P. (2008). A systematic review of the success of sinus floor elevation and survival of implants inserted in combination with sinus floor elevation. *Journal of Clinical Periodontology* 35, 216–240.

Pretzl, B., Wiedemann, D., Cosgarea, R. et al. (2009). Effort and costs of tooth preservation in supportive periodontal treatment in a German population. *Journal of Clinical Periodontology* 36, 669–676.

Quaranta, A., Piemontese, M., Rappelli, G. et al. (2014). Technical and biological complications related to crown to implant ratio: A systematic review. *Implant Dentistry* 23, 180–187.

Regan, R., and Rogers, B. (2003). Delayed treatment of haemoglobin neurotoxicity. *Journal of Neurotrauma* 20, 111–120.

Renouard, F., and Nisand, D. (2006). Impact of implant length and diameter on survival rates. *Clinical Oral Implants Research* 17 (Suppl. 2), 35–51.

Renton, T., and Yilmaz, Z. (2012). Managing iatrogenic trigeminal nerve injury: A case series and review of the literature. *International Journal of Oral and Maxillofacial Surgery* 41, 629–637.

Renvert, S., and Polyzois, I. (2015). Risk indicators for peri-implant mucositis: A systematic literature review. *Journal of Clinical Periodontology* 42, S172–S186.

Renvert, S., and Quirynen, M. (2015). Risk indicators for peri-implantitis: A narrative review. *Clinical Oral Implants Research* 26, 15–44.

Renvert, S., Roos-Jansåker, A.M., and Claffey, N. (2008). Non-surgical treatment of peri-implant mucositis and peri-implantitis: A literature review. *Journal of Clinical Periodontology* 35 (Suppl. 8), 305–315. doi:10.1111/j.1600-051X.2008.01276.x.

Renvert, S., Samuelsson, E., Lindahl, C., and Persson, G.R. (2009). Mechanical non-surgical treatment of peri-implantitis: A double-blind randomized longitudinal clinical study. *I: Clinical results. Journal of Clinical Periodontology* 36, 604–609. doi:10.1111/j.1600-051X.2009.01421.x.

Rocchietta, I., Fontana, F., and Simion, M. (2008). Clinical outcomes of vertical bone augmentation to enable dental implant placement: A systematic review. *Journal of Clinical Periodontology* 35, 203–215.

Roccuzzo, M., Bonino, L., Dalmasso, P., and Aglietta, M. (2014). Long-term results of a three arms prospective cohort study on implants in periodontally compromised patients: 10-year data around sandblasted and acid-etched (SLA) surface. *Clinical Oral Implants Research* 25, 1105–1112.

Schwartz-Arad, D., Herzberg, R., and Dolev, E. (2004). The prevalence of surgical complications of the sinus graft procedure and their impact on implant survival. *Journal of Periodontology* 75, 511–516.

Schwarz, F., Papanicolau, P., Rothamel, D. et al. (2006). Influence of plaque biofilm removal on reestablishment of the biocompatibility of contaminated titanium surfaces. *Journal of Biomedical Material Research* 77, 437–444.

Schwarz, F., Sahm, N., Schwarz, K., and Becker, J. (2010). Impact of defect configuration on the clinical outcome following surgical regenerative therapy of peri-implantitis. *Journal of Clinical Periodontology* 37, 449–455.

Seddon, H.J. (1942). *A classification of nerve injuries. British Medical Journal* 2, 237–239.

Sousa, V., Mardas, N., Farias, B. et al. (2016a). A systematic review of implant outcomes in treated periodontitis patients. *Clinical Oral Implants Research* 27: 787–844.

Sousa, V., Mardas, N., Spratt, D. et al. (2016b). Experimental models for contamination of titanium surfaces and disinfection protocols. *Clinical Oral Implants Research* 27, 1233–1242.

Srinivasan, M., Vazquez, L., Rieder, P. et al. Survival rates of short (6 mm) micro-rough surface implants: A review of literature and meta-analysis. *Clinical Oral Implants Research* 25, 539–545.

Stanford, C.M. (2010). Surface modification of biomedical and dental implants and the processes of inflammation, wound healing and bone formation. *International Journal of Molecular Sciences* 11, 354–369. doi:10.3390/ijms11010354.

Summers, R. (1998). Sinus floor elevation with osteotomes. *Journal of Esthetic Dentistry* 10, 164–171.

Tan, W.C., Lang, N.P., Zwahlen, M., and Pjetursson, B.E. (2008). A systematic review of the success of sinus floor elevation and survival of implants inserted in combination with sinus floor elevation. Part II: Transalveolar technique. *Journal of Clinical Periodontology* 35(Suppl. 8), 241–254.

Tepper, G., Haas, R., Zechner, W. et al. (2002) Three-dimensional finite element analysis of implant stability in the atrophic posterior maxilla: A mathematical study of the sinus floor augmentation. *Clinical Oral Implants Research* 13, 657–665.

Thoma, D.S., Zeltner, M., Hüsler, J. et al.; EAO Supplement Working Group 4 (2015). Short implants versus sinus lifting with longer implants to restore the posterior maxilla:

A systematic review. *Clinical Oral Implants Research* 26 (Suppl. 11), 154–169.

Timmenga, N.M., Raghoebar, G.M., Boering, G., and van Weissenbruch, R. (1997). Maxillary sinus function after sinus lifts for the insertion of dental implants. *Journal of Oral and Maxillofacial Surgery* 55, 936–939.

Timmenga, N.M., Raghoebar, G.M., Boering, G. et al. (2003). Maxillary sinus floor elevation surgery: A clinical, radiographic and endoscopic evaluation. *Clinical Oral Implants Research* 14, 322–328.

Toffler, M. (2004). Osteotome-mediated sinus floor elevation: A clinical report. *International Journal of Oral and Maxillofacial Implants* 19, 266–273.

Ueda, M., and Kaneda, T. (1992). Maxillary sinusitis caused by dental implants: Report of two cases. *Journal of Oral and Maxillofacial Surgery* 50, 285–287.

van den Bergh, J.P., Bruggenkate ten, C.M., Disch, F.J., and Tuinzing, D.B. (2000). Anatomical aspects of sinus floor elevations. *Clinical Oral Implants Research* 11, 256–265.

van Steenberghe, D., Quirynen, M., Molly, L., and Jacobs, R. (2003). Impact of systemic diseases and medication on osseointegration. *Periodontology 2000* 33, 163–171.

Velloso, G.R., Vidigal, G.M., de Freitas, M.M. et al. (2006). Tridimensional analysis of maxillary sinus anatomy related to sinus lift procedure. *Implant Dentistry* 15, 192–196.

Wallace, S.S., and Froum, S.J. (2003). Effect of maxillary sinus augmentation on the survival of endosseous dental implants: A systematic review. *Annals of Periodontology* 8, 328–343.

Wang, H.-L., Burgett, F.G., Shyr, Y., and Ramfjord, S. (1994). The influence of molar furcation involvement and mobility on future clinical periodontal attachment loss. *Journal of Periodontology* 65, 25–29.

Wiltfang, J., Schultze-Mosgau, S., Merten, H.A. et al. (2000). Endoscopic and ultrasonographic evaluation of the maxillary sinus after combined sinus floor augmentation and implant insertion. *Oral Surgery, Oral Medicine, Oral Pathology, Oral Radiology, Endodontology* 89, 288–291.

Winwood, K., Zioupos, P., Currey, J.D. et al. (2006). The importance of the elastic and plastic components of strain in tensile and compressive fatigue of human cortical bone in relation to orthopaedic biomechanics. *Journal of Musculoskeletal and Neuronal Interactions* 6, 134–141.

Yacoub, N., Ismail, Y.H., and Mao, J.J. (2002). Transmission of bone strain in the craniofacial bones of edentulous human skulls upon dental implant loading. *Journal of Prosthetic Dentistry* 88, 192–199.

Zitzmann, N.U., and Berglundh, T. (2008). Definition and prevalence of peri-implant diseases. *Journal of Clinical Periodontology* 35, 286–291.

Zitzmann, N.U., Scherrer, S.S., Weiger, R. et al. (2011). Preferences of dental care providers in maintaining compromised teeth in relation to their professional status: Implants instead of periodontally involved maxillary molars? *Clinical Oral Implants Research* 22, 143–150.

Chapter 12

Is it Worth it? Health Economics of Furcation Involvement

Falk Schwendicke[1] and Christian Graetz[2]

[1] Department of Operative and Preventive Dentistry, Charité-Universitätsmedizin Berlin, Berlin, Germany
[2] Clinic for Conservative Dentistry and Periodontology, Christian-Albrechts-University, Kiel, Germany

12.1 Health Economic Relevance of Furcation Involvement

A growing number of patients keep the majority of their teeth throughout their life, with even multi-rooted teeth being retained. In Germany, for example, around one-third of adults aged 65 years or older retain all their first or second molars (Jordan and Micheelis 2016). This high number of retained teeth generates periodontal treatment needs (Jordan and Micheelis 2016; Holtfreter et al. 2010; Kassebaum et al. 2014). On the other hand, those who loose teeth are more likely to have them replaced nowadays than in the past, mainly because the demand for replacements is growing while replacement via implant-supported crowns is widely available (Micheelis and Schiffer 2006; Roos-Jansaker et al. 2006).

Both tooth retention and replacement generate costs, which are relevant not only for patients (when they bear them on their own) but also for public or private insurers (who need to weigh incurring costs against the resulting health benefit and the demand from patients for such costly procedures; that is, their justifiability in both the public and private domain). Treatment costs are also relevant from an equity perspective, since they might determine the utilization of services, with those who cannot afford treatment avoiding it, increasing existing health disparities (Zhong 2010).

In general, systematic periodontal treatment seems to allow long-term retention of most periodontally compromised teeth (Hatch et al. 2001; Loesche et al. 2002; Fardal et al. 2004; Chambrone and Chambrone 2006; Eickholz et al. 2008; Graetz et al. 2017a,b, 2011, 2013, 2015; Johansson et al. 2013; Salvi et al. 2014). In many cases, such retention of teeth in subjects with periodontitis seems affordable, with costs for supportive periodontal therapy (SPT) being limited (Pretzl et al. 2009; Fardal and Grytten 2013; Schwendicke et al. 2016b).

In contrast, for multi-rooted teeth with furcation involvement (FI) – that is, mainly compromised molars – long-term retention might be more difficult to achieve, with survival times being possibly correlated with the degree of FI (Checchi et al. 2002; König et al. 2002; Dannewitz et al. 2006a; Johansson et al. 2013; Graetz et al. 2015), as discussed in Chapter 5. As a result, more complex and expensive treatments and more frequent SPT visits are often needed for retaining such teeth, which might have an impact on the costs of tooth retention (Pretzl et al., 2009; Lee et al. 2012; Schwendicke et al. 2014).

Diagnosis and Treatment of Furcation-Involved Teeth, First Edition. Edited by Luigi Nibali.
© 2018 John Wiley & Sons Ltd. Published 2018 by John Wiley & Sons Ltd.
Companion website: www.wiley.com/go/nibali/diagnosis

Given the growing demand for retaining or replacing molars and the wide availability of both options in most developed dental settings, costs come into focus. In rationalized healthcare settings, where funding is limited and competition for it between sectors is high, it is important to quantify both the costs of a disease and the cost-effectiveness of different treatment options. For molars with FI, this means estimating the annual retention costs, and comparing them with the alternative costs for tooth replacement via implant-supported crowns, or fixed or removal dental prostheses. Such cost estimation should best account not only for periodontal but also endodontic, restorative, and prosthetic treatments. Moreover, the functionality (or other kind of utility) of retained versus replaced or even missing furcation-involved molars needs to be known to weigh it against the expected costs. Last, the evaluation of costs and utilities (or any other kind of health benefit) should be performed in time horizons relevant to payers and consumers; that is, long term.

12.2 Health Economic Analyses

Health economic analyses are typically defined according to the evaluated outcome (Vernazza et al. 2012):

- *Cost-of-disease studies* investigate the required treatment efforts for managing or resolving a disease or its symptoms. Such costs are usually termed direct costs. Cost-of-disease studies further measure indirect costs (e.g. those for getting to the doctor or dentist) and opportunity costs (e.g. those for not being able to work during this time).
- *Cost-effectiveness studies* measure costs against the effectiveness of a treatment. Effectiveness usually means a clinical outcome (survival time of a tooth, retention time of a restoration), as determined in a real-life setting or in rather artificial (randomized controlled) settings. Note that while the latter is termed 'efficacy', no

such strict separation is done for health economic studies.

- *Cost-utility analyses* measure costs against the resulting utility, like quality- or disability-adjusted life years. They involve the subjective value placed by someone (usually patients) on a certain health state. One needs to elicit these utilities, which is not always easy and has not been widely done so far with regard to tooth values. (What is the utility of a filled tooth against a sound one? What that of a periodontally impaired but asymptomatic molar against a non-compromised molar?)
- *Cost–benefit analyses* transform effectiveness or utility – that is, the health outcome – into a monetary value. They theoretically allow comparison of effort and outcome on the same scale, but their methodology is not fully accepted and has only very sparsely been applied in dentistry so far.

All these types of analyses can be performed in one of two ways. The first involves the (re-)use of primary data, for example from cohort or controlled studies. For example, cohort studies allow estimation of the exact costs incurred for staff (via recording staff hours and factorizing them with the costs per hour for different staff) or materials (factorizing unit price and used units). This micro-costing allows very detailed and realistic cost estimation. In addition, these studies can estimate the effectiveness of the performed treatments (how long a tooth was retained etc.). Randomized controlled trials also often collect cost data, allowing comparison of different treatment strategies (like scaling and root planing versus open-flap debridement).

The second way also involves re-use of data, although not in the original framework of a clinical study, but rather in a mathematical model. Modelling studies construct a hypothetical path of a tooth or patients ('the model') reflecting the clinical (natural) pathway. Teeth or patients can translate from one to another health status (e.g. molar with FI without furcation caries → molar with FI with furcation caries), with the chance of such translation depending on transition probabilities. For each translation, a treatment is assumed (e.g. application of fluoride varnish to arrest a lesion, or restoration), generating costs. Many of these models are analysed via Monte Carlo micro-simulations, which allow parameter uncertainty to be introduced. This is done via simulating a number of patients (e.g. 1000), with transition probabilities (or other uncertain parameters) being randomly sampled from a certain range of the parameter. The sampling of this population is then simulated again for a series of times (e.g. 1000), allowing estimation of both the per-patient and per-population variance. In general, such models allow investigation of several groups over a longer time than most clinical trials (randomized trials rarely follow up patients for decades), with high validity given that most data are from reviews and meta-analyses. They have, however, limited applicability to other settings than the one analysed, and are only as valid as the assumptions made. They need validation via sensitivity analyses, assessing the impact the uncertainties have on the finding of a study.

The available health economic studies on molars with FI are mainly cost-of-disease studies, with data collection in prospectively or retrospectively assessed cohorts, or cost-effectiveness studies, using models to demonstrate the costs and cost-effectiveness of different strategies of retaining or replacing furcation-involved molars.

12.3 The Costs of Furcation Involvement

Several clinical studies have attempted to measure the costs of retaining furcation-involved molars. Most of these have followed molars after successful active periodontal treatment (APT), which were regularly retreated as part of the SPT.

For example, a German study retrospectively assessed molars in patients who all had received initial or follow-up periodontal treatments, including subgingival debridement (Graetz et al. 2015). The therapeutic strategy for these molars was aimed at improving access to furcations, allowing regular individual and professional oral hygiene in these areas (Figure 12.1).

Conservative scaling and root planing (SRP) had been performed for molars with probing pocket depths (PPDs) < 5 mm without bleeding on probing, and open-flap surgery including furcation debridement if PPD ≥ 5 mm plus bleeding or PPD ≥ 6 mm regardless of bleeding was present (Kocher and Plagmann 1999). Root-resection therapy or tunnelling was mainly provided in molars with advanced bone loss which had received endodontic treatment, as well as for molars with furcation caries (Figure 12.2).

Tunnelling was only performed for lower molars with both lingual and buccal FI degree II, or FI degree III with limited access for oral hygiene, often combined with persistent inflammation, if resection was not possible. Different retrospective studies demonstrated long-term stability for molars with such a treatment strategy during regular SPT (Graetz et al. 2017b, 2013, 2015; Figure 12.3).

Costs were assessed in the context of German healthcare. As such, any costs occurring to payers (regardless if this was the statutory insurance, the patient, or their private insurer) were estimated using fee items of German item catalogues. The authors quantified the resources provided based on the number of periodontal, restorative, endodontic, or prosthetic treatments, which had been ascertained via case records. Resources and fee item–based costs were calculated per tooth. Services provided to more than one tooth (e.g. examination, antibiotics) were distributed among the teeth present. Items charged per tooth (like SRP) were not distributed.

The study (Schwendicke et al. 2016a) assessed 2306 molars in 379 patients (mean initial age 45.7, standard deviation [SD] 10.0 years). The majority of molars (72.8%) had no PPD > 4 mm after APT. Molars were followed up for 16.5 (SD 6.8) years. Over this period of SPT, a mean of 0.07 (SD 0.12) SRP

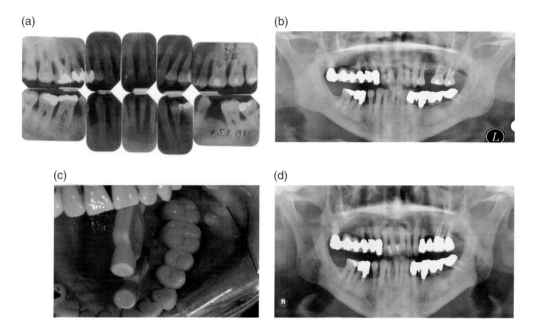

Figure 12.1 Man, aged 42 years and non-smoker, diagnosed with chronic periodontitis and horizontal bone loss in both jaws with furcation involvement degree II up to III (Hamp et al. 1975) on all first and second molars (a: initial status). He received scaling and root planing and open-flap debridement of all posterior teeth. After 22 years of regular supportive periodontal therapy (b), endodontic treatment was required, with trisection of the upper right molars and prosthetic reconstruction being performed. Afterwards, furcation cleaning with interdental brushes (c) was possible. The situation remained stable for a further seven years (d, last observation).

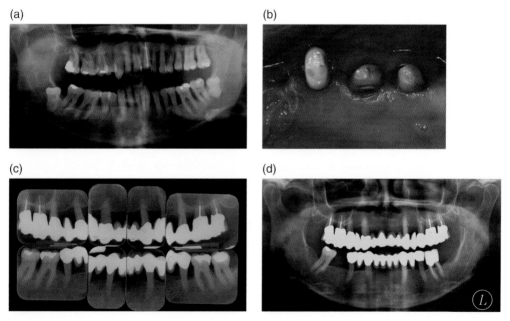

Figure 12.2 Woman, aged 36 years and non-smoker, diagnosed with aggressive periodontitis and horizontal bone loss in both jaws and furcation involvement degree III (Hamp et al. 1975) of all upper molars and tooth 14 (UR4), as well as degree II (Hamp et al. 1975) of all lower molars (a: initial status). Initial periodontal therapy with scaling and root planing was followed by open-flap debridement of all premolars and molars. After re-evaluation, supportive periodontal therapy was commenced and after 1.5 years the buccal roots of all upper molars were resected and fixed dental prostheses provided (b). Two (c) and 17 years later (d), no further attachment loss was noted. Tooth 46 (LR6) had to be extracted due to a fracture.

(a)

(b)

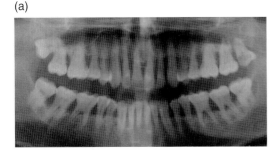
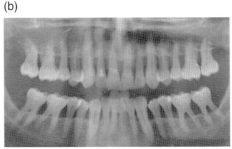

Figure 12.3 Man, aged 47 years and smoker; chronic periodontitis and horizontal bone loss in both jaws with furcation involvement degree II (Hamp et al. 1975) on all upper molars and right lower molars, as well as degree III (Hamp et al. 1975) on all left lower molars (a: initial status). Open-flap debridement of all molars, including tunnelling of the left lower molars, was provided. The patient stopped smoking after the 8th year during SPT. After 28 years of regular supportive periodontal therapy (b), the periodontal situation remained stable.

had been provided per year (Table 12.1). Similarly, a mean of 0.04 (SD 0.11) flap debridements (FD) had been provided per year. This number was increased in older subjects, molars with PPD ≥ 5 mm, mobile molars, and those with prosthetic treatment initially present. Resections had been mainly performed in upper molars, molars with mobility grade 3, FI degree III, bone loss, and those with endodontic treatment, periapical lesions, or previous prosthetic treatment. Few molars received endodontic, restorative, or prosthetic treatments, with prosthetically restored molars being more likely to receive endodontic therapy or prosthetic retreatment. The last component assessed was SPT, with a mean of 2.49 (SD 0.12) SPT visits per year and per patient.

Based on these estimates for the resources used, annual costs per molar were €18.28 (SD 16.91) for all treatments and €13.04 (SD 9.58) for periodontal treatments only (Table 12.2). The robustness of these estimates was demonstrated by calculating costs for patients with different health insurances (which allows for different charges being claimed by dentists). Total treatment costs increased significantly for molars with FI, PPD ≥ 5 mm, bone loss, endodontic or prosthetic treatment, and periapical lesions. If analysed on a patient level, mean costs per year were

€137.86 (SD 370.03). There was a significant association between these costs and smoking status (costs being higher in current smokers than non-smokers).

Another study assessed the tooth-retention efforts in periodontally compromised but successfully treated subjects over 10 years of SPT, again within German healthcare (Pretzl et al. 2009). This study found that 0.34 SRP had been provided over the 10 years (including the first SRP). What can be seen from both studies is the low number of treatments needed to retain compromised molars. Total periodontal treatment costs for tooth retention ranged between €6 and €13, which is low given the costs of alternative options (like implants or fixed dental prostheses). What was further shown was that periodontal treatment costs made up around two-thirds of the total long-term costs; that is, most molars did not generate significant costs for endodontic or restorative treatment (furcation caries, for example, was found in only 2% of teeth over the whole observation period). In both studies, the periodontal treatment efforts were higher in teeth with bone loss, severe FI, prosthetic abutment status, and maxillary molars, but not patients with aggressive versus chronic periodontitis. Practitioners should be aware of these predictors, as they determine not only the

Table 12.1 Mean (SD) number of treatments provided per year of retention. Differences of number of treatments between groups are indicated in bold (p < 0.05, ANOVA). For more than two groups, different superscript letters indicate a significantly different number of treatments according to the Bonferroni post-hoc test (p < 0.05).

Parameter	N	Deep scaling/ root planing	Surgical flap debridement	Root resection	Supportive therapy	Endodontic treatment	Restorative treatment	Prosthetic treatment
Patients' age at T0								
<50	738	**0.09 (0.17)**	**0.04 (0.09)**	0.01 (0.04)	**2.48 (0.12)**	0.01 (0.04)	0.00 (0.01)	0.01 (0.03)
≥50	1568	**0.06 (0.08)**	**0.05 (0.12)**	0.01 (0.04)	**2.51 (0.12)**	0.01 (0.04)	0.00 (0.01)	0.01 (0.03)
Gender								
Male	950	0.07 (0.10)	0.04 (0.12)	0.01 (0.05)	2.48 (0.12)	0.01 (0.05)	0.00 (0.01)	0.01 (0.03)
Female	1356	0.07 (0.10)	0.04 (0.11)	0.01 (0.03)	2.49 (0.13)	0.01 (0.03)	0.00 (0.01)	0.01 (0.03)
Diagnosis								
Aggressive periodontitis	453	0.07 (0.13)	0.04 (0.12)	0.01 (0.03)	2.49 (0.10)	0.01 (0.04)	0.00 (0.01)	0.01 (0.03)
Chronic periodontitis	1853	0.06 (0.09)	0.05 (0.09)	0.01 (0.04)	2.49 (0.10)	0.01 (0.04)	0.00 (0.01)	0.01 (0.03)
Number of teeth at T0								
≥24	1760	0.06 (0.12)	0.04 (0.10)	0.01 (0.03)	2.49 (0.10)	0.01 (0.04)	0.00 (0.01)	0.01 (0.03)
<24	546	0.08 (0.12)	0.05 (0.11)	0.01 (0.06)	2.50 (0.10)	0.01 (0.04)	0.00 (0.01)	0.01 (0.03)
Smoking status								
Non-smoker	1458	0.07 (0.09)	0.04 (0.10)	0.00 (0.04)	2.48 (0.11)	0.01 (0.04)	0.00 (0.01)	0.01 (0.03)
Former smoker	547	0.07 (0.13)	0.05 (0.15)	0.00 (0.06)	2.49 (0.15)	0.01 (0.04	0.00 (0.01)	0.01 (0.03)
Smoker	301	0.07 (0.10)	0.05 (0.11)	0.00 (0.02)	2.50 (0.11)	0.01 (0.02	0.00 (0.01)	0.01 (0.03)
Jaw								
Maxilla	1108	0.07 (0.14)	0.05 (0.11)	**0.01 (0.06)**	2.49 (0.13)	0.01 (0.05)	0.00 (0.01)	0.01 (0.03)
Mandible	1198	0.07 (0.09)	0.03 (0.11)	**0.00 (0.02)**	2.48 (0.12)	0.01 (0.03)	0.00 (0.01)	0.01 (0.03)
Maximum PPD at T1								
<5 mm	1678	**0.06 (0.08)**	**0.03 (0.108)**	0.01 (0.03)	**2.47 (0.09)**	0.01 (0.03)	0.00 (0.01)	0.01 (0.03)
≥5 mm	628	**0.09 (0.19)**	**0.08 (0.16)**	0.01 (0.06)	**2.52 (0.17)**	0.01 (0.05)	0.00 (0.01)	0.01 (0.03)

	N								
Mobility at T0									
0	1833	0.07 (0.13)	**0.03 (0.07)**[a]	**0.00 (0.02)**[a]	**2.48 (0.09)**[a]	0.01 (0.04)	0.00 (0.01)	0.00 (0.01)	0.01 (0.03)
1	332	0.06 (0.09)	**0.07 (0.16)**[b]	**0.01 (0.05)**[b]	**2.50 (0.15)**[b]	0.01 (0.05)	0.00 (0.01)	0.00 (0.01)	0.02 (0.03)
2	77	0.05 (0.07)	**0.11 (0.27)**[c]	**0.01 (0.03)**[b]	**2.52 (0.26)**[b]	0.01 (0.04)	0.00 (0.00)	0.00 (0.00)	0.01 (0.03)
3	64	0.08 (0.12)	**0.15 (0.27)**[c]	**0.04 (0.19)**[c]	**2.61 (0.27)**[c]	0.01 (0.04)	0.00 (0.02)	0.00 (0.02)	0.01 (0.03)
FI at T1									
0	1105	0.07 (0.13)	**0.03 (0.09)**[a]	**0.00 (0.04)**[a]	**2.47 (0.11)**[a]	**0.01 (0.03)**[a]	**0.00 (0.01)**[a]	**0.00 (0.01)**[a]	**0.01 (0.02)**[a]
1	652	0.07 (0.10)	**0.04 (0.06)**[a]	**0.01 (0.03)**[a]	**2.48 (0.07)**[a]	**0.01 (0.04)**[a]	**0.00 (0.01)**[a]	**0.00 (0.01)**[a]	**0.01 (0.03)**[a]
2	356	0.07 (0.11)	**0.07 (0.13)**[b]	**0.01 (0.03)**[a]	**2.51 (0.14)**[b]	**0.01 (0.03)**[a]	**0.00 (0.01)**[a]	**0.00 (0.01)**[a]	**0.01 (0.03)**[a]
3	193	0.06 (0.12)	**0.11 (0.23)**[b]	**0.03 (0.11)**[b]	**2.54 (0.22)**[b]	**0.03 (0.08)**[b]	**0.01 (0.02)**[b]	**0.01 (0.02)**[b]	**0.02 (0.05)**[b]
Bone loss at T0									
>50%	980	0.07 (0.15)	0.06 (0.14)	**0.01 (0.06)**[a]	**2.50 (0.15)**[a]	**0.01 (0.05)**[a]	0.00 (0.01)	0.00 (0.01)	0.01 (0.03)
25-50%	882	0.07 (0.10)	0.04 (0.10)	**0.00 (0.02)**[b]	**2.48 (0.11)**[b]	**0.01 (0.03)**[b]	0.00 (0.01)	0.00 (0.01)	0.01 (0.03)
<25%	444	0.07 (0.06)	0.02 (0.04)	**0.00 (0.02)**[b]	**2.46 (0.06)**[b]	**0.01 (0.03)**[b]	0.00 (0.01)	0.00 (0.01)	0.01 (0.03)
Endodontic treatment									
Not present	2163	0.07 (0.12)	0.04 (0.11)	**0.01 (0.02)**	**2.48 (0.12)**	**0.01 (0.04)**	0.00 (0.01)	0.00 (0.01)	**0.01 (0.03)**
Present	143	0.07 (0.10)	0.04 (0.16)	**0.06 (0.14)**	**2.52 (0.16)**	**0.01 (0.02)**	0.00 (0.01)	0.00 (0.01)	**0.02 (0.04)**
Periapical lesion									
Not present	2243	0.07 (0.12)	0.05 (0.11)	**0.01 (0.04)**	2.49 (0.12)	0.01 (0.04)	0.00 (0.01)	0.00 (0.01)	**0.01 (0.03)**
Present	63	0.05 (0.10)	0.03 (0.18)	**0.04 (0.10)**	2.53 (0.13)	0.01 (0.04)	0.00 (0.01)	0.00 (0.01)	**0.03 (0.07)**
Prosthetic treatment									
Not present	1460	0.07 (0.13)	**0.04 (0.12)**	**0.00 (0.02)**	2.49 (0.13)	**0.01 (0.04)**	0.00 (0.01)	0.00 (0.01)	**0.00 (0.00)**
Present	846	0.07 (0.10)	**0.09 (0.09)**	**0.01 (0.06)**	2.48 (0.10)	**0.01 (0.05)**	0.00 (0.01)	0.00 (0.01)	**0.03 (0.04)**

ANOVA = analysis of variance; FI = furcation involvement; N = number of molars; PPD = probing pocket depth; SD = standard deviation; T = time.

Table 12.2 Mean (SD) periodontal and total treatment costs per retention year. Base case (privately insured patient) and sensitivity (publically insured patient) analyses are shown. Differences of costs between groups are indicated in bold (p < 0.05, ANOVA). For more than two groups, different superscript letters indicate significantly different costs according to the Bonferroni post-hoc test (p < 0.05).

Parameter	N	Base case analysis		Sensitivity analysis	
		Total treatment costs per year	Periodontal treatment costs per year	Total treatment costs per year	Periodontal treatment costs per year
Patients' age at T0					
<50	738	19.45 (17.71)	13.74 (11.98)	21.08 (21.77)	15.99 (16.66)
≥50	1568	17.70 (16.52)	12.62 (8.22)	18.44 (17.22)	14.05 (10.23)
Gender					
Male	950	17.44 (16.83)	12.61 (7.25)	18.48 (16.91)	14.18 (8.66)
Female	1356	18.82 (16.90)	13.26 (10.90)	19.83 (19.99)	15.01 (14.84)
Diagnosis					
Aggressive periodontitis	453	17.11 (13.64) 18.51 (17.59)	13.25 (6.41)	18.15 (13.99)	14.81 (7.99)
Chronic periodontitis	1853		12.93 (10.25)	19.55 (19.79)	14.64 (13.52)
Number of teeth at T0					
≥24	1760	17.33 (16.20)	**12.61 (8.99)**	18.23 (17.99)	**14.10 (14.66)**
<24	546	21.19 (18.74)	**14.20 (11.23)**	22.82 (20.91)	**16.55 (14.97)**
Smoking status					
Non-smoker	1458	18.33 (17.51)	12.91 (10.39)	19.32 (19.82)	14.58 (14.14)
Former smoker	547	17.64 (16.51)	13.28 (8.97)	19.10 (18.29)	15.07 (10.82)
Smoker	301	18.73 (14.49)	12.90 (5.89)	19.40 (14.02)	14.41 (6.55)
Jaw					
Maxilla	1108	19.04 (18.49)	13.60 (11.12)	20.51 (21.19)	15.56 (15.00)
Mandible	1198	17.50 (15.33)	12.50 (7.86)	18.15 (16.27)	13.88 (9.91)
Maximum PPD at T1					
<5 mm	1678	**17.34 (15.69)**	**12.38 (9.26)**	**17.96 (17.12)**	**13.82 (12.49)**
≥5 mm	628	**20.62 (19.50)**	**14.71 (10.32)**	**22.92 (22.33)**	**16.96 (12.98)**
Mobility at T0					
0	1833	**17.33 (14.27)**[a]	**12.38 (6.49)**[a]	**17.96 (14.60)**[a]	**13.82 (8.60)**[a]
1	332	**21.12 (21.17)**[a]	**14.41 (12.23)**[b]	**22.82 (23.39)**[b]	**16.61 (15.78)**[b]
2	77	**21.00 (22.45)**[a]	**15.59 (13.01)**[b]	**23.27 (26.46)**[b]	**17.29 (14.03)**[b]
3	64	**26.98 (37.77)**[b]	**20.12 (32.67)**[c]	**37.01 (54.486**[c]	**27.77 (47.66)**[c]
FI at T1					
0	1105	**16.50 (13.27)**[a]	**11.95 (6.75)**[a]	**17.04 (14.69)**[a]	**13.19 (8.91)**[a]
1	652	**16.72 (11.72)**[a]	**12.49 (5.12)**[a]	**17.64 (11.36)**[a]	**14.00 (6.45)**[b]
2	356	**20.60 (16.99)**[b]	**14.20 (9.07)**[b]	**22.06 (18.29)**[b]	**16.04 (11.14)**[b]
3	193	**29.07 (35.69)**[c]	**18.64 (23.59)**[c]	**33.69 (42.37)** [c]	**23.35 (32.62)**[c]

Table 12.2 (Continued)

Parameter	N	Base case analysis		Sensitivity analysis	
		Total treatment costs per year	Periodontal treatment costs per year	Total treatment costs per year	Periodontal treatment costs per year
Bone loss at T0					
>50%	980	**19.71 (19.25)**[a]	**14.28 (13.02)** [a]	**21.74 (23.54)**[a]	16.55 (17.51)
25-50%	882	**17.68 (16.47)**[b]	**12.51 (6.49)**[b]	**18.15 (16.14)**[b]	13.81 (8.12)
<25%	444	**16.15 (11.00)**[b]	**11.16 (3.23)**[b]	**16.25 (9.13)**[b]	12.34 (3.55)
Endodontic treatment					
Not present	2163	**17.52 (14.84)**	**12.50 (6.23)**	**18.25 (15.09)**	13.83 (7.42)
Present	143	**29.28 (33.97)**	**21.20 (28.77)**	**35.84 (45.82)**	27.95 (40.89)
Peri-apical lesion					
Not present	2243	**17.70(14.66)**	**12.74 (7.68)**	**18.67 (15.92)**	14.28 (9.78)
Present	63	**36.19 (49.92)**	**22.15 (34.36)**	**42.75 (60.09)**	29.50 (49.65)
Prosthetic treatment					
Not present	1460	**13.80 (12.71)**	12.99 (10.05)	**15.90 (17.53)**	14.58 (13.30)
Present	846	**25.91 (20.25)**	13.04 (8.89)	**25.14 (19.43)**	14.81 (11.41)

ANOVA = analysis of variance; FI = furcation involvement; N = number of molars; PPD = probing pocket depth; SD = standard deviation; T = time.

chance of clinical success, but also the efforts needed to ensure this success, and should guide decision making towards retaining or replacing teeth. It should be noted that prosthetically involved molars were generally found to be more expensive to retain, which indicates not only periodontal treatment needs, but also the necessity of retreating prosthetically (due to caries, fractures, porcelain chippings) or endodontically (Goodacre et al. 2003; Walton 2013; see also Figure 12.4).

(a) (b) (c)

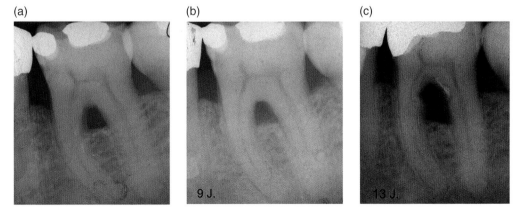

Figure 12.4 First lower molar with furcation involvement degree III (Hamp et al. 1975) after treatment with tunnelling for cleaning at home (a). The situation remained stable for over 9 years (b), while after 13 years (c) a carious lesion in the furcation developed, leading to endodontic involvement and, eventually, extraction.

Such increased risks of reinterventions for prosthetically restored teeth was shown mainly if prosthetics had been placed prior to periodontitis treatment (Pretzl et al. 2008; Graetz et al. 2013), while prosthetics inserted after successful initial therapy and during systematic SPT were not necessarily found to generate more treatment efforts and costs (Yi et al. 1995; Lulic et al. 2007; Fardal and Linden 2010; Graetz et al, 2013; see also Figure 12.5).

Overall, the very limited available evidence finds retention of FI molars to require more effort than non-molar or non-FI teeth, which has impacts on the costs required for retention. This is truer in molars with severe

(a)

(b)

(c)

(d)

(e)

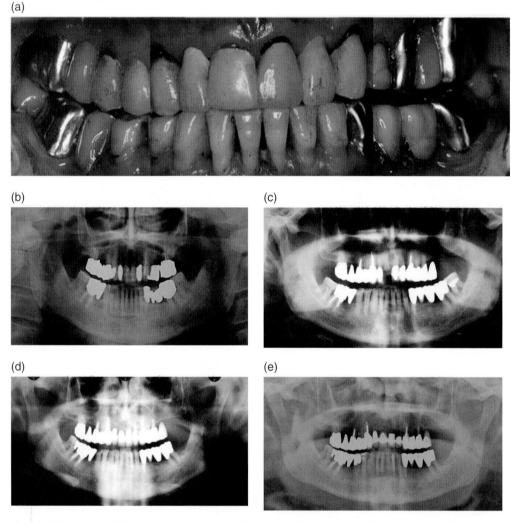

Figure 12.5 Man, aged 59 years and non-smoker, diagnosed with generalized chronic periodontitis and horizontal bone loss up to one-quarter of the root length in both jaws and furcation involvement degree I (lower molars) and II (upper molars) (Hamp et al. 1975) (a and b). Initial periodontal therapy using scaling and root planing followed by open-flap debridement of all pre/molars with extraction of tooth 17 (UR7) (as a result of a root carious lesion) was provided. After re-evaluation, a regular supportive periodontal therapy was started and after one year a fixed dental prosthesis was fitted. Seven years later, tooth 11 fractured (c) and a fixed dental prosthesis was provided in the front (d). This situation remained stable for 29 years (e, last observation).

furcation involvement (FI degree III), but not necessarily for FI degree I. More important, however, is the fact that overall retention costs were very limited, with only a few euros per year being required to retain such molars. Based on this finding, it is now relevant to compare these costs with those generated by other, alternative treatments.

12.4 Cost-effectiveness of Retaining Furcation-involved Molars

There are only very few data comparing the cost-effectiveness of different strategies to retain molars with FI. One recent study (Schwendicke et al. 2014) used a mathematical model to assess the cost-effectiveness of treatment alternatives for periodontally affected, vital molars with furcation FI, comparing tooth-retaining strategies with tooth removal and replacement via implant-supported crowns (ISCs). Categories of tooth-retaining strategies were

- Conservative, non-surgical furcation therapy involving SRP.
- SRP with surgical access (i.e. FD).
- For teeth with FI degree II or III, root resection (RR; i.e. hemisection, trisection, or amputation), as well as
- Guided tissue regeneration (GTR, including insertion of bone-substitute material and placement of a resorbable membrane), and
- Tunnelling (TU, for mandibular molars only).

Tooth-retaining strategies were compared with the removal and replacement of teeth via ISCs.

This study assessed cost-effectiveness as lifetime treatment costs (initial plus follow-up treatments) per retention time of the tooth or implant (in years). All analyses were performed separately for molars with FI degree I, lower molars with F degree II/III, and upper molars with FI degree II/III, again in the context of German healthcare.

The study simulated an initially 50-year-old male patient with an average remaining life expectancy of 29.7 years. The model used consisted of the initial and various follow-up health states (Figure 12.6), simulating the natural history of a periodontally affected tooth or an ISC.

As to the costs assessed, the following assumptions had been made:

- All initial therapies comprised full case assessment including oral hygiene assessment, advice and motivation, radiographs, scale and polish, re-evaluation, and the necessary treatment as already outlined, including anaesthesia, possible endodontic, surgical, or prosthetic procedures, and short-term post-operative care.
- Supportive periodontal or implant treatment involved biannual re-revaluation, scale and polish, subgingival retreatment, and antiseptic irrigation, as well as radiographic reassessment every two years. For teeth but not implants, fluoridation of root surfaces was assumed to be additionally performed.
- Modelling involved fatal complications – that is, those leading to loss of the tooth or implant (for example periodontal complications or untreatable root caries, or untreatable peri-implantitis or implant fracture, respectively) – and non-fatal complications – for instance treatable caries at restoration margins, treatment-responsive peri-implantitis, or loss of crowns or abutments. Mending of complications was assumed to generate costs, and involved repair or renewal of restorations, recementation or refixing of crowns or abutments, and peri-implant treatment (Mombelli and Lang, 1998).

For molars with FI degree I, SRP was both less costly and more effective than ISC. Compared with FD, ISC was always more costly, but also more effective (i.e. implants were retained longer). Regardless of the dental arch, treating molars with FI degree II/III via tooth-retaining options was found to be more

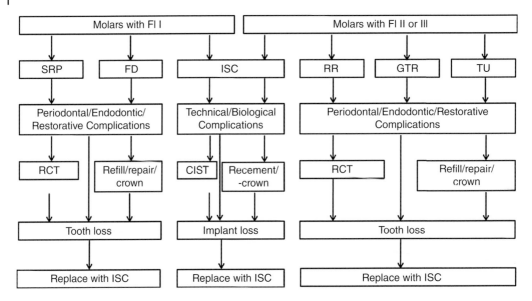

Figure 12.6 State transition diagram. Molars with furcation involvement (FI) degrees I and II/III were analysed separately, with different treatments being compared. All periodontal treatments were compared with implant-supported crowns (ISC). For all teeth, periodontal, endodontic, and restorative complications were modelled, with fatal (leading to tooth loss) and non-fatal (mendable) complications being simulated separately. For implants, we modelled technical (loss of crowns, abutment fracture, implant fracture) and biological complications (peri-implantitis), again with separate simulation of fatal and non-fatal failures. If complications were mendable, teeth and implants were allocated to follow-up treatments, which generated costs. In case these treatments were not final, i.e. another retreatment was possible (for example re-restoration after repair), this was modelled as well. Eventually, lost teeth or implants were assumed to be replaced using implant-supported crowns. Note that within base case analysis, all failed teeth or implants were assumed to be (re-)replaced. To explore the effects of this assumption, sensitivity analyses were performed. CIST = cumulative supportive interceptive therapy; FD = flap debridement; GTR = guided tissue regeneration; RCT = root canal treatment; RR = root resection; SRP = scaling and root planing; TU = tunnelling.

effective and less costly than tooth removal and replacement via ISC (Figure 12.7).

This cost-effectiveness ranking – with implants being more costly than tooth-retaining strategies – did hold even under the worst-case assumptions modelled, and was also stable regardless of how costs were estimated.

Retaining teeth was significantly less costly than removing and replacing them, mainly as ISCs are so costly initially, but also as retreatments on ISCs (which are not needed very frequently) are relatively costly. For example, treating peri-implantitis is not only challenging but costly, as is mending non-biological complications (ceramic chippings, crown decementations, fractures), which usually involve costly materials and often generate further staff costs for dental technicians.

This finding is in line with a number of observational studies from another health-care setting as well (Fardal and Grytten 2013; Martin et al. 2014).

More specifically, it is unlikely that removing and replacing molars with FI degree I will be cost-effective (the 10-year survival rate for molars treated via SRP and SPT was 97% in this study). This is in line with FI degree I being found to have only limited impact on tooth success when compared with FI degree 0 (Salvi et al. 2014; Graetz et al., 2015), but also to only limited impact on required treatment efforts (as has been shown already and in Tables 12.1 and 12.2). FD seems less effective than ISCs, while being more costly than SRP. It is therefore doubtful if such a strategy can be more cost-effective than SRP in molars with FI degree I (Heitz-Mayfield et al. 2002).

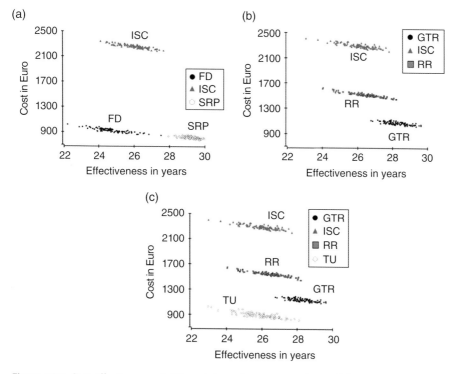

Figure 12.7 Cost-effectiveness of different strategies to treat molars with furcation involvement (FI). For FI degree I, we compared conservative scaling and root planing (SRP) and flap debridement and SRP (FD) with implant-supported crowns (ISC). For molars with FI degrees II or III, root resection (RR), guided tissue regeneration (GTR), and tunnelling (TU, for lower molars) were compared with ISC. The presented cost-effectiveness planes (a, b, c) demonstrate the discounted lifetime costs (y-axis) per effectiveness (in years of tooth or implant retention). In the case of FI degree I (a), SRP was more effective and less costly than ISC, while FD was both less effective and less costly than ISC. For upper (b) or lower (c) molars with FI degree II or III, ISC was dominated by all tooth-retaining strategies.

In general, there is debate around the cost-effectiveness of FD versus SRP, as the effectiveness gain seems limited (also in non-FI degree I teeth) while the additional costs are substantial (Antczak-Bouckoms and Weinstein 1987). There is, however, some indication that the need for maintenance visits seems reduced after FD compared with SRP, which could offset initially higher treatment costs (Miremadi et al. 2015).

There is greater uncertainty as to how best to treat molars with FI degree II or III (or whether to replace them). Treatment options have been discussed extensively in this book (mainly in Chapters 7, 8, and 9). RR especially was relatively costly, as costs occur not only for the periodontal procedure, but also root canal treatment (note that – as discussed

already – RR might be mainly applied to molars which had received endodontic therapy earlier) and crown placement (Carnevale et al. 1991; Huynh-Ba et al. 2009; Schwendicke et al. 2013). When considering the range of estimated survival rates for RR – 91% after 10 years in Schwendicke et al. (2013); 93% after 3.5 years in Helldén et al. (1989); 68% after 10 years in Blomlöf et al. (1997); and 83% after 7 years in Little et al. (1995; reviewed in Chapter 8), it remains uncertain whether the high costs for RR are truly justified.

What is clear from the existing studies is that one cannot really attempt to compare most periodontal treatments with one another, since their indications differ (RR will not be applied to the same teeth as SRP etc.).

What should be further borne in mind is that different periodontal treatments require different degrees of patient motivation and compliance. For example, tunnelling might require highly motivated patients to maintain the tunnel and prevent root caries (Hamp et al. 1975). That said, doubts remain regarding the postulated high risk of caries within tunnels (Little et al. 1995; Dannewitz et al. 2006b; Feres et al. 2006), as was seen in the German cohort study discussed, which reported such caries in only 2% of molars over 16.5 years (Schwendicke et al. 2016a). Lastly, retention and replacement are not the only viable options for treating molars with FI; shortened dental arches might also yield sufficient functionality and subjective oral health (Wolfart et al. 2014), while generating limited initial and long-term costs (Faggion et al. 2011; Wolfart et al. 2012). Here again, the available data are insufficient to assign monetary or utility values to missing, replaced, or retained teeth, which would allow different strategies to be properly compared.

12.5 Research Gaps

Adhesive dentistry increases the number of options for dealing with furcation-involved teeth. Splinting of different teeth or (resected) roots, or even using extracted teeth as adhesive bridge pontic, has been performed not only in the anterior region, but also posteriorly (Figures 12.8 and 12.9). Clinical experience allows the hypotheses that using glass fibre–enforced ribbons could allow similar retention periods to be achieved to conventional adhesive (Maryland) bridges used normally in the front, with similar complications of debonding and fracture (Miettinen and Millar 2013). However, reliable efficacy data and any data on cost-effectiveness or the value patients place on such treatments are missing at present.

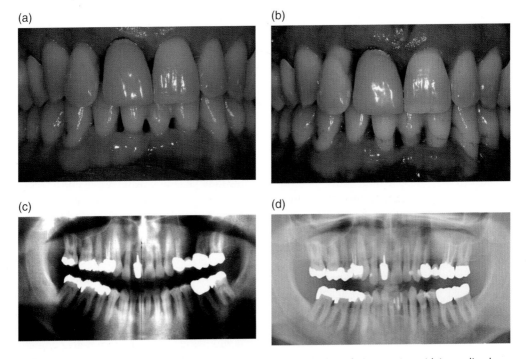

(a) (b) (c) (d)

Figure 12.8 Man, aged 46 years, with generalized chronic periodontitis after extraction with immediately re-fixation of tooth 31 (LL1) (a, b: before extraction) and long-term stability of the situation during supportive periodontal therapy over 10 years (c, d).

(a)

(b)

(c)

(d)

(e)

(f)

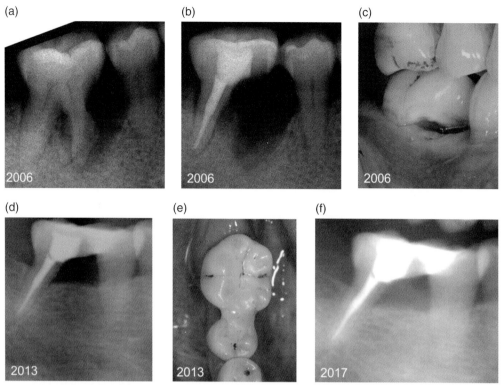

Figure 12.9 Woman, aged 47 years, with generalized chronic periodontitis and root resorption of the mesial root of tooth 46 (LR6) (a). After successful endodontic treatment and resection of the mesial root (b), a fibre-enforced pontic was directly placed (c), allowing splinting of teeth 46 and 45 (LR5). Long-term stability was achieved during supportive periodontal therapy over 11 years (d–f).

In general, there are growing data on cost-effectiveness, largely stemming from either cohort or modelling studies. Recording of efficiency data alongside randomized trials is not common at present and can be recommended. Cost–utility or cost–benefit analyses are even less common, mainly since the subjective value that patients place on single retained, replaced, or missing teeth is not known at present.

12.6   Conclusions

Given both the demographic changes in many rich countries as well as the epidemiological shift in older populations – who retain more teeth than ever before – retaining molars with FI is highly relevant from a public health and health economic perspective.

A range of study types has been employed in this field, mainly to describe the costs of retaining these molars, but also to compare the cost-effectiveness of different retention and replacement strategies. Based on these studies, retaining molars with FI might require more effort than retaining non-FI teeth. However, the resulting annual treatment costs are nevertheless very limited. The larger proportion of these costs is for periodontal, not other (restorative, endodontic, prosthetic) treatments. There are a number of factors which are associated with greater effort being needed, resulting in higher costs, like bone loss, severe FI, mobility, or status as prosthetic abutment. Dentists should consider these factors in treatment decisions. If comparing different strategies for managing molars with FI, tooth retention seems   probably   less   costly   than   tooth replacement via ISC. This is mainly because implant placement but also maintenance is relatively costly compared to costs for tooth retention.

In conclusion, dentists should not focus only on the reported success or survival rates of certain treatments (which are, for example, very high for implants). Instead, they should consider the long-term consequences and extent of possible retreatments, as well as their feasibility and costs. Retaining molars with FI is likely to be both achievable and cost-effective.

Summary of Evidence

- Teeth with furcation involvement (FI) can be retained in the long term, but at higher costs than teeth without FI.
- These costs increase with higher degrees of FI, bone loss, and mobility.
- However, removing and replacing teeth using implant-supported crowns does not seem to be less costly.
- Dentists should consider these risk factors and the required treatment needs for planning the retention or removal of teeth.

References

Antczak-Bouckoms, A.A., and Weinstein, M.C. (1987). Cost-effectiveness analysis of periodontal disease control. *Journal of Dental Research* 66, 1630–1635.

Blomlof, L., Jansson, L., Appelgren, R. et al. (1997). Prognosis and mortality of root-resected molars. *International Journal of Periodontics and Restorative Dentistry* 17, 190–201.

Carnevale, G., Di Febo, G., Tonelli, M.P. et al. (1991). A retrospective analysis of the periodontal-prosthetic treatment of molars with interradicular lesions. *International Journal of Periodontics and Restorative Dentistry* 11, 189–205.

Chambrone, L.A., and Chambrone, L. (2006). Tooth loss in well-maintained patients with chronic periodontitis during long-term supportive therapy in Brazil. *Journal of Clinical Periodontolpgy* 33, 759–764. doi:10.1111/j.1600-051X.2006.00972.x.

Checchi, L., Montevecchi, M., Gatto, M.R., and Trombelli, L. (2002). Retrospective study of tooth loss in 92 treated periodontal patients. *Journal of Clinical Periodontology* 29, 651–656.

Dannewitz, B., Krieger, J.K., Husing, J., and Eickholz, P. (2006a) Loss of molars in periodontally treated patients: A retrospective analysis five years or more after active periodontal treatment. *Journal of Clinical Periodontology* 33, 53–61. doi:10.1111/j.1600-051X.2005.00858.x.

Dannewitz, B., Krieger, J.K., Hüsing, J., and Eickholz, P. (2006b). Loss of molars in periodontally treated patients: A retrospective analysis five years or more after active periodontal treatment. *Journal of Clinical Periodontology* 33, 53–61. doi:10.1111/j.1600-051X.2005.00858.x.

Eickholz, P., Kaltschmitt, J., Berbig, J. et al. (2008). Tooth loss after active periodontal therapy. 1: Patient-related factors for risk, prognosis, and quality of outcome. *Journal of Clinical Periodontology* 35, 165–174. doi:10.1111/j.1600-051X.2007.01184.x.

Faggion, C.M., Jr, Giannakopoulos, N.N., and Listl, S. (2011). How strong is the evidence for the need to restore posterior bounded edentulous spaces in adults? Grading the quality of evidence and the strength of recommendations. *Journal of Dentistry* 39, 108–116. doi:10.1016/j.jdent.2010.11.002.

Fardal, O., and Grytten, J. (2013). A comparison of teeth and implants during maintenance therapy in terms of the number of disease-free years and costs: An in vivo internal control study. *Journal of Clinical Periodontology* 40, 645–651. doi:10.1111/jcpe.12101.

Fardal, O., Johannessen, A.C., and Linden, G.J. (2004). Tooth loss during maintenance following periodontal treatment in a periodontal practice in Norway. *Journal of Clinical Periodontology* 31, 550–555. doi:10.1111/j.1600-051X.2004.00519.x.

Fardal, O., and Linden, G.J. (2010). Long-term outcomes for cross-arch stabilizing bridges in periodontal maintenance patients: A retrospective study. *Journal of Clinical Periodontology* 37, 299–304. doi:10.1111/j.1600-051X.2009.01528.x.

Feres, M., Araujo, M.W., Figueiredo, L.C., and Oppermann, R.V. (2006). Clinical evaluation of tunneled molars: A retrospective study. *Journal of the International Academy of Periodontology* 8, 96–103.

Goodacre, C J., Bernal, G., Rungcharassaeng, K., and Kan, J.Y. (2003). Clinical complications in fixed prosthodontics. *Journal of Prosthetic Dentistry* 90, 31–41. doi:10.1016/s0022391303002142.

Graetz, C., Dörfer, C.E., Kahl, M. et al. (2011). Retention of questionable and hopeless teeth in compliant patients treated for aggressive periodontitis. *Journal of Clinical Periodontology* 38, 707°714. doi:10.1111/j.1600-051X.2011.01743.x.

Graetz, C., Schutzhold, S., Plaumann, A. et al. (2015). Prognostic factors for the loss of molars: An 18-years retrospective cohort study. *Journal of Clinical Periodontology* 42, 943–950. doi:10.1111/jcpe.12460.

Graetz, C., Schwendicke, F., Kahl, M. (2013). Prosthetic rehabilitation of patients with history of moderate to severe periodontitis: A long-term evaluation. *Journal of Clinical Periodontology* 40, 799–806. doi:10.1111/jcpe.12124.

Graetz, C., Sälzer, S., Plaumann, A., Schlattmann, P., Kahl, M., Springer, C., Dörfer, C., and Schwendicke, F. (2017a). Tooth loss in generalized aggressive periodontitis: Prognostic factors after 17 years of supportive periodontal treatment. *J Clin Periodontol* 44, 612–619. doi:10.1111/jcpe.12725.

Graetz, C., Plaumann, A., Schlattmann, P., Kahl, M., Springer, C., Sälzer, S., Gomer, K.,

Dörfer, C., and Schwendicke, F. (2017b). Long-term tooth retention in chronic periodontitis – results after 18 years of a conservative periodontal treatment regimen in a university setting. *J Clin Periodontol* 44, 169–177. doi:10.1111/jcpe.12680.

Hamp, S.E., Nyman, S., and Lindhe, J. (1975). Periodontal treatment of multirooted teeth: Results after 5 years. *Journal of Clinical Periodontology* 2, 126–135.

Hatch, J.P., Shinkai, R.S., Sakai, S. et al. (2001). Determinants of masticatory performance in dentate adults. *Archives of Oral Biology* 46, 641–648.

Heitz-Mayfield, L.J., Trombelli, L., Heitz, F. et al. (2002). A systematic review of the effect of surgical debridement vs non-surgical debridement for the treatment of chronic periodontitis. *Journal of Clinical Periodontology* 29 (Suppl. 3), 92–102; discussion 160–162.

Helldén, L.B., Elliot, A., Steffensen, B., and Steffensen, J.E. (1989). The prognosis of tunnel preparations in treatment of class III furcations: A follow-up study. *Journal of Periodontology* 60, 182–187. doi:10.1902/jop.1989.60.4.182.

Holtfreter, B., Kocher, T., Hoffmann, T. et al. (2010). Prevalence of periodontal disease and treatment demands based on a German dental survey (DMS IV). *Journal of Clinical Periodontology* 37, 211–219. doi:10.1111/j.1600-051X.2009.01517.x.

Huynh-Ba, G., Kuonen, P., Hofer, D. et al. (2009). The effect of periodontal therapy on the survival rate and incidence of complications of multirooted teeth with furcation involvement after an observation period of at least 5 years: A systematic review. *Journal of Clinical Periodontology* 36, 164–176. doi:10.1111/j.1600-051X.2008.01358.x.

Johansson, K.J., Johansson, C.S., and Ravald, N. (2013). The prevalence and alterations of furcation involvements 13 to 16 years after periodontal treatment. *Swedish Dental Journal* 37, 87–95.

Jordan, A.R., and Micheelis, W. (2016). Fünfte Deutsche Mundgesundheitsstudie (DMS V). Köln: Deutscher Ärzte-Verlag.

Kassebaum, N.J., Bernabe, E., Dahiya, M. et al. (2014). Global burden of severe periodontitis in 1990–2010: A systematic review and meta-regression. *Journal of Dental Research* 93, 1045–1053. doi:10.1177/0022034514552491.

Kocher, T., and Plagmann, H.C. (1999). Root debridement of molars with furcation involvement using diamond-coated sonic scaler inserts during flap surgery: A pilot study. *Journal of Clinical Periodontology* 26, 525–530.

König, J., Plagmann, H.C., Rühling, A., and Kocher, T. (2002). Tooth loss and pocket probing depths in compliant periodontally treated patients: A retrospective analysis. *Journal of Clinical Periodontology* 29, 1092–1100. doi:cpe291208 [pii].

Lee, K.L., Corbet, E.F., and Leung, W.K. (2012). Survival of molar teeth after resective periodontal therapy: A retrospective study. *Journal of Clinical Periodontology* 39, 850–860. doi:10.1111/j.1600-051X.2012.01918.x.

Little, L.A., Beck, F.M., Bagci, B., and Horton, J.E. (1995). Lack of furcal bone loss following the tunnelling procedure. *Journal of Clinical Periodontology* 22, 637–641.

Loesche, W.J., Giordano, J.R., Soehren, S., and Kaciroti, N. (2002). The nonsurgical treatment of patients with periodontal disease: Results after five years. *Journal of the American Dental Association* 133, 311–320.

Lulic, M., Bragger, U., Lang, N.P. et al. (2007). Ante's (1926) law revisited: A systematic review on survival rates and complications of fixed dental prostheses (FDPs) on severely reduced periodontal tissue support. *Clinical Oral Implants Research* 18 (Suppl. 3), 63–72. doi:10.1111/j.1600-0501.2007.01438.x.

Martin, J.A., Fardal, O., Page, R.C. et al. (2014). Incorporating severity and risk as factors to the Fardal cost-effectiveness model to create a cost-benefit model for periodontal treatment. *Journal of Periodontology* 85, e31–e39. doi:10.1902/jop.2013.130237.

Micheelis, W., and Schiffer, U. (2006). *Vierte Deutsche Mundgesundheitsstudie (DMS-IV)*. Köln: Deutscher Zahnärzte.

Miettinen, M., and Millar, B.J. (2013). A review of the success and failure characteristics of resin-bonded bridges. *British Dental Journal* 215, E3. doi:10.1038/sj.bdj.2013.686.

Miremadi, S.R., De Bruyn, H., Steyaert, H. et al. (2015). A randomized controlled trial comparing surgical and non-surgical periodontal therapy: A 3-year clinical and cost-effectiveness analysis. *Journal of Clinical Periodontology* 42, 740–747. doi:10.1111/jcpe.12434.

Mombelli, A., and Lang, N.P. (1998). The diagnosis and treatment of peri-implantitis. *Periodontology 2000* 17, 63–76.

Pretzl, B., Kaltschmitt, J., Kim, T.S. et al. (2008). Tooth loss after active periodontal therapy. 2: Tooth-related factors. *Journal of Clinical Periodontology* 35, 175–182. doi:10.1111/j.1600-051X.2007.01182.x.

Pretzl, B., Wiedemann, D., Cosgarea, R. et al. (2009). Effort and costs of tooth preservation in supportive periodontal treatment in a German population. *Journal of Clinical Periodontology* 36, 669–676. doi:10.1111/j.1600-051X.2009.01409.x.

Roos-Jansaker, A.M., Lindahl, C., Renvert, H., and Renvert, S. (2006). Nine- to fourteen-year follow-up of implant treatment. Part II: Presence of peri-implant lesions. *Journal of Clinical Periodontology* 33, 290–295. doi:10.1111/j.1600-051X.2006.00906.x.

Salvi, G.E., Mischler, D.C., Schmidlin, K. et al. (2014). Risk factors associated with the longevity of multi-rooted teeth: Long-term outcomes after active and supportive periodontal therapy. *Journal of Clinical Periodontology* 41, 701–707. doi:10.1111/jcpe.12266.

Schwendicke, F., Graetz, C., Stolpe, M., and Dorfer, C.E. (2014). Retaining or replacing molars with furcation involvement: A cost-effectiveness comparison of different strategies. *Journal of Clinical Periodontology* 41, 1090–1097. doi:10.1111/jcpe.12315.

Schwendicke, F., Plaumann, A., Stolpe, M. et al. (2016a). Retention costs of periodontally compromised molars in a German population. *Journal of Clinical Periodontology* 43, 261–270. doi:10.1111/jcpe.12509.

Schwendicke, F., Stolpe, M., Meyer-Lueckel, H. et al. (2013). Cost-effectiveness of one- and two-step incomplete and complete excavations. *Journal of Dental Research* 90, 880–887.

Schwendicke, F., Stolpe, M., Plaumann, A., and Graetz, C. (2016b). Cost-effectiveness of regular versus irregular supportive periodontal therapy or tooth removal. *Journal of Clinical Periodontology* 43, 940–947. doi:10.1111/jcpe.12595.

Vernazza, C., Heasman, P., Gaunt, F., and Pennington, M. (2012). How to measure the cost-effectiveness of periodontal treatments. *Periodontology* 2000 60, 138–146. doi:10.1111/j.1600-0757.2011.00406.x.

Walton, T.R. (2013). The up to 25-year survival and clinical performance of 2,340 high gold-based metal-ceramic single crowns. *International Journal of Prosthodontics* 26, 151–160. doi:10.11607/ijp.3136.

Wolfart, S., Marre, B., Wostmann, B. et al. (2012). The randomized shortened dental arch study: 5-year maintenance. *Journal of Dental Research* 91, 65 s–71 s. doi:10.1177/0022034 512447950.

Wolfart, S., Muller, F., Gerss, J. et al. (2014). The randomized shortened dental arch study: Oral health-related quality of life. *Clinical Oral Investigations* 18, 525–533. doi:10.1007/s00784-013-0991-6.

Yi, S.W., Ericsson, I., Carlsson, G.E., and Wennstrom, J.L. (1995). Long-term follow-up of cross-arch fixed partial dentures in patients with advanced periodontal destruction: Evaluation of the supporting tissues. *Acta Odontologica Scandinavica* 53, 242–248.

Zhong, H. (2010). On decomposing the inequality and inequity change in health care utilization: Change in means, or change in the distributions? *International Journal of Health Care Finance and Economics* 10, 369–386. doi:10.1007/s10754-010-9085-z.

Chapter 13

Deep Gaps between the Roots of the Molars: A Patient's Point of View

Luigi Nibali

Centre for Immunobiology and Regenerative Medicine, Centre for Oral Clinical Research, Institute of Dentistry, Barts and the London School of Medicine and Dentistry, Queen Mary University of London (QMUL), London, UK

13.1 Introduction

Dentistry is moving towards a more patient-centred approach, with more attention paid to the patient's point of view and striving to improve the patient's quality of life. Ultimately, as treating clinicians we should realize that reduction of probing pocket depths and bleeding on probing are just surrogate measures of disease progression and they do not necessarily mirror the patient's aims and needs. Furthermore, every patient is different and what works for one patient may not work for another. However, it is interesting to note how most studies in the periodontal literature have focused so much on clinical measurements, leaving aside aspects such as costs and effects on the patient's quality of life. Equally, previous chapters of this book have focused on clinical parameters, bone levels, and 'success' as defined by the treating periodontist, but not based on the patient's perceptions. This chapter aims to review studies focusing on patient quality-of-life measures relative to furcation involvement. Given the paucity of data on this, anecdotally the feedback from some patients treated for furcation involvement will be presented, in order to give the reader a perspective from people who are on the receiving end of the treatment discussed in this book.

13.2 Patient-reported Outcome Measures in Periodontology

Socio-environmental measures such as function and psychological well-being have been applied to dentistry in the last few decades (Locker 1988). These measures aim to assess parameters related to the impact of oral health which are not objectively measurable by the treating clinician. The World Health Organization (WHO) defines quality of life as individuals' perception of their position in life in the context of the culture and value systems in which they live and in relation to their goals, expectations, standards, and concerns (WHOQOL Group 1994). It is a broad-ranging concept affected in a complex way by the person's physical health, psychological state, level of independence, social relationships, personal beliefs, and relationship to salient features of their environment. The American Dental Association emphasized the importance of quality-of-life measures by stating: 'Oral health is a functional, structural, aesthetic, physiologic and psychosocial state of well-being and is essential to an individual's general health and quality of life' (Glick and Meyer 2014; Glick et al. 2017).

Over the last decade, patient-reported outcome measures (PROMs) have increasingly

Diagnosis and Treatment of Furcation-Involved Teeth, First Edition. Edited by Luigi Nibali.
© 2018 John Wiley & Sons Ltd. Published 2018 by John Wiley & Sons Ltd.
Companion website: www.wiley.com/go/nibali/diagnosis

been recognized as a research priority and incorporated in periodontal research studies (Aslund et al. 2008; Buset et al. 2016). PROMs are defined as standardized measures used to capture the subjective effect of a disease or treatment on a patient's life, including daily activities and well-being (US Department of Health and Human Services et al. 2009). Health-related quality of life (HRQoL) and oral health–related quality of life (OHRQoL) are often used as measures of PROMs in medicine and more specifically dentistry. While the related questionnaires provide data about health or disease status (structure/function/activity/participation), other questionnaires such as the Oral Impacts on Daily Performance (OIDP) and the Oral Health Impact Profile (OHIP-14) assess the impacts of oral diseases on daily life (disease prevention/dysfunction/failure) in a pre-determined period (Adulyanon et al. 1996; Slade 1997). These are generic OHRQoL measures, so they are not specifically designed for patients with periodontitis. In other words, they measure the oral impacts of oral conditions in general, not attributing them to particular diseases/conditions. However, they have been used in studies of periodontal patients with the underlying – but largely untested – assumption that in such a patient sample most of the reported oral impacts would be due to that specific oral condition; that is, a periodontal condition in this case. Among the generic OHRQoL measures, the OIDP allows also for a condition-specific version, whereby patients attribute the reported oral impacts to specific 'causes', in other words conditions. Furthermore, while most of these measures assess the frequency of oral impacts (i.e. how often they were experienced), the OIDP measures both the frequency and the severity of oral impacts. Despite their differences, all these questionnaires tend to focus on covering the physical, psychological, and social aspects of the oral impacts on daily life.

The relevant literature goes beyond the oral health field and extends to generic HRQoL measures. The EuroQol Questionnaire (EQ-5D-5L) is a measure of HRQoL including self-assessments of mobility, pain/discomfort, self-care, anxiety/depression, and usual activities, recorded by patients on an ordinary scale with five levels (Herdman et al. 2011). It is unclear whether the valuations would refer to periodontal disease or to any other condition coexisting in the same person (or their combination, for that matter). Using the EuroQol Questionnaire, a cross-sectional study on a random sample of 709 45- to 54-year-old Australians was able to differentiate the impacts of varying degrees of periodontal diseases (from gingivitis to periodontitis; Brennan et al. 2007). For example, having a pocket depth of $\geq 6\,mm$ was associated with a prevalence of pain/discomfort in 25.8% of cases, compared with 6.1% pain/discomfort for patients with gingivitis. In a separate study, when OHIP-14 and OIDP structured interviewer-administered questionnaires, global self-report, and perceived need for dental treatment questions were administered to 264 patients, the majority (61.0%) rated their oral health status poorly and 203 (76.9%) perceived a need for treatment, highlighting the importance of patient-driven treatment needs (Lawal et al. 2015).

A systematic review on the impact of periodontitis on OHRQoL suggested that, although most studies showed a negative impact of periodontitis, it is difficult to draw definitive conclusions due to the heterogeneity of methods and reporting and confounding by other oral conditions (Al-Harthi et al. 2013). A more recent systematic review found a relationship between clinical periodontal disease extent and severity and OHRQoL (Buset et al. 2016). No specific studies on furcation treatment were detected among those included in these reviews.

Some studies have attempted to investigate the effects of periodontal treatment on patient-centred outcomes. In a study on periodontitis patients in the UK, the OIDP index was administered to 45 patients at baseline and one month after treatment (Tsakos et al. 2010); 17 of the patients received intensive and 28 received 'conservative' periodontal care. Both the generic and condition-specific versions of the OIDP for periodontal conditions were used, and one of the aims of the study was to estimate the minimally important difference for this measure among periodontal patients. The mean OIDP score after treatment was significantly lower than at baseline, indicating improvements in quality of life, with no differences between treatment groups. In general, the generic and condition-specific versions of the OIDP performed similarly, but the differences were more distinct, with a higher effect size, when the condition-specific version was used. This provided evidence in favour of the condition-specific version, even in a population of patients with severe periodontitis where no such difference would be expected, as almost all oral impacts would be due to the periodontal condition (rather than any other oral condition). A difference of five points in the OIDP was estimated to correspond to clinically meaningful differences, thereby providing context for changes in OHRQoL when using this measure (Tsakos et al. 2010).

In a randomized controlled clinical trial, both the OIDP and OHRQoL questionnaires were given to 90 patients divided into two groups: scaling and root planing (SRP, n = 45) and one-stage 'full-mouth disinfection' (FMD, n = 45). All patients were then reassessed at two time points: 30 days and 180 days after treatment. Patients treated by both SRP and FMD showed improvement in all periodontal clinical parameters and OHRQoL after treatment, with no significant differences between treatment groups (Santuchi et al. 2016). In a study by Makino-Oi and co-workers (2016), improvements in OHRQoL (in the domains pain and eating/chewing function) mirrored clinical improvements after non-surgical and then surgical treatment of moderate to severe chronic periodontitis. A greater improvement was noted following surgical therapy, with no further improvements during maintenance care. A randomized controlled trial evaluating two educational programmes including

87 patients with chronic periodontitis assessed OHRQoL with two different generic measures: the General Oral Health Assessment Index (GOHAI), which assesses the presence of symptoms, and the UK oral health-related quality-of-life measure (OHQoL-UK), which assesses the impact of oral health using a conceptualization of health beyond the absence of disease. Improvements in OHRQoL for both the GOHAI and the OHQoL-UK were detected after non-surgical periodontal therapy in both study groups, without any significant difference between the two groups. This research also assessed the minimally important difference for these measures, again providing some context for the differences observed (Jonsson and Öhrn 2014). An earlier systematic review investigated the effect of surgical periodontal therapy on OHRQoL. At that time, only three studies qualified following full-text screening and the results were conflicting. Again, no specific assessment of furcation intervention was tested (Shanbhag et al. 2012).

13.3 Patient-reported Outcome Measures in Furcation Involvement

Helldén and co-workers (1989) presented clinical and patient-reported outcomes from a retrospective study on molars with furcation involvement treated with tunnel preparations. A total of 156 teeth among 107 patients had been treated surgically with tunnel preparations from 1977 to 1985. In 1986, all patients were asked to return for a re-evaluation, and 102 attended. All teeth involved were affected by degree III furcation involvement and were treated with tunnelling surgery. In particular, following elevation of full-thickness flaps, the furcations were widened by round burs at the entrance and then by bone files to create space for post-surgical inter-radicular plaque control, after which the flaps were apically positioned, sutured, and covered with surgical dressing.

After removal of the dressing, the patients were shown how to use interdental brushes inside the tunnelled area. The majority of the patients rinsed with 0.1% chlorhexidine for 4–6 weeks and at each post-surgical visit a fluoride varnish was applied to the teeth. Following three- to six-monthly maintenance visits for two years, the patients returned to their referring dentists for continued follow-up. On average, patients were re-examined 37.5 months after surgery. Before the clinical re-evaluation, the following five questions were asked of patients about their experience with the furcation-involved teeth (Helldén et al. 1989):

1) Do you have any discomfort from the tunnel area?
2) Does the gingiva bleed in the tunnel area?
3) Is the tooth sensitive to cold or warm temperatures?
4) Do you easily get access to the tunnel area for cleaning?
5) What kind of oral hygiene aids do you use in the tunnel areas?

At the end of the follow-up period, 10 of 102 teeth had been extracted and 7 had been hemisected or root resected, while 11 had developed incipient root caries and 12 teeth showed established caries lesions. Based on patient feedback, most cases were not associated with any discomfort (92%), gingival bleeding (72%), or sensitivity to cold or warm temperatures (95%). Most patients used a common toothbrush (98%) for the outer part of the tooth and an interdental brush for the tunnel areas (80%). Although plaque removal presented some difficulties, most such areas (70%) were found to be easily accessible for cleaning procedures by patients. The study by Helldén and co-workers represented a pioneering attempt to obtain information on subjective perceptions in patients affected by furcation involvement, although without a validated questionnaire. A systematic review on periodontal regeneration of furcation defects by the American Academy of Periodontology

recently reported that none of the reviewed studies had included any patient-reported outcomes. The authors highlighted the need to introduce this aspect in furcation research (Avila-Ortiz et al. 2015).

13.4   Patient Feedback

Given the paucity of data on PROMs relative to furcation involvement, some patients treated by the author were asked to provide feedback on their experience with furcation treatment. These are provided in this section.

Patient Feedback 1 (70-year-old Female, 10 Years After Tunnelling Surgery)

'I was made aware of the gap between the roots of my bottom right last tooth 10 years ago when I had a surgical procedure on it. Now I feel that, as I go through the process of cleaning my teeth, I automatically clean inside the roots and it doesn't feel any different than cleaning the other teeth. Occasionally I get some food stuck on that tooth. I come regularly to see the hygienist and periodontist and I am used to it now.'

Patient Feedback 2 (65-year-old Male, 12 Years After Tunnelling Surgeries)

'When I first saw a periodontist my mouth was in a poor state. Whenever I brushed my teeth my gums bled, and I was afraid of losing my teeth but I did not know how to make them better. At that stage I did not realize that bone loss caused by gum disease meant that the gaps between the furcations in the roots were hard or impossible to clean, and were providing a gathering place for bacteria causing the disease to continue and worsen. The periodontist performed a couple of operations to open up the gums to enable me to clean into these gaps, and showed me how to do the cleaning using little interdental brushes. From that time on I have been able to clean my teeth fully without any bleeding, and the disease has gone. I still lost some of my teeth; three of them have been replaced by implants, and these together with what remains of my natural teeth are sufficient for me to eat effectively. I have always dreaded the idea of having dentures, which seemed inevitable, but more than 12 years later I am keeping the disease and decay at bay and I remain hopeful of avoiding dentures for the foreseeable future.'

Patient Feedback 3 (60-year-old Male, 10 Years After Tunnelling Surgery)

'Having undergone surgery to my right upper teeth to combat gum disease some years ago I am very fortunate to say that after several years I am being able to maintain a reasonable level of health in this area. Following the surgery I took the view that I would work hard to maintain the situation and by diligence have, it seems, managed to do so. I have a cleansing regime that I adhere to rigidly and includes both morning and night a process which takes me approximately 15 minutes each time. And includes cleansing with an interdental brush, flossing, cleansing with 'sensitive' toothpaste and good quality electric brush and more work with the interdental brush to finish off. At times when the mouth is sensitive I brush with a specific gel. Although this takes some time and I have to exercise some personal discipline I believe it is time well spent and will do anything to prevent the loss of further teeth. The health of my mouth in general has also improved greatly. I also believe that my general health has improved as a result of this improvement in my oral health. I am very grateful that through this regular

care and this regime I have managed to extend the life of these teeth. May this continue!'

Patient Feedback 4 (50-year-old Male, 6 Years After Tunnelling Surgery on One Molar and Extraction and Implant Placement on the Contralateral Molar)

'Following treatment by my dentist whereby I had a tooth extraction on my right lower jaw and surgery to keep a tooth on my left lower jaw. With reference to my right jaw and tooth extraction I allowed the bone in that area of extraction to grow back before having an implant to secure and strengthen the teeth in that area. The additional surgery I had on my left jaw meant that my tooth was saved. My dentist inserted a small piece of tube between the two roots to enable the cleaning of the tooth and root area. All I do now on a daily basis is clean in between my teeth and roots using interdental brushes which is totally pain free and easy to do.'

Patient Feedback 5 (45-year-old Female, 10 Years After Root-resection Surgery)

'Soon after I was referred to the periodontist for treatment for my gums, a very fact-facing appointment, back tooth removed and three operations to clean the roots and I started to realize that there was a serious chance that I would lose some if not all my teeth, if I did not make a change. I then started on an ongoing treatment plan of seeing the periodontist every six months and the hygienist every alternative six months, but at this point I was still smoking. I was eventually able to give up smoking. Treatment is ongoing, I still have most of my teeth and I plan to keep them. I wish there was a once and for all cure, but am resigned to having ongoing maintenance treatment.'

Patient Feedback 6 (63-year-old Male, 5 Years After Molar Extraction and Implant Placement)

'Given my experience as a dental patient, I consider myself an expert. I've had caries, gum disease and extractions, followed by crowns and bridges. I work very hard at my dental hygiene, but I recognize I could probably do better. Over the years I've had problems around my crowns and bridges on my back teeth, both aesthetic concerns and several flare-ups with inflammation and discomfort. I think that this is because plaque gets stuck under the crown and bridgework. Some years ago, one of my molars was finally extracted and replaced with an implant. I've had to wait a few months after the extraction to finally have a crown on the implant, but I understand that is normal procedure. I feel the implant like a normal tooth, like it's always been there and I've no longer had any discomfort or inflammation'.

13.5 Reflections on Patient Feedback

While accepting that this is by no means a representative patient sample and that reporting feedback for the treating clinician may be seen as a biased exercise, several important items emerged from this feedback. It is clear that these patients were highly motivated and made a long-term commitment to the survival of their teeth. They effectively decided to change their dental health behaviour, including giving up smoking ('I eventually gave up smoking') and working hard on their oral hygiene ('I have a cleansing regime that I adhere to rigidly and includes both morning and night a process which takes me approximately 15 minutes each time'). In some cases this did not appear to be a burden on the patient ('All I do now on a daily basis is clean in between my teeth and roots using interdental brushes which is totally pain free and easy to do'), while in other cases it did ('am resigned to having ongoing maintenance treatment').

The specific act of cleaning inside a tunnelled furcation area was described as a relatively easy task by these patients ('I automatically clean inside the roots and it doesn't feel any different than cleaning the other teeth').

The patients' perception of the treatment carried out is also very interesting, ranging from what seems like a good understanding of the surgical tunnelling procedure ('the gaps between the furcations in the roots were hard or impossible to clean, and were providing a gathering place for bacteria causing the disease to continue and worsen. The periodontist performed a couple of operations to open up the gums to enable me to clean into these gaps') to a rather more imaginative interpretation ('My dentist inserted a small piece of tube between the two roots to enable the cleaning of the tooth and root area'). The experience of having a dental implant to replace a molar previously affected by severe periodontal disease was also seen as very positive ('I've had problems around my crowns and bridges on my back teeth, both aesthetic concerns and several flare-ups with inflammation and discomfort. … one of my molars was finally extracted and replaced with an implant. … I feel the implant like a normal tooth, like it's always been there and I've no longer had any discomfort or inflammation').

13.6 Implementation of PROMs in Furcation Treatment

Given the increased recognition of the importance of patient-reported outcomes in medicine, the future should see the use of OHRQoL measures in studies investigating furcation treatment. The pioneering effort by Helldén and co-workers (1989, see earlier discussion) to investigate patient perceptions should be extended by using validated OHRQoL measures, and potentially by developing a condition-specific validated questionnaire which also takes into account items such as sensitivity, ease of cleaning inside the furcation area, and the alternatives of extraction with or without replacement. The development of such a condition-specific measure would need to be driven by qualitative research highlighting the main concerns of patients with furcation involvement.

More importantly, it would be ideal to use PROMs as outcomes in long-term randomized controlled trials testing different modalities of furcation treatment (for example conservative treatment vs root resection vs extraction and implant therapy). This could provide answers on the effects of these procedures on patients' quality of life and, together with clinical and financial considerations, could help design furcation treatment guidelines. In the everyday clinical reality, an assessment of patient perceptions related to periodontal treatment needs to accompany purely clinical and financial considerations. This could be considered in the treatment planning stages as well as being an outcome measure to assess the effectiveness of interventions.

Acknowledgements

The invaluable help and advice of Dr George Tsakos, University College London, in the preparation and revision of this chapter is gratefully acknowledged.

Summary of Evidence

- The attention to patients' preferences and points of view needs to take centre stage in treatment planning. As such, patient-reported outcome measures (PROMs) are fast becoming essential outcomes of any periodontal research study.
- There is a paucity of data on PROMs in patients with furcation involvement.
- Investigation of PROMs relative to furcation involvement should, together with clinical and financial considerations, form the basis of furcation treatment planning.

References

Adulyanon, S., Vourapukjaru, J., and Sheiham, A. (1996). Oral impacts affecting daily performance in a low dental disease Thai population. *Community Dentistry and Oral Epidemiology* 24, 385–389.

Al-Harthi, L.S., Cullinan, M.P., Leichter, J.W., and Thomson, W.M. (2013). The impact of periodontitis on oral health-related quality of life: A review of the evidence from observational studies. *Australian Dental Journal* 58, 274–277.

Aslund, M., Suvan, J., Moles, D.R. et al. (2008). Effects of two different methods of non-surgical periodontal therapy on patient perception of pain and quality of life: A randomized controlled clinical trial. *Journal of Periodontology* 79,1031–1040.

Avila-Ortiz, G., De Buitrago, J.G., and Reddy, M.S. (2015). Periodontal regeneration – furcation defects: A systematic review from the AAP Regeneration Workshop. *Journal of Periodontology* 86 (Suppl. 2), S108–S130.

Brennan, D.S., Spencer, A.J., and Roberts-Thomson, K.F. (2007). Quality of life and disability weights associated with periodontal disease. *Journal of Dental Research* 86, 713–717.

Buset, S.L., Walter, C., Friedmann, A. et al. (2016). Are periodontal diseases really silent? A systematic review of their effect on quality of life. *Journal of Clinical Periodontology* 43, 333–344.

Glick, M., and Meyer, D.M. (2014). Defining oral health: A prerequisite for any health policy. *Journal of the American Dental Association* 145, 519–520.

Glick, M., Williams, D.M., Kleinman, D.V. et al. (2017). Reprint of: A new definition for oral health supported by FDI opens the door to a universal definition of oral health. *Journal of Dentistry* 57, 1–3.

Helldén, L.B., Elliot, A., Steffensen, B., and Steffensen, J.E.M. (1989). Prognosis of tunnel preparations in treatment of class III furcations: A follow-up study. *Journal of Periodontology* 60, 182–187.

Herdman, M., Gudex, C., Lloyd, A. et al. (2011). Development and preliminary testing of the new five-level version of EQ-5D (EQ-5D-5L). *Quality of Life Research* 20, 1727–1736.

Jönsson, B., and Öhrn, K. (2014). Evaluation of the effect of non-surgical periodontal treatment on oral health-related quality of life: Estimation of minimal important differences 1 year after treatment. *Journal of Clinical Periodontology* 41, 275–282.

Lawal, F.B., Taiwo, J.O., and Arowojolu, M.O. (2015). Comparison of two oral health-related quality of life measures among adult dental patients. *Oral Health and Preventative Dentistry* 13, 65–74.

Locker, D. (1988). Measuring oral health: A conceptual framework. *Community Dental Health* 5, 3–18.

Makino-Oi, A., Ishii, Y., Hoshino, T. et al. (2016). Effect of periodontal surgery on oral health-related quality of life in patients who have completed initial periodontal therapy. *Journal of Periodontal Research* 51, 212–220.

Santuchi, C.C., Cortelli, J.R., Cortelli, S.C. et al. (2016). Scaling and root planing per quadrant versus one-stage full-mouth disinfection: Assessment of the impact of chronic periodontitis treatment on quality of life – a clinical randomized, controlled trial. *Journal of Periodontology* 87, 114–123.

Shanbhag, S., Dahiya, M., and Croucher, R. (2012). The impact of periodontal therapy on oral health-related quality of life in adults: A systematic review. *Journal of Clinical Periodontology* 39, 725–735.

Slade, G.D. (1997) Derivation and validation of a short-form oral health impact profile. *Community Dentistry and Oral Epidemiology* 25, 284–290.

Tsakos, G., Bernabé, E., D'Aiuto, F. et al. (2010). Assessing the minimally important difference in the oral impact on daily performances index in patients treated for periodontitis. *Journal of Clinical Periodontology* 37, 903–909.

U.S. Department of Health and Human Services, Food and Drug Administration, Center for Drug Evaluation and Research (CDER) et al. (2009). *Guidance for industry: Patient-reported outcome measures: Use in medical product development to support label claims*. Rockville, MD: FDA.

WHOQOL Group (1994). Development of the WHOQOL: Rationale and current status. *International Journal of Mental Health* 23, 24–56.

Chapter 14

Assessment of Two Example Cases Based on a Review of the Literature

Luigi Nibali

Centre for Immunobiology and Regenerative Medicine, Centre for Oral Clinical Research, Institute of Dentistry, Barts and the London School of Medicine and Dentistry, Queen Mary University of London (QMUL), London, UK

In an attempt to apply the knowledge gained throughout this book to the treatment of cases with furcation involvement, two example cases are presented. They will be discussed in light of the evidence gained in each of the previous 13 chapters.

14.1 Case 1 (Maxillary)

A 50-year-old male patient presented with a complaint of bleeding on brushing and gum recessions. He was medically healthy, never smoked, and was not aware of any family history of periodontal disease. His oral hygiene was good, with full mouth plaque scores < 10%; he had generalized gingival recessions and localized probing pocket depths (PPD) > 4 mm only on upper molars. The case will be dissected based on the evidence provided in each of the previous chapters before reaching a treatment planning decision.

14.1.1 Anatomy (Chapter 1)

The maxillary first and second right and left molars in Figure 14.1 present a relatively 'normal' anatomy, with three roots each, all apparently distally curved to varying degrees. The root trunks appear reasonably small, in favour of longer root cones. High root divergence appears on teeth 16 (UR6) and 26 (UL6), while the roots of 17 (UR7) and 27 (UL7) are less divergent. Among predisposing factors described in Chapter 1, bifurcation ridges, enamel projections, and enamel pearls do not seem to be present.

14.1.2 Diagnosis (Chapter 2)

Although two-dimensional radiographic examination is not completely reliable for furcation diagnosis, the areas of radiolucency between roots, coupled with interproximal bone levels apical to the furcation entrances, indicate a likely *triple through-and-through furcation involvement (FI) for teeth 16, 17, and 27*. Doubts exist about possible FI on tooth 26. Clinical examination with a curved Nabers probe confirms this, with a diagnosis of triple (buccal, mesial, and distal) degree III FI on teeth 16, 17, and 27 (Hamp et al. 1975). The same diagnosis would be given when using the Glickman (1953) classification and the classification modified by Ammons and Harrington (2006; see Table 2.4). Degree I FI was recorded only distal of 26. Vertical subclassification (Tarnow and Fletcher 1984) is reported in Table 14.1. The comprehensive diagnosis system in the table summarizes clinical and radiographic findings on example tooth 16.

Diagnosis and Treatment of Furcation-Involved Teeth, First Edition. Edited by Luigi Nibali.
© 2018 John Wiley & Sons Ltd. Published 2018 by John Wiley & Sons Ltd.
Companion website: www.wiley.com/go/nibali/diagnosis

(a)

(b)

(c)

(d)

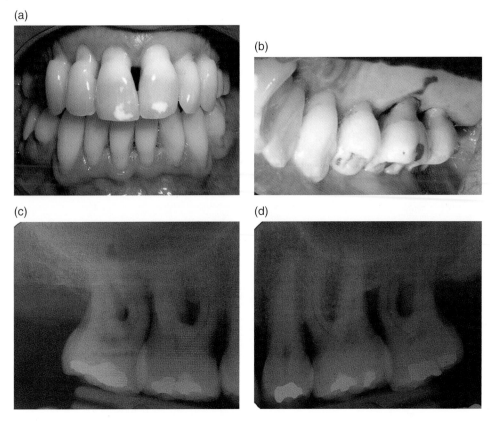

Figure 14.1 Case 1, clinical photograph of frontal (a) and upper right palatal (b), followed by baseline periapical radiographs of upper molars (c and d), the only teeth with probing pocket depth > 4 mm at first visit.

14.1.3 Initial Therapy (Chapter 3)

Most furcation areas, including probably those in this case, have narrow entrances (<0.75 mm). *Ultrasonic scalers, especially with slimline tips, have been shown to be better suited than hand instruments for the debridement of narrow furcation areas* (Matia et al. 1986; Sugaya et al. 2002), particularly in degree II and III FI (Leon and Vogel 1987). *Micro Mini Five® Gracey curettes could also be helpful in narrow furcation entrances* (see Chapter 3 for details). However, interproximal FI is likely to respond less favourably to mechanical debridement compared to buccal furcations (Del Peloso Ribeiro et al. 2007) and more residual calculus will be left with a closed (non-surgical) approach compared to an open approach (Matia et al. 1986; Fleischer et al. 1989). Although this patient exhibits very good oral

hygiene levels, it is crucial that *further oral hygiene reinforcements are given as part of initial periodontal therapy.* Research shows that in interproximal sites, bristled or rubber interdental brushes remove more plaque than flossing or brushing alone (Christou et al. 1998; Abouassi et al. 2014). Therefore, the use of interdental brushes of the correct size and shape in the molar region should be encouraged and discussed with the patient.

14.1.4 Endodontics (Chapter 4)

Although all four maxillary molars have restorations, they are not large enough to endanger the endodontic status of the teeth. However, accessory canals in the furcation region are frequent and might represent a communication pathway between endodontic and periodontal pathologies through

Table 14.1 Case 1, diagnosis of furcation on 16 based on Muller and Eger (1999).

Patient PL (age 50)				Tooth 16	
Mobility (0, 1, 2, 3)				0	
Elongation (0, 1)				0	
Sensibility testing (1: positive, 2: negative)				1	
Endodontic dx (0: OK, 1: revision necessary)				0	
Caries/restorations (0: caries free, 1: small caries or filling, 2: extended caries, large filling, 3: artificial crown)				1	

Rx diagnosis	Mesial root		Distal root		Palatal root	
	M	D	M	D	M	D
Bone loss	2	2	2	2	1	1
	m/d roots	m/p roots	d/p roots			
Separation degree	1	1	1			
Degree of divergence	1	1	1			

Clinical diagnosis						
	mb	b	db	mp	p	dp
BOP (0,1)	1	0	1	1	0	0
Plaque (0,1)	0	0	0	0	0	1
PPD	6	6	6	6	3	7
vCAL	7	7	8	9	6	9
hCAL	–	6	–	6	–	6
Degree	–	III B	–	III B	–	III C

Bone loss: 0 (≤ ⅓ root length), 1 (⅓–⅔ root length), 2 (≥ ⅔ root length); separation degree: 0 (< ⅓), 1 (> ⅓); degree of divergence: 0 (≤30°), 1(>30°).
B = buccal; BOP = bleeding on probing; CAL = clinical attachment loss; D = distal; h = horizontal; M = mesial; P = palatal; PPD = probing pocket depth; v = vertical.

the induction of inflammatory responses. Furthermore, a small radiolucency area seems to be present on 17 (palatal root). Therefore, it is always advisable to test tooth vitality. *Vitality testing was positive for all tested molars (16, 17, 26, and 27).* Hence no endodontic treatment was required, but retesting during treatment and maintenance therapy was recommended.

14.1.5 Long-term Prognosis (Chapter 5)

Molars with FI have a higher risk of tooth loss than molars with no FI (twice as likely to be lost up to 15 years of follow-up), following comprehensive periodontal treatment (non-surgical and surgical). For degree III FI, the relative risk of tooth loss is approximately three times that of degree I FI molars and twice compared with degree II FI molars (Nibali et al. 2016). In a follow-up maintenance programme varying from 5 to 53 years, 30% of degree III FI molars are lost (Nibali et al. 2016). Meta-analyses providing specific data for maxillary degree III FI molars, or specifically for first or second molars, are lacking. *Based on these data, it may be considered worth trying to maintain this tooth.* Treatment options need to be assessed in the following sections. *A strict post-treatment maintenance programme including three- to four-monthly periodontal charting, supra- and subgingival debridement, and oral hygiene reinforcement and motivation is recommended* based on the available literature (Nibali et al. 2016).

14.1.6 Regeneration (Chapters 6 and 7)

The first aim of periodontal treatment, where possible, should be to regenerate the lost periodontal support. However, despite some successful reports of regeneration of degree III FI molars in animal models (Chapter 6), human studies do not support the use of regeneration in maxillary degree III FI molars (Chapter 7). In particular, one randomized controlled trial with split-mouth design with 11 patients compared guided tissue regeneration (GTR) and open-flap debridement (OFD) in the treatment of maxillary interproximal degree III furcation defects (Pontoriero and Lindhe 1995). Baseline and six-month examinations were performed by re-entry after flap elevation. Neither GTR nor OFD led to even partial closure of the 22 degree III furcations. Based on these data, *these teeth are not suitable for regenerative treatment of their FI.*

14.1.7 Resective Therapy (Chapter 8)

Common sense would suggest that if you cannot close the furcation by regeneration, at least you should eliminate it surgically or make it cleansable. The options of root separation, root amputation, and root resection could be considered in a case of advanced FI, as for the molars in this case. However, these options are more suitable when, for example, one root is affected to a greater extent than the others. Furthermore, particular caution should be taken when the teeth are intact, because this is an invasive procedure involving a considerable biological cost that must always be carefully evaluated. For this reason, in this case, *inadequate residual attachment on the remaining roots and tooth vitality*

do not make root resection the preferred treatment option for teeth 16, 17, and 27.

14.1.8 Tunnelling (Chapter 9)

The furcation tunnelling procedure should be considered at stable (no more than mobility grade I) furcation-involved molars with advanced inter-radicular bone loss (preferably degree III FI) when accessibility to the furcation area for plaque removal is difficult. As a rule of thumb, the alveolar bone support should be of equal amounts at all roots and at least cover one-third of the root length, with *mainly horizontal bone loss.* The length of the root trunk should not exceed 4 mm and the diameter of the furcation entrance should be at least 0.5 mm. Fulfilment of these criteria for teeth 17, 16, and 27, this patient's full cooperation, *good oral hygiene dexterity and attitude, and a relatively low caries risk make tunnelling surgery an attractive treatment option in this case.* However, we should bear in mind that very few reports of long-term success of triple maxillary tunnels exist in the literature (Helldén et al. 1989).

14.1.9 Innovative and Adjunctive Therapy (Chapter 10)

In order to maximize the efficacy of non-surgical therapy of FI on the molars presented here, adjunctive systems such as an endoscope, lasers, photodynamic therapy, air-polishing devices, antimicrobials, or probiotics could be considered. However, this should be carefully weighed in the light of *costs and the so far poor evidence for their efficacy specific to furcations* (de Andrade et al. 2008; Ribeiro Edel et al. 2010; Tomasi and Wennstrom 2011; Eickholz et al. 2016).

14.1.10 Extraction and Implant Placement (Chapter 11)

Given the extensive loss of periodontal support and FI and the perceived low predictability of furcation treatment, teeth 17, 16, and

27 could be considered hopeless by some treating clinicians based on published prognostic systems (Becker et al. 1984; Machtei et al. 1989). If a decision was made to extract them, the options of a shortened dental arch, partial dentures, or implants could be considered. Bearing in mind the high long-term survival rates of implant-supported restorations (Moraschini et al. 2015) and the relatively young age and motivation of the patient, implant placement was discussed as his main alternative option to tooth retention. However, as discussed in Chapter 11, *reduced quantity of bone, proximity to maxillary sinus, need for grafting, and previous history of periodontitis may result in reduced implant-survival rates in this case* (Becker et al. 1999; Drago 1992; Graziani et al. 2004; Pjetursson et al. 2008). The option of extraction, socket preservation, and short implants could also be considered, provided enough residual bone was available to allow implant placement (Thoma et al. 2015).

14.1.11   Health Economics (Chapter 12)

A handful of studies have now shown that *treating molars with degree III FI via tooth-retaining options was more effective and less costly than tooth removal and replacement via implant-supported restorations* (Fardal and Grytten 2013; Martin et al. 2014; Schwendicke et al. 2014). Among possible treatment options, considering that all molars are still vital, it remains uncertain whether the high costs for root-resective therapy could be truly justified (Little et al. 1995; Blomlof et al. 1997; see Chapter 12 for more details).

14.1.12   Patient's Point of View (Chapter 13)

In the absence of data on patient-reported outcomes on treatment of degree III FI, some suggestions could be drawn from the paper on tunnelling discussed in Chapter 13 (Helldén et al. 1989). Most cases treated with tunnelling were not associated with any discomfort, gingival bleeding, or sensitivity. Although plaque removal presented some difficulties, most furcation areas were found to be easily accessible for cleaning procedures by patients with interdental brushes. In this specific case, *the patient expressed his wish to maintain these teeth for as long as possible, and he showed very good oral hygiene and commitment.*

14.1.13   Treatment Decision

Based on all these considerations, backed when possible by data from the literature, it was decided to maintain the molars affected by FI and to carry out non-surgical debridement and oral hygiene reinforcement. Following re-evaluation two months later, residual pockets and FI were detected on the affected molars and it was decided to proceed with tunnelling surgeries for 16, 17, and 27, followed by strict supportive periodontal therapy (see Chapter 9 for a step-by-step guide on the furcation tunnelling surgical technique). Post-operative photos and radiographs are presented in Chapter 15 (Figure 15.8). The main reasons for this choice are summarised in Table 14.2).

Table 14.2 Case 1, main reasons for treatment choice (tunnelling surgery).

	Factors
TOOTH	Good root divergence
	Short root trunk
	Prevalently horizontal bone loss affecting all roots
	Tooth vitality and no restorative concerns
	Importance in masticatory function
PATIENT	Clear medical history
	Non-smoker
	Motivation to keep teeth
	No financial or other concerns for surgical treatment
	Good oral hygiene dexterity

14.2 Case 2 (Mandibular)

A 47-year-old male patient presented with a complaint of occasional bleeding on brushing and discomfort from the lower left gingivae. He was medically healthy, he used to smoke (10 a day for 20 years, and gave up 10 years before the first examination), and was not aware of any family history of periodontal disease. His oral hygiene was fair, with full mouth plaque scores of 40% (generalized interproximal plaque), localized gingival recessions, and localized probing pocket depths > 4 mm only on the lower left first molar (LL6). The case will be dissected based on the evidence provided in each of the previous chapters before reaching a treatment planning decision.

14.2.1 Anatomy (Chapter 1)

The mandibular left first molar (LL6) in Figure 14.2 presents a relatively 'normal' anatomy, with two roots (mesial and distal). The mesial root is slightly distally tilted towards the apex. The root trunks and root cones appear to be of average length and root divergence seems normal. Among the predisposing factors described in Chapter 1, bifurcation ridges, enamel projections, and enamel pearls do not seem to be present.

14.2.2 Diagnosis (Chapter 2)

Although two-dimensional radiographic examination is not completely reliable for furcation diagnosis, the area of radiolucency between mesial and distal roots, coupled with distal interproximal bone levels apical to the furcation entrances, suggests a *likely through-and-through furcation involvement (FI)*. However, clinical examination with a curved Nabers probe only resulted in degree II buccal and lingual FI (Hamp et al. 1975) and a possible degree III when using the Glickman (1953) classification and the classification modified by Ammons and Harrington (2006; see Table 2.4). Probing pocket depths are reported in Table 14.3.

Table 14.3 Case 2, evaluation.

Tooth 36 (LL6)	v-PPD	CAL	h-PPD
Mesio-buccal	2	2	–
Buccal	8	10	5
Disto-buccal	12	15	–
Mesio-lingual	3	3	–
Lingual	7	7	4
Disto-lingual	10	11	–

CAL = clinical attachment loss; h-PPD = horizontal probing pocket depth; v-PPD = vertical probing pocket depth.

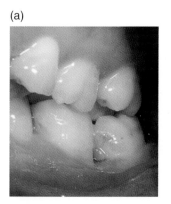 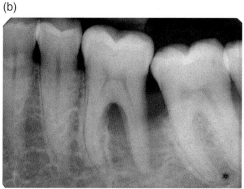

Figure 14.2 Case 2, clinical photograph (a) of left mandibular first molar, followed by baseline periapical radiograph (b).

On vertical probing, degree C FI was diagnosed (exceeding 6 mm in both buccal and lingual furcations; Tarnow and Fletcher 1984). Therefore, a degree II C diagnosis was given to both furcations, but with doubt on possible degree III through-and-through. It is important to note that the furcation defect is combined with a very deep distal intrabony defect, reaching the apex of the distal root, with some reduced bone support also on the mesial aspect of neighbouring tooth 37 (LL7).

In this case, due to the difficulty in probing the furcation, it may be worth considering a three-dimensional radiograph to ascertain the presence of residual alveolar bone by the furcation fornex for treatment planning purposes.

14.2.3 Initial Therapy (Chapter 3)

As discussed for Case 1, due to narrow furcation entrances *ultrasonic scalers with slimline tips, possibly complemented by Micro Mini Five® Gracey curettes*, are particularly suited for the debridement of FI. It is likely that residual calculus might be left with a closed (non-surgical) approach compared to the open approach (Matia et al. 1986; Fleischer et al. 1989), although probably not as much as in interproximal furcations. Particular attention needs to be paid to the difficult-to-reach concavity around the furcation fornix. An improvement in oral hygiene levels is necessary for this patient, with the introduction of *large interdental brushes* for cleaning the interproximal area between LL6 and LL7.

14.2.4 Endodontics (Chapter 4)

Although the tooth is non-restored, due to extensive FI and a distal intrabony defect reaching the apex, a neuro-vascular bundle damage may have occurred (Langeland et al. 1974). Therefore, it is advisable to test tooth vitality. *Vitality testing was positive for 36.* Some authors have even advocated that since

pulp necrosis might occur during periodontal healing, root canal treatment could be preventively performed to avoid any interference with the regeneration process in case of periodontal bone loss to the apex (Cortellini and Tonetti 2001). However, this was not considered necessary in this case. Instead, retesting of vitality after treatment was planned.

14.2.5 Long-term Prognosis (Chapter 5)

According to the evidence discussed in Chapter 5, following comprehensive periodontal treatment, as a furcation-involved molar this tooth has a higher risk of tooth loss than a molar with no FI (twice as likely to be lost up to 15 years of follow-up). According to a recent systematic review (Nibali et al. 2016), 18% of degree II FI molars are lost in a follow-up maintenance programme varying from 5 to 53 years, and this tooth's relative risk of needing extraction is 1.67 compared with degree I FI molars. The risk could actually be higher for this tooth, affected at least by double degree II FI and possibly by degree III FI. *Based on these data, it may be worth trying to maintain this tooth.* Treatment options need to be assessed, as in the following sections. *A strict post-treatment maintenance programme including three- to four-monthly periodontal charting, supra- and subgingival debridement, and oral hygiene reinforcement and motivation are recommended* based on the available literature (Nibali et al. 2016).

14.2.6 Regeneration (Chapters 6 and 7)

Tooth 36 seems to be affected by degree II FI, although a degree III FI cannot be ruled out. Despite some successful reports of regeneration of degree III furcation-involved molars in animal models, according to the literature reviewed in Chapter 7, human studies do not support the use of regeneration in maxillary degree III FI molars. However, *in case of mandibular FI II, the chances are good of achieving at least a partial fill of the furcation defect*, converting the degree II to a degree I FI. Treatment with either guided tissue regeneration (GTR) or enamel matrix derivative (EMD) has produced histological evidence of regeneration (Stoller et al. 2001; Nevins et al. 2003) and consistently more favourable clinical outcomes (reduction to degree I or closure) compared with access flaps in degree II mandibular furcations (Jepsen et al. 2002, 2004). The high bone support on the mesial root of 36 (above the furcation fornix) as well as on the mesial root of the adjacent 37 (next to the distal intrabony defect of 36) would have a beneficial impact on the regeneration potential, provided that good soft-tissue closure of the defect could be achieved post-operatively. Therefore, if degree II FI was confirmed intra-surgically, according to the evidence reviewed in Chapter 7, this molar appears to be suitable to benefit from regenerative furcation therapy, although, due to the bilateral degree II FI (in the best-case scenario), the results of regenerative therapy might be less predictable than in a single degree II FI.

14.2.7 Resective Therapy (Chapter 8)

The options of root separation, root amputation, and root resection could be considered in cases of advanced FI, like this one. *The options of root amputation* (removing the distal root and leaving the crown intact) *or root resection* (removing the distal root and the relative section of the crown) *are particularly suitable when one root is affected to a greater extent than the others*, which is the case for the tooth in question. Although the distal root has a significantly smaller root surface area than the mesial one (Dunlap and Gher 1985), the mesial root has a deep concavity, which makes it more difficult to endodontically treat and properly prepare and restore. The reported long-term survival of root-resected molars is in the 60–90% range for studies up to 10 years (Langer et al. 1981; Carnevale et al. 1998; reviewed in Chapter 8).

However, caution should be employed, as the tooth presented here is not restored, hence a root-resection procedure would involve a considerable biological cost.

14.2.8 Tunnelling (Chapter 9)

As seen for Case 1, the furcation tunnelling procedure should be considered for furcation-involved molars with advanced interradicular bone loss (preferably FI degree III) when accessibility to the furcation area for plaque removal is difficult. Indications for tunnelling are mainly good oral hygiene dexterity and motivation, and horizontal bone loss covering at least one-third of the root length. Therefore, this case does not seem suitable for tunnelling surgery.

14.2.9 Innovative and Adjunctive Therapy (Chapter 10)

As discussed for Case 1, adjunctive therapy to non-surgical periodontal treatment could be considered, but should be carefully balanced with *costs and the so far poor evidence for their efficacy specific to furcations* (de Andrade et al. 2008; Ribeiro Edel et al. 2010; Tomasi and Wennstrom 2011; Eickholz et al. 2016).

14.2.10 Extraction and Implant Placement (Chapter 11)

Given the extensive loss of periodontal support to the apex and FI, tooth 36 might be considered hopeless based on published prognostic systems (Becker et al. 1984; Machtei et al. 1989; Cortellini et al. 2011). *Reduced bone quantity on the distal aspect of the tooth may mean that there might be need for bone grafting after extraction; a previous history of periodontitis might result in a reduced implant-survival rate in this case* (Drago 1992; Becker et al. 1999; Graziani et al. 2004; Pjetursson et al. 2008). However, it is not inconceivable to think that, instead of distal root resection, extraction of the tooth and replacement could be an option here.

14.2.11 Health Economics (Chapter 12)

As discussed earlier, studies have now shown that *treating molars with degree II and III FI via tooth-retaining options was more effective and less costly than tooth removal and replacement via implant-supported restorations* (Fardal and Grytten 2013; Martin et al. 2014; Schwendicke et al. 2014). However, this may not apply if the more invasive and expensive options of root resection, endodontic therapy, and restoration are chosen for tooth retention (Little et al. 1995; Blomlof et al. 1997).

14.2.12 Patient's Point of View (Chapter 13)

In the absence of data on patient-reported outcomes on treatment of furcation-involved molars (in particular degree II, as in this case), patient preferences are very important. In this specific case, *the patient was very keen to maintain 36 for as long as possible.*

14.2.13 Treatment Decision

Based on all these considerations, backed when possible by data from the literature, it was decided to maintain 36 and to carry out non-surgical debridement and oral hygiene instructions. Following re-evaluation two months later, residual pockets, bleeding on probing, and FI were detected on this tooth (see Table 14.4).

Given the residual FI and residual deep pockets, associated with a high risk of future tooth loss (Matuliene et al. 2008; Nibali et al. 2016), a decision to attempt surgical exploration and if possible regenerative surgery was made. No through-and through FI could be detected intra-surgically, although probably only a very limited layer of bone may have been present. Therefore, regenerative therapy with EMD was provided (see Chapter 7 for a step-by-step guide to the furcation regenerative surgical technique). Post-operative photos and radiographs are presented in Chapter 15 (Figure 15.5). The main reasons for this choice are summarized in Table 14.5.

Table 14.4 Case 2, re-evaluation.

Tooth 36 (LL6)	v-PPD	CAL	h-PPD
Mesio-buccal	2	2	–
Buccal	6	8	4
Disto-buccal	10	13	–
Mesio-lingual	3	3	–
Lingual	6	6	4
Disto-lingual	9	11	–

CAL = clinical attachment loss; h-PPD = horizontal probing pocket depth; v-PPD = vertical probing pocket depth.

Table 14.5 Case 2, main reasons for treatment choice (regenerative therapy with enamel matrix derivative).

	Factors
TOOTH	Good mesial bone support Good bone support on neighbouring tooth 37 Reduced tooth divergence Intrabony defect affecting distal root and furcation Tooth vitality and no restorative concerns Importance in masticatory function
PATIENT	Clear medical history Non-smoker Motivation to keep the tooth No financial or other concerns for surgical treatment

References

Abouassi, T., Woelber, J.P., Holst, K. et al. (2014). Clinical efficacy and patients' acceptance of a rubber interdental bristle: A randomized controlled trial. *Clinical Oral Investigations* 18, 1873–1880. doi:10.1007/s00784-013-1164-3.

Ammons, W.F., and Harrington G.W. (2006). Furcation: Involvement and treatment. In: *Carranza's Clinical Periodontology* (ed. M.G. Newman, H.H. Takei, P.R. Klokkevold, and F.A. Carranza), 991–1004. St. Louis, MO: Saunders Elsevier.

Becker, W., Becker, B.E., Alsuwyed, A., and Al-Mubarak, S. (1999). Long-term evaluation of 282 implants in maxillary and mandibular molar positions: A prospective study. *Journal of Periodontology* 70, 896–901.

Becker, W., Becker, B.E., and Berg, L.E. (1984). Periodontal treatment without maintenance: A retrospective study in 44 patients. *Journal of Periodontology* 55, 505–509.

Blomlöf, L., Jansson, L., Appelgren, R. et al. (1997). Prognosis and mortality of root-resected molars. *International Journal of Periodontics and Restorative Dentistry* 17, 190–201.

Carnevale, G., Pontoriero, R., and di Febo, G. (1998). Long-term effects of root-resective therapy in furcation-involved molars: A 10-year longitudinal study. *Journal of Clinical Periodontology* 25, 209–214.

Christou, V., Timmerman, M.F., Van der Velden, U., and Van der Weijden, F.A. (1998). Comparison of different approaches of interdental oral hygiene: Interdental brushes versus dental floss. *Journal of Periodontology* 69, 759–764. doi:10.1902/jop.1998.69.7.759.

Cortellini, P., Stalpers, G., Mollo, A., and Tonetti, M.S. (2011). Periodontal regeneration versus extraction and prosthetic replacement of teeth severely compromised by attachment loss to the apex: 5-year results of an ongoing randomized clinical trial. *Journal of Clinical Periodontology* 38, 915–924.

Cortellini, P., and Tonetti, M.S. (2001). Evaluation of the effect of tooth vitality on regenerative outcomes in infrabony defects. *Journal of Clinical Periodontology* 28, 672–679.

de Andrade, A.K., Feist, I.S., Pannuti, C.M. et al. (2008). Nd:YAG laser clinical assisted in class II furcation treatment. *Lasers in Medical Science* 23, 341–347. doi:10.1007/s10103-007-0482-6.

Del Peloso Ribeiro, E., Bittencourt, S., Nociti, F.H., Jr et al. (2007). Comparative study of ultrasonic instrumentation for the non-surgical treatment of interproximal and non-interproximal furcation involvements. *Journal of Periodontology* 78, 224–230. doi:10.1902/jop.2007.060312.

Drago, C.J. (1992). Rates of osseointegration of dental implants with regard to anatomical location. *Journal of Prosthodontics* 1, 29–31.

Dunlap, R.M., and Gher, M.E. (1985). Root surface measurements of the mandibular first molar. *Journal of Periodontology* 56, 234–248.

Eickholz, P., Nickles, K., Koch, R. et al. (2016). Is furcation class involvement affected by adjunctive systemic amoxicillin plus metronidazole? A clinical trial's exploratory subanalysis. *Journal of Clinical Periodontology* 43, 839–848.

Fardal, O., and Grytten, J. (2013). A comparison of teeth and implants during maintenance therapy in terms of the number of disease-free years and costs: An in vivo internal control study. *Journal of Clinical Periodontology* 40, 645–651. doi:10.1111/jcpe.12101.

Fleischer, H.C., Mellonig, J.T., Brayer, W.K. et al. (1989). Scaling and root planing efficacy in multirooted teeth. *Journal of Periodontology* 60, 402–409. doi:10.1902/jop.1989.60.7.402.

Glickmann, I. (1953). *Clinical Periodontology.* Pennsylvania, PA: Saunders.

Graziani, F., Donos, N., Needleman, I. et al. (2004). Comparison of implant survival following sinus floor augmentation procedures with implants placed in pristine posterior maxillary bone: A systematic review. *Clinical Oral Implants* 15, 677–682.

Hamp, S.E., Nyman, S., and Lindhe, J. (1975). Periodontal treatment of multirooted teeth: Results after 5 years. *Journal of Clinical Periodontology* 2, 126–135.

Helldén, L.B., Elliot, A., Steffensen, B., and Steffensen, J.E.M. (1989). Prognosis of tunnel preparations in treatment of class III furcations: A follow-up study. *Journal of Periodontology* 60, 182–187.

Jepsen, S., Eberhard, J., Herrera, D., and Needleman, I. (2002). A systematic review of guided tissue regeneration for periodontal furcation defects: What is the effect of guided tissue regeneration compared with surgical debridement in the treatment of furcation defects? *Journal of Clinical Periodontology* 29 (Suppl. 3), 103–116.

Jepsen, S., Heinz, B., Jepsen, K. et al. (2004). A randomized clinical trial comparing enamel matrix derivative and membrane treatment of buccal Class II furcation involvement in mandibular molars. Part I: Study design and results for primary outcomes. *Journal of Periodontology* 75, 1150–1160.

Joseph, I., Varma, B.R., and Bhat, K.M. (1996). Clinical significance of furcation anatomy of the maxillary first premolar: A biometric study on extracted teeth. *Journal of Periodontology* 67, 386–389.

Langeland, K., Rodrigues, H., and Dowden, W. (1974). Periodontal disease, bacteria, and pulpal histopathology. *Oral Surgery, Oral Medicine, Oral Pathology* 37, 257–270.

Langer, B., Stein, S.D., and Wagenberg, B. (1981). An evaluation of root resections: A ten-year study. *Journal of Periodontology* 52, 719–722.

Leon, L.E., and Vogel, R.I. (1987). A comparison of the effectiveness of hand scaling and ultrasonic debridement in furcations as evaluated by differential dark-field microscopy. *Journal of Periodontology* 58, 86–94. doi:10.1902/jop.1987.58.2.86.

Little, L.A., Beck, F.M., Bagci, B., and Horton, J.E. (1995). Lack of furcal bone loss following the tunnelling procedure. *Journal of Clinical Periodontology* 22, 637–641.

Machtei, E.E., Zubrey, Y., Yehuda, A.B., and Soskolne, W.A. (1989). Proximal bone loss adjacent to periodontally 'hopeless' teeth with and without extraction. *Journal of Periodontology* 60, 512–515.

Martin, J.A., Fardal, O., Page, R.C. et al. (2014). Incorporating severity and risk as factors to the Fardal cost-effectiveness model to create a cost–benefit model for periodontal treatment. *Journal of Periodontology* 85, e31–e39. doi:10.1902/jop.2013.130237.

Matia, J.I., Bissada, N.F., Maybury, J.E., and Ricchetti, P. (1986). Efficiency of scaling of the molar furcation area with and without surgical access. *International Journal of Periodontics and Restorative Dentistry* 6, 24–35.

Matuliene, G., Pjetursson, B.E., Salvi, G.E. et al. (2008). Influence of residual pockets on progression of periodontitis and tooth loss: Results after 11 years of maintenance. *Journal of Clinical Periodontology* 35, 685–695.

Moraschini, V., Poubel, L.A., Ferreira, V.F., and Barboza Edos, S. (2015). Evaluation of survival and success rates of dental implants reported in longitudinal studies with a follow-up period of at least 10 years: A systematic review. *International Journal of Oral and Maxillofacial Surgery* 44, 377–388.

Muller, H.P., and Eger, T. (1999). Furcation diagnosis. *Journal of Clinical Periodontology* 26, 485–498.

Nevins, M., Camelo, M., Nevins, M.L. et al. (2003). Periodontal regeneration in humans using recombinant human platelet-derived growth factor-bb (rhPDGF-BB) and allogenic bone. *Journal of Periodontology* 74, 1282–1292.

Nibali, L., Zavattini, A., Nagata, K. et al. (2016). Tooth loss in molars with and without furcation involvement: A systematic review and meta-analysis. *Journal of Clinical Periodontology* 43, 156–166.

Pjetursson, B.E., Tan, W.C., Zwahlen, M., and Lang, N.P. (2008). A systematic review of the success of sinus floor elevation and survival of implants inserted in combination with sinus floor elevation. *Journal of Clinical Periodontology* 35, 216–240.

Pontoriero, R., and Lindhe, J. (1995). Guided tissue regeneration in the treatment of degree III furcation defects in maxillary molars. *Journal of Clinical Periodontology* 22, 810–812.

Ribeiro Edel, P., Bittencourt, S., Sallum, E.A. et al. (2010). Non-surgical instrumentation associated with povidone-iodine in the treatment of interproximal furcation involvements. *Journal of Applied Oral Sciences* 18, 599–606.

Schwendicke, F., Graetz, C., Stolpe, M., and Dorfer, C.E. (2014). Retaining or replacing molars with furcation involvement: A cost-effectiveness comparison of different strategies. *Journal of Clinical Periodontology* 41, 1090–1097.

Stoller, N.H., Johnson, L.R., and Garrett, S. (2001). Periodontal regeneration of a class II furcation defect utilizing a bioabsorbable barrier in a human: A case study with histology. *Journal of Periodontology* 72, 238–242.

Sugaya, T., Kawanami, M., and Kato, H. (2002). Effects of debridement with an ultrasonic furcation tip in degree II furcation involvement of mandibular molars. *Journal*

of the International Academy of Periodontology 4, 138–142.

Tarnow, D., and Fletcher, P. (1984). Classification of the vertical component of furcation involvement. *Journal of Periodontology* 55, 283–284.

Thoma, D.S., Zeltner, M., Hüsler, J. et al. (2015). EAO Supplement Working Group 4 – EAO CC 2015. Short implants versus sinus lifting with longer implants to restore the posterior maxilla: A systematic review. *Clinical Oral Implant Research* 26 (Suppl. 11), 154–169.

Tomasi, C., and Wennstrom, J.L. (2011). Locally delivered doxycycline as an adjunct to mechanical debridement at retreatment of periodontal pockets: Outcome at furcation sites. *Journal of Periodontology* 82, 210–218. doi:10.1902/jop.2010.100308.

Chapter 15

Furcations: A Treatment Algorithm

Luigi Nibali

Centre for Immunobiology and Regenerative Medicine, Centre for Oral Clinical Research, Institute of Dentistry, Barts and the London School of Medicine and Dentistry, Queen Mary University of London (QMUL), London, UK

15.1 Introduction

What do you do when facing a molar with furcation involvement (FI)? Extract? Ignore? Treat? And how? Regeneration? Root resection? Several papers in the periodontal literature have covered the treatment of molars with FI. Previous chapters of this book have reviewed and carefully scrutinized the evidence for no treatment, and for conservative, regenerative, and resective therapy. But how do we approach decision-making? How can we merge the patient's preferences and needs with the financial considerations and the clinical criteria discussed in this book to achieve a favourable outcome? We embark on this chapter with a scientific evidence-based approach to try to answer these questions. However, in the absence of randomized controlled trials comparing different management options for molars with varying degrees of FI, pragmatic considerations and experience will complement the evidence in order to obtain treatment guidelines. The main points to consider are highlighted in what follows.

15.2 First Things First: Proper Diagnosis

Diagnosis is the first step towards treatment. As in any other field of medicine, every effort needs to be expended for a correct diagnosis of the problem (Khullar et al. 2015). Most of the mistakes I have made in my professional career or have seen made by students or colleagues were due to incorrect diagnosis. This is particularly important for furcations, since diagnosis is not straightforward. Therefore, spending more time and effort for diagnostic purposes before rushing to pick up blade or forceps is recommended.

Furcation diagnosis has been covered by Eickholz and Walter in Chapter 2. Their clear message is that *clinical and radiographic diagnoses need to be combined* to obtain a correct measure of the involvement of the furcation area. *A curved Nabers probe is vital* for measuring the bone loss in the furcation area, although the difference between degrees II and III might be difficult to ascertain, especially in maxillary molars. Three-dimensional radiography may also be needed for treatment planning purposes in some cases.

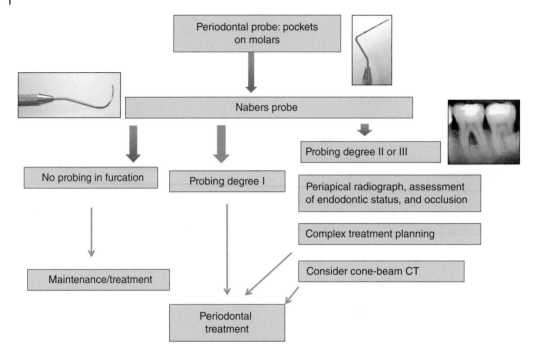

Figure 15.1 Proposed algorithm for furcation diagnosis.

Figure 15.1 shows a furcation diagnosis algorithm, essential for treatment planning. It is suggested that a Nabers probe is used in all cases of probing pocket depths > 4 mm in molars, to establish a furcation diagnosis. In the case of FI degree II or III, further diagnostic tests, including periapical radiographs and endodontic and occlusal assessments, may be necessary for treatment planning. When the diagnosis and extent of FI are not clear, posing doubts about the best treatment plan, cone-beam computed tomography (CBCT) may be justifiable as a useful diagnostic adjunct, especially for maxillary molars (Walter et al. 2016; see Chapter 2 for more details).

The main differential diagnostic elements to consider for complex treatment planning are briefly highlighted in Table 15.1.

Bearing in mind all the factors discussed, treatment guidelines for different degrees of FI are proposed in the following sections. These cannot be applied as 'blanket' treatment guidelines, but need to be adapted to every different patient and every different molar.

15.3 Degree I Furcation Involvement

The evidence from the literature, summarized in a recent systematic review and discussed in Chapter 5, suggests that increasing FI degree is associated with an increased risk of tooth loss (Nibali et al. 2016). The long-term risk of tooth loss appears minimal in degree I FI molars undergoing regular care compared with molars with no FI. In fact, re-examining data from that systematic review, it appears that *molars with degree I FI undergoing regular supportive periodontal therapy (SPT) have an identical tooth loss rate to molars with no FI* (0.01 teeth/patient/year; Nibali et al. 2016). For this reason, the consensus opinion at present is that degree I FI is not suitable for complex treatment such as periodontal regeneration. Authors of a previous systematic review had also concluded that degree I FI could be successfully managed by non-surgical mechanical debridement (Huynh-Ba et al. 2009).

Less is known about FI degree I molars not undergoing regular periodontal care. Data

Table 15.1 Main differential diagnostic elements to consider for complex furcation treatment planning.

	Factors	Thresholds/grades
ANATOMY	Endodontic status	Degree 1–5 (Ørstavik et al. 1986)
	Restorability	Class I–III (Esteves et al. 2011)
	Degree of furcation involvement	I–III (Hamp et al. 1975)
	Number of furcation involvements	Single, double, or triple
	Vertical probing	A–C (Tarnow and Fletcher 1984)
	Degree of separation (root divergence)	30° (Muller and Eger 1999)
	Separation degree	⅓ (Muller and Eger 1999)
	Bone loss	⅓, ⅔ of root length (Muller and Eger 1999)
	Position of furcation fornix relative to bone crest and interproximal bone levels	Coronal or apical (Bowers et al. 2003)
	Furcation width	Narrow or wide (Horwitz et al. 2004)
	Other anatomical features	Length of root cone, root trunk etc.
PATIENT	Medical history	Healthy vs medically compromised
	Smoking	Current/former/never
	Preferences/motivation	Refusal to undergo surgery
	Financial	Inability/unwillingness to pay for complex treatment
	Oral hygiene dexterity	Inability to access furcation entrance
OPERATOR	Ability/experience	
STRATEGY	Abutment	
	Functional	
RISK	Anatomical risks, surgical risks	
ALTERNATIVES	Replacement with implant, prosthetic bridge, removable denture	

from SHIP (Study for Health In Pomerania) show an incidence rate ratio (IRR) for molar loss of 1.73 (95% confidence interval [CI] 1.34–2.23, $p < 0.001$) for degree I FI versus no FI after 11 years of follow-up, suggesting that *'no treatment' worsens the prognosis of molars with FI degree I* (Nibali et al. 2017a).

Therefore, it could be suggested that oral hygiene instructions and non-surgical therapy represent the treatment of choice for degree I FI, irrespective of location or other factors. Odontoplasty might complement this treatment in cases where the furcation entrance anatomy might contribute to the presence of a degree I FI and might interfere with oral hygiene manoeuvres (see Figure 15.2).

15.4 Degree II Furcation Involvement

The real complexity starts when considering *degree II FI*, as this *seems to be the threshold at which the risk of tooth loss sharply increases* (Nibali et al. 2016, 2017a). Therefore, treatment is needed to reduce the impact of such FI in determining tooth loss. The main treatment goal should be the reduction of degree

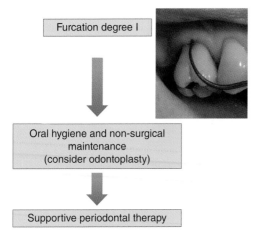

Furcation degree I

↓

Oral hygiene and non-surgical maintenance
(consider odontoplasty)

↓

Supportive periodontal therapy

Figure 15.2 Proposed algorithm for furcation treatment (degree I furcation involvement).

II FI to degree I FI or to no FI (ideal). It is implied that oral hygiene instructions and non-surgical therapy (with or without adjuncts) are a prerequisite for this treatment algorithm, and they should always represent the starting point. In some occasions, oral hygiene instructions and non-surgical therapy can already lead to the reduction of degree II FI to degree I FI through mechanisms including reduction of gingival oedema, epithelial reattachment, reduced probe penetration, and potentially radiographic bone fill (see the case in Figure 15.3). However, residual degree II FI after causal therapy needs to be further addressed.

15.4.1 Mandibular Degree II Furcations

Except for cases of degree II FI after initial periodontal therapy where odontoplasty and/or surgical osteoplasty could lead to a reduction to degree I FI, reduction of degree II FI could be achieved via regenerative therapy. Chapters 6 and 7 have presented the evidence for the efficacy of regeneration in furcations. Based on the discussion in these chapters, an important differentiation needs to be made between maxillary and mandibular degree II furcations. Figure 15.4 shows a

(a)   (b)

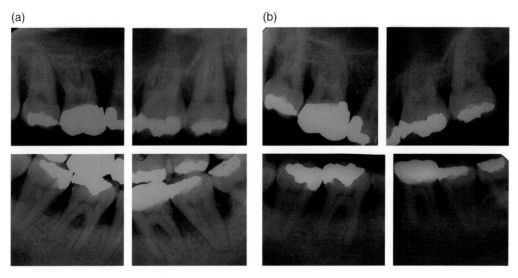

Figure 15.3 (a) Periapical radiographs of molars of a female 32-year-old aggressive periodontitis patient at periodontal diagnosis. Radiolucency inside the furcation areas is visible, particularly for UR6 and 7 (both degree II clinical furcation involvement [FI] diagnosis), UL6 and 7 (degree I FI), LL6 (degree I FI), and LR6 (degree II FI), often associated with intrabony defects. (b) Periapical radiographs of the same molars one year after initial periodontal therapy (oral hygiene instructions and supra- and subgingival debridement with adjunctive systemic antibiotics and extraction of UL8), showing radiographic bone fill in furcation defects and intrabony defects, associated with clinical reduction of FI degrees (now only degree I for UR6 and 7, UL6 and 7, and LR6).

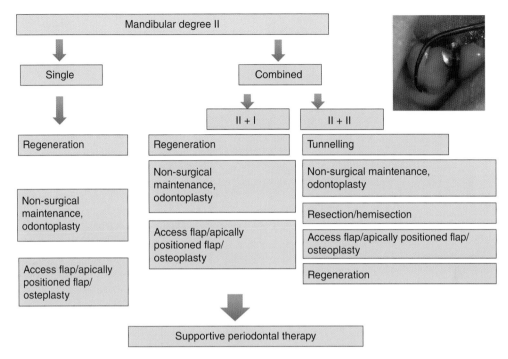

Figure 15.4 Proposed algorithm for furcation treatment (degree II mandibular furcation involvement).

proposed algorithm for the treatment of mandibular degree II FI. A hierarchy is presented starting from the preferred choice at the top, although this is rather arbitrary and not strictly evidence based.

Another important differentiation to be drawn is based on whether the furcation is single (e.g. only buccal or only lingual) or double (both buccal and lingual). In a case of single degree II mandibular FI following initial therapy, regeneration seems to be the preferred choice. The evidence reviewed by Jepsen and Jepsen in Chapter 7 shows that, although *complete furcation closure in degree II FI is not a predictable outcome*, treatment with either guided tissue regeneration (GTR) or enamel matrix derivative (EMD) has produced histological evidence of regeneration (Stoller et al. 2001; Nevins et al. 2003) and consistently more favourable clinical outcomes (reduction to degree I or closure) compared with access flaps, especially in mandibular furcations (Jepsen et al. 2002, 2004). Alternatives to regenerative therapy

are non-surgical maintenance/SPT, access flap with or without osteoplasty, or apically positioned flap (APF), to improve access for professional cleaning of the furcation region. Similar treatment options are recommended for combined degree II and I mandibular furcations.

However, when double degree II mandibular furcations are present, regeneration becomes much less predictable, albeit not impossible (see Figure 15.5, in relation to Case 2 described in Chapter 14).

In contrast, tunnelling comes into play as probably the preferred option. Tunnelling surgery can improve access to self-performed, as well as professional, cleaning of the furcation area, so it could be indicated too in cases of double degree II mandibular FI. Studies with 5–10 years follow-up show success rates varying between 51 and 93% (Hamp et al. 1975; Dannewitz et al. 2006). Patient selection (good oral hygiene and motivation, low caries risk) and tooth selection (short root trunk, favourable root divergence; Muller

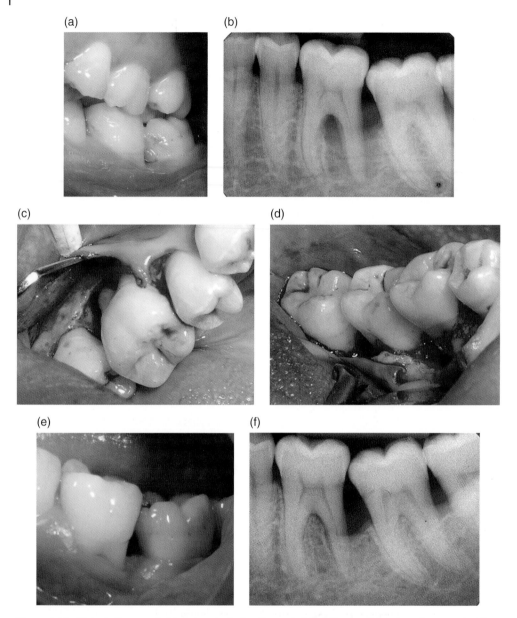

Figure 15.5 Clinical photograph (a) and periapical radiograph (b) of 47-year-old patient diagnosed with chronic periodontitis and affected by double degree II furcation involvement and distal intrabony defect (disto-buccal and disto-lingual probing pocket depth [PPD] 12 mm) on tooth 36 (LL6). Following non-surgical periodontal therapy, regenerative surgery with enamel matrix derivative was carried out (c and d, buccal and lingual intra-operative views after full-thickness flaps elevation), with favourable outcomes at five years after surgery, with reduction of PPD to 4 mm and only degree I furcation lingual (e) and fill of intrabony and furcation defect (f).

and Eger 1999) are vital for tunnelling, and for access reasons mandibular furcations are clearly more suitable.

Other options such as non-surgical maintenance/odontoplasty, root resection/ hemisection, or access flap (or APF) are also realistic. We should bear in mind that root-resection studies with follow-ups at 5–10 years showed success rates of 62–100% (Carnevale et al. 1998; Dannewitz et al. 2006) and, with the exception of three studies, the average survival rate of the molars treated with root separation/resection was close to 90% (see Chapter 8). Access flap (or APF) with or without ostectomy could improve access for professional cleaning of the furcation area and lead to reduction of probing pocket depths and inflammation (Wang et al. 1994).

15.4.2 Single Maxillary Degree II Buccal Furcations

Maxillary molars with degree II FI after initial periodontal therapy present probably the most challenging scenario in terms of potential treatment choices and expected outcome. Again, in the absence of randomized controlled trials comparing all options, we need to draw guidelines mainly based on low-evidence studies, experience, and common sense. Figure 15.6 shows options for degree II maxillary furcations.

Favourable results could be achieved with GTR therapy and EMD in maxillary degree II furcations (Yukna and Yukna 1996; Casarin et al. 2010), but the evidence suggests that

such results are more predictable in buccal sites (Pontoriero and Lindhe 1995a). Therefore, regeneration could be a good alternative to non-surgical maintenance, odontoplasty, and access flap surgery in order to reduce the buccal furcation to degree I or to achieve complete closure. The decision for regenerative therapy would depend on factors mentioned in the previous section (see Table 15.1), such as smoking and financial considerations, as well as good interproximal bone levels, reduced vertical furcation component, and reduced furcation width, all shown to favour regeneration in animal and human studies (Pontoriero et al. 1992; Bowers et al. 2003; Horwitz et al. 2004).

15.4.3 Single Maxillary Degree II Interproximal Furcations

Overall, the application of GTR, EMD, or combination therapy (EMD/bone grafts) to proximal furcations in maxillary molars achieved some furcation closures, but was not as favourable as that in mandibular furcations or buccal maxillary furcations

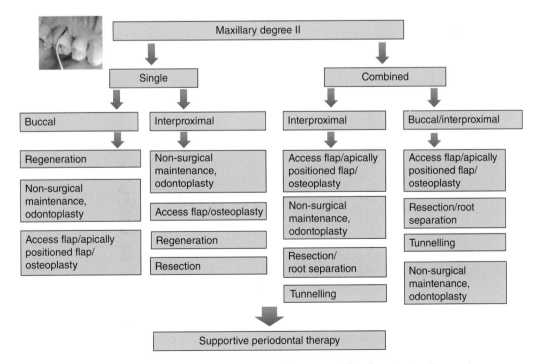

Figure 15.6 Proposed algorithm for furcation treatment (degree II maxillary furcation involvement).

(Pontoriero and Lindhe 1995a; Avera et al. 1998; Casarin et al. 2010; Peres et al. 2013). Therefore, non-surgical maintenance/odontoplasty, access flap/osteoplasty (or APF), and potentially also root resection could be valid alternatives. The latter could be particularly suitable for previously endodontically treated molars.

15.4.4 Combined Maxillary Degree II Furcations

Although regenerative periodontal therapy may be a viable option for degree II maxillary molars, this would be probably only limited to single degree II maxillary defects, as the unpredictability would certainly increase several-fold in multiple degree II maxillary FI (which often could hide a true degree III FI). Therefore, root resection, access flap, and tunnelling procedures are probably the best alternatives to choose from in these cases.

As previously discussed for mandibular degree II furcations, root-resective surgery and access flap/APF with or without ostectomy could be good potential alternatives (Wang et al. 1994; Carnevale et al. 1998). Root resection/separation is mainly recommended for previously endodontically treated maxillary molars with combined furcations degree II, particularly when the worst-affected root is the disto-buccal. Tunnelling, given the correct patient and molar selection, could be another appropriate treatment choice in selected cases.

When for patient or tooth reasons these options are not feasible or not worth pursuing, non-surgical maintenance with frequent SPT recalls based on a patient risk profile (Lang and Tonetti 2003) remains a valid option, with the clear limitation of difficulties in achieving proper debridement of the furcation area (Fleischer et al. 1989).

Root resection and tunnelling options may be more indicated in cases of combined buccal/interproximal degree II furcations, rather than when both are interproximal. The reasons for this are that resecting the palatal root (in cases of mesial and distal

degree II FI) is less favourable owing to anatomical features (see Chapter 8), and that access to the furcation tunnel for self-performed hygiene is easier from a buccal access (see Chapter 9). Therefore, a slightly different hierarchy of choice is presented in Figure 15.6, with root resection and tunnelling considered to have more 'worth' for combined buccal–interproximal FI, and more conservative options probably indicated for combined interproximal furcations.

The unlikely case of triple non-through-and-through degree II furcation involvement could be considered within the degree III FI treatment options.

15.5 Degree III Furcation Involvement

When bone loss in the furcation area goes through and through, from one root-separation area to another on the same tooth, we are faced with degree III FI. The main treatment challenge here derives from the limitations of regenerative therapy in such cases. *No clinical study in humans has so far reported any degree III furcation closures with GTR, EMD, or both combined*, but only clinical reductions in furcation degree in some very limited cases (Pontoriero et al. 1989; Pontoriero and Lindhe 1995b; Eickholz et al. 1998, 1999; Jepsen et al. 2002; Donos et al. 2004). Jepsen and Jepsen in Chapter 7 reviewed the available evidence to conclude that degree III FI cannot be improved predictably by regenerative therapy, until new developments in regenerative material and techniques are available (discussed in Chapter 6). Therefore, it would be difficult to justify the use of regenerative surgery on degree III FI at present. The persistence of a degree III furcation defect which is not regenerable and is difficult to clean (see Chapter 3) equals a higher risk of future tooth loss than for degree I and degree II FI molars (Nibali et al. 2016). Hence the need to find a solution to manage these cases and to reduce the risk of tooth loss. The treatment options are presented in

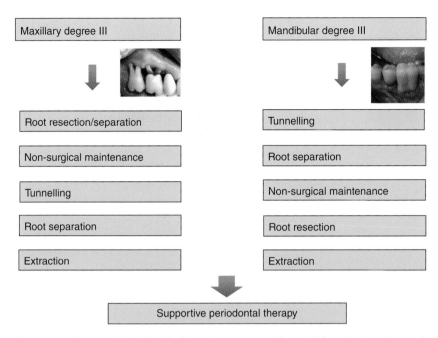

Figure 15.7 Proposed algorithm for furcation treatment (degree III furcation involvement).

Figure 15.7, divided between maxillary and mandibular molars.

The difference, clearly, is that maxillary molars, with three furcation entrances, could potentially have three through-and-through furcation lesions, making the access for cleaning (both professional and self-performed) very challenging. On the other hand, mandibular degree III FI molars can only have one through-and-through furcation lesion, with access both buccally and lingually. While bearing in mind the evidence of success for tunnelling and root-resection procedures in long-term clinical trials (Helldén et al. 1989; Carnevale et al. 1998), we need to stress the importance of proper diagnosis and patient and molar selection. The factors highlighted in Table 15.1 need again to be kept in mind in order to ensure long-term success.

avoided in cases with high caries risk, high tooth sensitivity, poor compliance, or poor manual dexterity, as lack of proper oral hygiene defies the purpose of this therapy. Molars with a short root trunk, high degree of separation (root divergence), and a large band of keratinized gingiva are particularly suitable for this procedure (see Chapter 9). When tunnelling is not indicated, root separation (premolarization) could be considered a valid alternative, especially in cases of good residual bone support in the distal aspect of the distal root and in the mesial aspect of the mesial root. This would again aim to improve cleaning (by removal of the furcation region), but would entail extensive restorative work. Long-term non-surgical maintenance (preceded or not by surgical access) and root resection represent possible alternatives if tooth survival is chosen.

15.5.1 Mandibular Degree III Furcations

Tunnelling could be considered the treatment of choice for mandibular degree III FI. As already mentioned, tunnelling should be

15.5.2 Maxillary Degree III Furcations

Root resection or non-surgical maintenance could be considered the treatment of choice for degree III FI maxillary molars. These two procedures have different indications, as root resection is generally more advisable in the case of a double degree III FI, mainly affecting one root. In this case, the resection of a root (preferably if it is the smallest disto-buccal root) could leave two easily maintainable roots with no FI. As Rotundo and Fonzar discussed in Chapter 6, root resection in a case of a triple degree III FI is less advisable, as it would anyway result in a residual difficult-to-clean furcation. In such a case (triple degree III FI), regular subgingival debridement seems the most reasonable option in cases where tooth survival is preferred. This could be preceded or not by surgical access for furcation debridement, shown to improve professional cleaning efficacy (see Chapter 3). Other factors mentioned earlier, such as patient preferences and financial considerations, play an important role in the decision of whether to maintain such teeth or not.

Under exceptional circumstances, tunnelling could be considered an option for triple degree III FI, mainly in cases of very compliant patients with good manual dexterity and low caries risk. Tunnelling can occur either naturally, by virtue of gingival recession, as a result of oral hygiene and non-surgical therapy, or can be created surgically. The main reason for the failure of tunnelling is not periodontal but restorative, linked with root caries following the exposure of the root surface (Helldén et al. 1989). Figure 15.8 shows a case of surgically created triple degree III FI in maxillary molars maintained for over 10 years with no clinical and radiographic signs of disease progression or caries (Case 1 described in Chapter 14).

Root separation is also a possible option for degree III maxillary molars, associated or not with root resection. Careful endodontic and prosthetic considerations are needed before deciding on this treatment option (Carnevale et al. 1998).

However, in making the decision on whether to extract or not, one should take into account that, despite a higher tooth loss risk, the majority of maxillary degree III FI molars could be maintained over at least a 10–15-year period of periodontal supportive care (Nibali et al. 2016), meaning that extraction of molars affected by degree III FI should not be a given.

15.6 Upper Premolars

Upper first premolars are normally two-rooted, while second maxillary premolars and mandibular canines are occasionally two-rooted. However, very little data exist in the literature about the treatment of non-molar teeth with FI (Hamp et al. 1975). As discussed in Chapter 7, the majority of maxillary first premolars have fused roots. In upper premolars with separated roots, the furcation entrance is on average 8 mm apical to the cemento-enamel junction and only 7–10% of furcation entrances are in the coronal third of the root (Joseph et al. 1996; Dababneh and Rodan 2013). Furthermore, root grooves and concavities are the norm in upper premolars. Owing to these anatomical features, root resection and tunnelling are not usually viable options for upper premolars with FI, and access flap and/or non-surgical maintenance should be preferred.

15.7 Innovative Treatment

Novel treatments for furcation-involved teeth were discussed in Chapter 10. Some of these, such as adjunctive photodynamic therapy, lasers, or air-polishing devices, could be added to the options discussed in this chapter, although more evidence needs to be gathered before routinely recommending these therapies.

15.8 So, When Should We Extract?

The emphasis of this chapter, and perhaps of the whole book, has been on tooth retention. However, there are cases where even the most

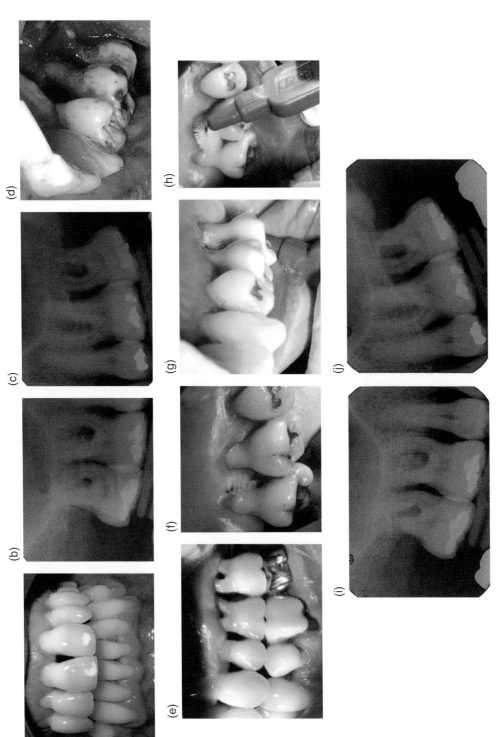

Figure 15.8 Clinical photograph (a) and periapical radiographs (b and c) of 50-year-old patient diagnosed with chronic periodontitis and affected by triple degree III furcation involvement on 17 (UR7), 16 (UR6), and 27 (UL7). Following non-surgical periodontal therapy, tunnelling surgery was carried out (d, intra-operative view after full-thickness flaps elevation and osteoplasty), with favourable outcomes at 12 years after surgery with probing pocket depths < 5 mm (e), continued good oral hygiene access to furcations (f, g, and h), and stable radiographic bone levels (i and j).

daring periodontist has to admit that a tooth is hopeless or irrational to treat, and extraction might be the best option. Several definitions of 'hopeless' have been proposed in the periodontal literature. Becker and colleagues (1984) reported a range of criteria for hopeless teeth, including degree III FI or bone loss > 75%. Machtei and co-workers (1989) defined as hopeless teeth with bone loss ≥ 50%, or radiographic evidence of total bone loss in the furcation area (grade III FI). In their landmark prognosis paper, McGuire and Nunn (1996) more vaguely identified as hopeless teeth with 'inadequate attachment'. Hopeless has also been defined as having loss of ≥ 70% bone height (Graetz et al. 2011) or as having bone loss to the apex (Cortellini et al. 2011).

We recently assigned an 'unfavourable' prognosis to teeth with ≥ 70% bone loss which were also either unrestorable (Esteves et al. 2011), with an endodontic periapical index

(PAI) score of 4 (Ørstavik et al. 1986), or with mobility grade III or FI degree III (Nibali et al. 2017b). This new prognostic system aims to be more conservative than previous proposals, based on the data discussed earlier showing that degree III FI alone should not qualify a tooth as hopeless (Nibali et al. 2016). In the reality of everyday practice, patient-related factors (e.g. risk of caries, compliance, and smoking), patient preferences, financial considerations, and overall strategic value need to accompany clinical and radiographic criteria in reaching a decision about maintaining or extracting. Further considerations on possible extraction and implant replacement can be found in Chapter 11.

Finally, it is important to remember that community-wide oral hygiene instruction and primary prevention programmes are the best measures for reducing oral diseases and tooth loss.

Summary of Evidence

- Furcation diagnosis is crucial for treatment planning purposes.
- Degree I, II, and III maxillary and mandibular molars have very different treatment indications.
- Degree I furcation involvement (FI) has a good long-term prognosis and does not represent a higher risk of tooth loss if under periodontal maintenance care.
- Degree II FI could benefit from periodontal regeneration or other conservative therapy (or root resection).
- Degree II interproximal maxillary FI is less suitable for regeneration.
- Degree III FI is linked with a higher risk of tooth loss and treatment options need to

be carefully considered before embarking on treatment or extraction.
- A holistic approach, including clinical and radiographic parameters but also overall strategic tooth value, financial considerations, and patient preferences, needs to be pursued in order to obtain the most satisfactory outcome of furcation therapy.
- General dentists should bear in mind that referral to a periodontist is advised for molars with severe FI, and that most molars with FI can be maintained functionally in the long term.
- Adherence to patient-tailored supportive periodontal therapy is crucial to reduce the long-term tooth loss risk.

References

Avera, J.B., Camargo, P.M., Klokkevold, P.R. et al. (1998). Guided tissue regeneration in class II furcation involved maxillary molars: A controlled study of 8 split-mouth cases. *Journal of Periodontology* 69, 1020–1026.

Becker, W., Becker, B.E., and Berg, L.E. (1984). Periodontal treatment without maintenance:

A retrospective study in 44 patients. *Journal of Periodontology* 55, 505–509.

Bowers, G.M., Schallhorn, R.G., McClain, P.K. et al. (2003). Factors influencing the outcome of regenerative therapy in mandibular class II furcations: Part I. *Journal of Periodontology* 74, 1255–1268.

Carnevale, G., Pontoriero, R., and di Febo, G. (1998). Long-term effects of root-resective therapy in furcation-involved molars: A 10-year longitudinal study. *Journal of Clinical Periodontology* 25, 209–214.

Casarin, R.C., Ribeiro Edel, P., Nociti, F.H., Jr et al. (2010). Enamel matrix derivative proteins for the treatment of proximal class II furcation involvements: A prospective 24-month randomized clinical trial. *Journal of Clinical Periodontology* 37, 1100–1109.

Cortellini, P., Stalpers, G., Mollo, A., and Tonetti, M.S. (2011). Periodontal regeneration versus extraction and prosthetic replacement of teeth severely compromised by attachment loss to the apex: 5-year results of an ongoing randomized clinical trial. *Journal of Clinical Periodontology* 38, 915–924.

Dababneh, R., and Rodan, R. (2013). Anatomical landmarks of maxillary bifurcated first premolars and their influence on periodontal diagnosis and treatment. *Journal of the International Academy of Periodontology* 15, 8–15.

Dannewitz, B., Krieger, J.K., Husing, J., and Eickholz, P. (2006). Loss of molars in periodontally treated patients: A retrospective analysis five years or more after active periodontal treatment. *Journal of Clinical Periodontology* 33, 53–61.

Donos, N., Glavind, L., Karring, T., and Sculean, A. (2004). Clinical evaluation of an enamel matrix derivative and a bioresorbable membrane in the treatment of degree III mandibular furcation involvement: A series of nine patients. *International Journal of Periodontics and Restorative Dentistry* 24, 362–369.

Eickholz, P., and Hausmann, E. (1999). Evidence for healing of class II and III furcations 24 months after GTR therapy: Digital subtraction and clinical measurements. *Journal of Periodontology* 70, 1490–1500.

Eickholz, P., Kim, T.-S., and Holle, R. (1998). Regenerative periodontal surgery with non-resorbable and biodegradable barriers: Results after 24 months. *Journal of Clinical Periodontology* 25, 666–676.

Esteves, H., Correia, A., and Araújo, F. (2011) Classification of extensively damaged teeth to evaluate prognosis. *Journal of the Canadian Dental Association* 77, 105.

Fleischer, H.C., Mellonig, J.T., Brayer, W.K. et al. (1989). Scaling and root planing efficacy in multirooted teeth. *Journal of Periodontology* 60, 402–409.

Graetz, C., Dorfer, C.E., Kahl, M. et al. (2011). Retention of questionable and hopeless teeth in compliant patients treated for aggressive periodontitis. *Journal of Clinical Periodontology* 38, 707–714.

Hamp, S.E., Nyman, S., and Lindhe, J. (1975). Periodontal treatment of multirooted teeth: Results after 5 years. *Journal of Clinical Periodontology* 2, 126–135.

Helldén, L.B., Elliot, A., Steffensen, B., and Steffensen, J.E.M. (1989). Prognosis of tunnel preparations in treatment of class III furcations: A follow-up study. *Journal of Periodontology* 60, 182–187.

Horwitz, J., Machtei, E.E., Reitmeir, P. et al. (2004). Radiographic parameters as prognostic indicators for healing of class II furcation defects. *Journal of Clinical Periodontology* 31, 105–111.

Huynh-Ba, G., Kuonen, P., Hofer, D. et al. (2009). The effect of periodontal therapy on the survival rate and incidence of complications of multirooted teeth with furcation involvement after an observation period of at least 5 years: A systematic review. *Journal of Clinical Periodontology* 36, 164–176.

Jepsen, S., Eberhard, J., Herrera, D., and Needleman, I. (2002). A systematic review of guided tissue regeneration for periodontal furcation defects: What is the effect of guided tissue regeneration compared with surgical debridement in the treatment of furcation defects? *Journal of Clinical Periodontology* 29 (Suppl. 3), 103–116.

Jepsen, S., Heinz, B., Jepsen, K. et al. (2004). A randomized clinical trial comparing enamel matrix derivative and membrane treatment of buccal class II furcation involvement in mandibular molars. Part I: Study design and results for primary outcomes. *Journal of Periodontology* 75, 1150–1160.

Joseph, I., Varma, B.R., and Bhat, K.M. (1996). Clinical significance of furcation anatomy of the maxillary first premolar: A biometric study on extracted teeth. *Journal of Periodontology* 67, 386–389.

Khullar, D., Jha, A.K., and Jena, A.B. (2015). Reducing diagnostic errors: Why now. *New England Journal of Medicine* 373, 2491–2493.

Lang, N.P., and Tonetti, M.S. (2003). Periodontal risk assessment for patients in supportive periodontal therapy (SPT). *Oral Health & Preventive Dentistry* 1, 7–16.

Machtei, E.E., Zubrey, Y., Yehuda, A.B., and Soskolne, W.A. (1989). Proximal bone loss adjacent to periodontally 'hopeless' teeth with and without extraction. *Journal of Periodontology* 60, 512–515.

McGuire, M.K., and Nunn, M.E. (1996). Prognosis versus actual outcome. III. The effectiveness of clinical parameters in accurately predicting tooth survival. *Journal of Periodontology* 67, 666–674.

Muller, H.P., and Eger, T. (1999). Furcation diagnosis. *Journal of Clinical Periodontology* 26, 485–498.

Nevins, M., Camelo, M., Nevins, M.L. et al. (2003). Periodontal regeneration in humans using recombinant human platelet-derived growth factor-BB (rhPDGF-BB) and allogenic bone. *Journal of Periodontology* 74, 1282–1292.

Nibali, L., Krajewski, A., Donos, N. et al. (2017a). The effect of furcation involvement on tooth loss in a population without regular periodontal therapy. *Journal of Clinical Periodontology* 44, 813–821.

Nibali, L., Sun, C., Akcalı, A. et al. (2017b). A retrospective study on periodontal disease progression in private practice. *Journal of Clinical Periodontology* 44, 290–297.

Nibali, L., Zavattini, A., Nagata, K. et al. (2016). Tooth loss in molars with and without furcation involvement: A systematic review and meta-analysis. *Journal of Clinical Periodontology* 43, 156–166.

Ørstavik, D., Kerekes, K., and Eriksen, H.M. (1986). The periapical index: A scoring system for radiographic assessment of apical periodontitis. *Endodontics & Dental Traumatology* 2, 20–34.

Peres, M.F.S., Ribeiro, E.D.P., Casarin, R.C.V. et al. (2013). Hydroxyapatite/β-tricalcium phosphate and enamel matrix derivative for treatment of proximal class II furcation defects: A randomized clinical trial. *Journal of Clinical Periodontology* 40, 252–259.

Pontoriero, R., and Lindhe, J. (1995a). Guided tissue regeneration in the treatment of degree II furcations in maxillary molars. *Journal of Clinical Periodontology* 22, 756–763.

Pontoriero, R., and Lindhe, J. (1995b). Guided tissue regeneration in the treatment of degree III furcation defects in maxillary molars. *Journal of Clinical Periodontology* 22, 810–812.

Pontoriero, R., Lindhe, J., Nyman, S. et al. (1989). Guided tissue regeneration in the treatment of defects in mandibular molars: A clinical study of degree III involvements. *Journal of Clinical Periodontology* 16, 170–174.

Pontoriero, R., Nyman, S., Ericsson, I., and Lindhe, J. (1992). Guided tissue regeneration in surgically-produced furcation defects: An experimental study in the beagle dog. *Journal of Clinical Periodontology* 19, 159–163.

Stoller, N.H., Johnson, L.R., and Garrett, S. (2001). Periodontal regeneration of a class II furcation defect utilizing a bioabsorbable barrier in a human: A case study with histology. *Journal of Periodontology* 72, 238–242.

Tarnow, D., and Fletcher, P. (1984). Classification of the vertical component of furcation involvement. *Journal of Periodontology* 55, 283–284.

Walter, C., Schmidt, J.C., Dula, K. et al. (2016). Cone beam computed tomography (CBCT) for diagnosis and treatment planning in periodontology: A systematic review. *Quintessence International* 47, 25–37.

Wang, H.L., Burgett, F.G., Shyr, Y., and Ramfjord, S. (1994). The influence of molar furcation involvement and mobility on future clinical periodontal attachment loss. *Journal of Periodontology* 65, 25–29.

Yukna, C.N., and Yukna, R.A. (1996). Multi-center evaluation of bioabsorbable collagen membrane for guided tissue regeneration in human class II furcations. *Journal of Periodontology* 67, 650–657.

Index

Page numbers in *italics* refer to illustrations; those in **bold** refer to tables

Diagnosis and Treatment of Furcation-Involved Teeth, First Edition. Edited by Luigi Nibali.
© 2018 John Wiley & Sons Ltd. Published 2018 by John Wiley & Sons Ltd.
Companion website: www.wiley.com/go/nibali/diagnosis